INNOVATIONS IN CLINICAL PRACTICE

Focus on Health and Wellness

A Volume in the *Innovations in Clinical Practice* Series

Edited by
LEON VANDECREEK
JEFFERY B. ALLEN

PROFESSIONAL RESOURCE PRESS
P.O. Box 15560
Sarasota, FL 34277-1560

EARN HOME STUDY CONTINUING EDUCATION CREDITS*

Professional Resource Exchange, Inc. offers a home study continuing education program as a supplement to *Innovations in Clinical Practice: Focus on Health and Wellness*. For further information, please call 1-800-443-3364, fax to 941-343-9201, write to the address below, or visit our website: http://www.prpress.com

*The Professional Resource Exchange, Inc. is approved by the American Psychological Association to offer Continuing Education for psychologists. The Professional Resource Exchange, Inc. maintains responsibility for the program. We are also recognized by the National Board of Certified Counselors to offer continuing education for National Certified Counselors. We adhere to NBCC Continuing Education Guidelines (Provider #5474). Home study CE programs are accepted by most state licensing boards. Please consult your board if you have questions regarding that body's acceptance of structured home study programs offered by APA-approved sponsors. Our programs have also been specifically approved for MFCCs and LCSWs in California and MFTs, LCSWs, and MHCs in Florida.

Published by Professional Resource Press
(An imprint of Professional Resource Exchange, Inc.)
Post Office Box 15560
Sarasota, FL 34277-1560

Copyright © 2005 by Professional Resource Exchange, Inc.

Printed in the United States of America.

Library of Congress Cataloging-in-Publication Data

Focus on health and wellness / edited by Leon VandeCreek, Jeffery B. Allen.
    p. cm. -- (Innovations in clinical practice)
    Includes bibliographical references and index.
    ISBN 1-56887-096-5 (alk. paper)
    1. Mental health services. 1. Primary care (Medicine) I. VandeCreek, Leon. II. Allen, Jeffery B. III. Innovations in clinical practice (Unnumbered)

RA790.5.F63 2005
362.2--dc22   2005050974

The copyeditor for this book was Patricia Rockwood, the managing editor was Debra Fink, the production coordinator was Laurie Girsch, and the typesetter was Richard Sullivan.

Preface

Volumes 1 through 20 in the *Innovations in Clinical Practice: A Source Book* series were not built around a particular theme. Instead, each of these volumes covered a wide range of topics of probable interest to clinicians. Our primary audience for these volumes was practicing mental health professionals. These practitioners consistently praised the timeliness of the topics that we covered, the highly applied focus and usefulness of the contributions, the expertise of contributors, and the quality of our editing.

Peter A. Keller was the senior editor of the series from its inception through Volume 10. Lawrence G. Ritt served as coeditor of the first five volumes and continues to consult about the development of subsequent volumes. Steven R. Heyman was coeditor of Volumes 6 to 10. Beginning with the 11th volume, Leon VandeCreek assumed the position of senior editor. Samuel Knapp served as associate editor for Volumes 11 through 16. Thomas L. Jackson has served as associate editor since Volume 11.

There are two other individuals who have made important contributions to the production of the original *Innovations* volumes. From the onset of this series, Debra Fink has supervised the final production of each volume and ensured careful attention to details that others might have missed. Laurie Girsch has ably assisted her since Volume 8. We appreciate their thoroughness and cooperative spirit. Each year they have become more important to the success of the series.

Other contributors to the preparation of these volumes include Patricia Rockwood and Jude Warinner, who have worked many hours copyediting and proofreading the manuscripts. Without their skilled assistance, this volume would not be a reality. We would also like to thank Jeff Klosterman and Krista Kauffman for their help in preparing the current volume for distribution.

CHANGES IN RECENT VOLUMES

Over the past several years, we began to notice a shift in interest (and sales) amongst our readers that appeared to correspond to changes that had occurred in their practices; namely, readers were reporting that their practices had become more "specialized" and they were now less interested in the broad range of topics that were included in each *Innovations* volume. They were also reporting lower incomes and a desire for less expensive books and other resources.

After reviewing responses to the survey questions in recent *Innovations* continuing education (CE) modules, reviewing the literature, and holding a series of focus groups and editorial conference calls, we decided to begin producing a series of somewhat smaller, less expensive, and more focused *Innovations* volumes to meet the current needs of the majority of our customers. The first four volumes are:

- *Innovations in Clinical Practice: Focus on Children and Adolescents*
- *Innovations in Clinical Practice: Focus on Violence Treatment and Prevention*
- *Innovations in Clinical Practice: Focus on Adults*
- *Innovations in Clinical Practice: Focus on Health and Wellness*

The Senior Editor, Leon VandeCreek, along with coeditors, Jeffery B. Allen, Frederick L. Peterson, Jr., and Jill Bley have already begun work on the next *Innovations* volumes; the tentative titles are *Innovations in Clinical Practice: Focus on Group, Couples, and Family Therapy* and *Innovations in Clinical Practice: Focus on Sexual Health*.

All of these new volumes will continue to follow the general format of prior *Innovations* volumes with timely, cutting-edge applied materials written with a "how to do it" emphasis, client handouts, forms, and informal instruments that clinicians can put to immediate use in their practices.

AN INVITATION TO SUBMIT A CONTRIBUTION

The editors are currently soliciting contributions for future volumes in the *Innovations* series. If you are doing something innovative in your work, please let us hear from you. Contact Dr. Leon VandeCreek, Senior Editor, Ellis Human Development Institute, 9 N. Edwin C. Moses Boulevard, Dayton, OH 45407, if you would like more detailed information on becoming a contributor.

CONTINUING EDUCATION

The Professional Resource Exchange is approved as a continuing education (CE) sponsor by several national and state organizations including the American Psychological Association and the National Board for Certified Counselors. CE credits are available to readers who are required to participate in CE programs, as well as by those who simply wish to validate their learning. To learn how to obtain home study continuing education credits through the *Innovations in Clinical Practice* series, please visit our website (www.prpress.com) or call 800-443-3364. These programs provide an economical means of obtaining continuing education credits while acquiring relevant clinical knowledge. Readers have been consistently positive about the experience of obtaining CE credits through this series.

COPYRIGHT POLICIES

Most of the material in this volume may be duplicated. You may photocopy materials (such as office forms and instruments) or reproduce them for use in your practice or share contributions with your students in the classroom; however, no part of this publication may be stored in a retrieval system, scanned, recorded, posted on an Internet website, or transmitted by any other means or in any form. For materials on which the Professional Resource Exchange holds the copyright, no further permission is required for noncommercial, professional, or educational uses. However, unauthorized duplication or publication for resale or large-scale distribution of any material in this volume is expressly prohibited.

Any material that you duplicate from this volume (with the exceptions mentioned below) must be acknowledged as having been reprinted from this volume and must note that copyright is held by the Professional Resource Exchange, Inc. The format and exact wording required in the acknowledgment are shown on the copyright page of this volume. The only exception to this policy is that clinical and office forms (not instruments) for use with clients in your own office may be reprinted without the acknowledgment mentioned above.

There are exceptions to our liberal copyright policy. We do not hold copyright on some of the materials included in this volume and, therefore, cannot grant permission to freely duplicate those materials. When copyright is held by another publisher or author, such copyright is noted on the appropriate page of the contribution. Unless otherwise noted in the credit and copyright citation, any reproduction or duplication of these materials is strictly and expressly forbidden without the consent of the copyright holder.

Leon VandeCreek
Wright State University

Jeffery B. Allen
Wright State University

Biographies

Leon VandeCreek, PhD, Senior Editor, is a licensed psychologist who is the past dean and current Professor in the School of Professional Psychology at Wright State University in Dayton, Ohio. He has been awarded the Diplomate in Clinical Psychology and he is a Fellow of several divisions of the American Psychological Association. His interests include professional training and ethical/legal issues related to professional education and practice. Dr. VandeCreek has served as President of the Pennsylvania Psychological Association, Chair of the APA Insurance Trust, Chair of the Board of Educational Affairs of the APA, and Treasurer of the Ohio Psychological Association. In 2005 he served as President of the Division of Psychotherapy of the APA. He has authored and coauthored about 150 professional presentations and publications, including 15 books. Since 1992, he has served as Senior Editor of the *Innovations in Clinical Practice: A Source Book* series, published by Professional Resource Press. Dr. VandeCreek may be contacted at the Ellis Human Development Institute, 9 N. Edwin C. Moses Boulevard, Dayton, OH 45407. E-mail: leon.vandecreek@wright.edu

Jeffery B. Allen, PhD, ABPP-CN, is currently a Professor in the School of Professional Psychology at Wright State University in Dayton, Ohio. Dr. Allen's professional experience includes a specialty internship in neuropsychology at Brown University and a focused postdoctoral fellowship at the Rehabilitation Institute of Michigan in Detroit. He is widely published in the areas of neuropsychology, head injuries, and memory in such sources as *Neuropsychologia*, *Brain Injuries*, and *Archives of Clinical Neuropsychology and Assessment*. His areas of teaching also include physiological psychology and clinical neuropsychology. His research interests include neurobehavioral disorders, quality of life in medical populations, cognitive and neuropsychological assessment, and outcome measurement in rehabilitation. He is Board Certified by the American Board of Professional Psychology in Clinical Neuropsychology and has recently published the text, *General Practitioner's Guide to Neuropsychological Assessment*, through the American Psychological Association. Dr. Allen can be reached at SOPP, Wright State University, 3640 Colonel Glenn Highway, Dayton, OH 45435-0001. E-mail: jeffery.allen@wright.edu

Table of Contents

Preface   iii

Biographies   v

Introduction to the Volume   1

SECTION I: CLINICAL ISSUES AND APPLICATIONS

Introduction to Section I   3

Optimizing Quality of Life When Treating Patients With Chronic Medical Illnesses
Jeremy M. Bottoms and Jeffery B. Allen   5

Understanding and Assessing Cognitive and
Psychological Deficits Accompanying Chronic Medical Disease
Tricia M. Giessler and Jeffery B. Allen   21

Assessment and Treatment of the Psychosocial Aspects of Breast Cancer
Nicole L. Glick and Maurice F. Prout   33

Psychosocial Aspects of Obstetrics, Gynecology, and Fertility
Ann Morrison and Brenda J. B. Roman   57

Psychosocial Manifestations of Organ Failure and Transplantation
Jerome J. Schulte, Jr.   73

Assessment and Treatment of Psychosocial Issues With Cardiac Patients
Mark A. Williams and M. Gillian Steele   85

Assessment and Treatment of Child and Adolescent Eating Disorders
Eve M. Wolf and Crystal S. Collier   105

Assessment and Treatment of Children With Disabilities Who Have Been Abused
Leo M. Orange and Martin G. Brodwin   131

SECTION II: PRACTICE MANAGEMENT AND PROFESSIONAL DEVELOPMENT

Introduction to Section II   143

Interventions for Bridging the Gaps in Minority Health
Tawanda M. Greer   145

The Development of a Sexual Health Component in Your Practice
Frederick L. Peterson, Jr. and Jill W. Bley   159

Designing a Mental Health Professional's Website: Practical and Ethical Issues
Anthony Ragusea   169

Problems and Solutions With Online Therapy
Paul A. Smiley and Leon VandeCreek   187

SECTION III: ASSESSMENT INSTRUMENTS AND CLIENT HANDOUTS

Introduction to Section III   199

Assessment Instruments

Quality of Life Rating (QOLR) Instrument
Jeffery B. Allen   201

Adolescent Suicide Assessment Protocol-20
William Fremouw, Julia M. Strunk, Elizabeth A. Tyner, and Robert (Bob) Musick   207

The Index of Race-Related Stress–Brief Version (IRRS-B)
Compiled by Tawanda M. Greer   225

Eating Behaviors and Body Image Test for Preadolescent Girls
Compiled by Eve M. Wolf   231

Client Handout

Coping With Serious Illness
American Psychological Association   239

Eating Disorder Handouts

Ten Things Parents Can Do to Prevent Eating Disorders
National Eating Disorders Association   243

Tips for Kids on Eating Well and Feeling Good About Yourself
National Eating Disorders Association   245

Helping Yourself
Harvard Eating Disorders Center   247

Helping Your Child
Harvard Eating Disorders Center   251

Helping Your Friend
Harvard Eating Disorders Center   253

SECTION IV: SELECTED TOPICS

Introduction to Section IV   255

Psychotherapist Wellness as an Ethical Imperative
Jeffrey E. Barnett, Lesley C. Johnston, and Deborah Hillard   257

Ethical and Professional Issues for Mental Health Providers in Corrections
Ron Bonner   273

Subject Index   287

Continuing Education Available for Home Study   291

INNOVATIONS IN CLINICAL PRACTICE

Focus on Health and Wellness

A Volume in the *Innovations in Clinical Practice* Series

Introduction
To the Volume

This volume of *Innovations in Clinical Practice* represents the fourth publication since we shifted from comprehensive books with about 35 contributions, to more focused volumes that provide more depth on specific topics. In this volume, the focus is on health and wellness. As in prior volumes, contributions are grouped into sections with common themes.

The first section, CLINICAL ISSUES AND APPLICATIONS, includes contributions that are related to new developments in theory, assessment, and treatment. The range of topics is quite broad; no unifying themes are present other than that the focus of each contribution is on working with health and wellness topics. We hope these chapters provide current information about new clinical techniques that practitioners can incorporate into their practices.

The second section includes chapters on PRACTICE MANAGEMENT AND PROFESSIONAL DEVELOPMENT. These contributions are presented to assist practitioners in building and managing their practices in effective ways. Two of the chapters address interfacing with the Internet, one on how to design a website, and the other on special issues that arise when conducting online therapy. The other chapters in this section address interventions for bridging the gaps in minority health and development of a sexual health component in your practice.

The third section, ASSESSMENT INSTRUMENTS AND CLIENT HANDOUTS, provides tools for practitioners to use to collect and organize information. The assessment tools are primarily informal and designed to assist clinicians in collecting information about their clients. Our goal is to publish screening instruments and forms that aid in the organization of data, rather than the making of formal inferences and diagnoses. The materials presented here should be useful to mental health professionals, with minimal potential for misuse. We assume that readers will be thoroughly familiar with any disorders or processes that they evaluate, and readers are advised to carefully review the introductory materials that accompany contributions to this section. We have included four assessment instruments. We have also included six handouts for use with your clients in this section. Five of the handouts address eating disorders.

The fourth section, SELECTED TOPICS, includes contributions that do not fit neatly into one of the other sections. We have selected two contributions for this section.

Introduction to Section I:
Clinical Issues and Applications

The CLINICAL ISSUES AND APPLICATIONS section includes contributions that are primarily related to new developments in theory, prevention, assessment, and treatment. No unifying themes are intended other than that the focus of each contribution is on working with health and wellness issues. This section provides a means for practitioners to access current information about new clinical techniques that might be incorporated into their practices, or to learn of new developments in specialized areas.

In the first contribution, Jeremy Bottoms and Jeffery Allen introduce readers to the role that quality of life plays in measuring treatment outcomes for chronic medical illness. Chronic medical illness impacts patients' everyday functioning, and physicians and mental health practitioners should take into account the various ways that their patients' chronic medical illnesses impact their quality of life. Caregivers also can take quality of life issues into account when they design treatments and monitor outcomes. The chapter also includes a summary sheet of additional health domains to include during clinical interviews. Accompanying this chapter is an assessment instrument entitled, "Quality of Life Rating (QOLR) Instrument" that is included in the ASSESSMENT INSTRUMENTS AND CLIENT HANDOUTS section of this volume.

When general clinicians encounter clients who have impaired cognitive or psychological functioning, it is important to know that such impairments may or may not be the result of actual functional psychiatric conditions. Chronic medical and psychological factors are interrelated with overall functioning and with the manner in which psychotherapeutic and other services are delivered. If a client exhibits deficits in cognitive functioning, those deficits could be the result of a developmental or psychological condition, a psychological condition that occurs in response to medical illness, or a chronic medical condition itself. In the second contribution to this section, Tricia Giessler and Jeffery Allen discuss a number of specific medical conditions that are both relatively frequent in the general public and accompanied by reasonably consistent patterns of cognitive deficits. They provide information to assist mental health professionals in conducting effective interviews and formal testing to assist in differential diagnosis and psychological intervention. Also included in this chapter is a form that can be used to make a neuropsychological referral and a form that guides clinicians in taking a neuropsychological history.

In the third contribution to this section, Nicole Glick and Maurice Prout offer readers an overview of the physiological and psychosocial impact of breast cancer throughout its progression from initial diagnosis to recovery and recurrence. They provide a summary of the risk factors, the types of breast cancer, screening procedures, staging, and treatments. They suggest that psychosocial treatments may be presented in a variety of modalities from psychoeducation to supportive-expressive and cognitive-behavioral therapies.

The health and wellness of women is often linked to reproduction. For some women disorders of the menstrual cycle and menopause can compromise mental well-being. In addition, certain phases and events in women's reproductive lives, such as pregnancy and the postpartum period, are times of increased vulnerability to mental distress. Similarly, complications of conceiving and pregnancy, such as infertility, multiple births, abortion, miscarriage, and stillbirth, may have psychological consequences. In the fourth contribution, Ann Morrison and Brenda Roman discuss the interface between women's reproductive health and mental health.

In the next contribution, Jerome Schulte examines the psychosocial experiences of patients in, and the process of, organ failure and transplantation. In spite of the hazards of organ transplantation, the opportunity also gives hope. The success of transplantation has created its own set of issues, the largest of which is the supply and demand imbalance. Between the time of being diagnosed with organ failure and the time of relative safety from organ rejection, patients experience the vicissitudes of the organ transplantation process. Each stage has its own trials and tribulations.

Cardiovascular disease is the leading cause of death for both men and women in the United States. Medical diagnoses and treatments have improved substantially in recent years and there is an important role for prevention efforts and rehabilitation. Areas of primary, secondary, and tertiary prevention and rehabilitation are best accomplished by the involvement of individuals from multiple professions. In the next contribution, Mark Williams and M. Gillian Steele show how mental health professionals can play a substantial role in the prevention, treatment, and rehabilitation of persons with heart disease.

In the next contribution, Eve Wolf and Crystal Collier summarize information on the assessment and treatment of feeding and eating disorders in children and adolescents. They provide information on diagnostic considerations, the role of cultural and developmental factors in understanding and treating eating disorders, assessment procedures tailored to children and adolescents, and key approaches to treatment. This chapter also includes the "Children's Body Image Scale." Later sections of this volume include the "Eating Behaviors and Body Image Test for Preadolescent Girls" which is a quick assessment tool, and several client handouts.

In the final contribution in this section, Leo Orange and Martin Brodwin describe assessment and treatment procedures for children with disabilities who have been abused. While every child is vulnerable to sexual abuse, it is generally believed that children with disabilities are abused more frequently than children in the general population. The authors describe the signs and symptoms to look for when assessing a child who may have been sexually abused and they provide a wellness approach to the topic of sexual abuse.

Optimizing Quality of Life When Treating Patients With Chronic Medical Illnesses

Jeremy M. Bottoms and Jeffery B. Allen

Chronic medical illness impacts a patient's everyday functioning in myriad ways, including physical, occupational, recreational, and relational. Primary care physicians, specialists, and mental health professionals must take into account the various ways that their patients' chronic medical illnesses impact their quality of life, and what this impact means for designing effective treatments and monitoring treatment outcomes.

This contribution addresses the role quality of life plays in measuring treatment outcomes. We define quality of life, discuss how to apply quality of life measures in treatment, and provide a brief overview of several quality of life measures. We review quality of life issues with particular chronic medical illness populations, and make recommendations for maximizing the use of quality of life measures in designing beneficial treatments and evaluating treatment outcomes.

DEFINING QUALITY OF LIFE

There has been no consensual definition of quality of life (QOL); however, there is general agreement among researchers regarding the factors that comprise QOL (World Health Organization Quality of Life Group [WHOQOL], 1995). Perhaps the most important area of agreement is an understanding of QOL as a subjective entity. Indeed, several authors (Lehman, 1983; Moinpour et al., 1995; Wenger et al., 1984; WHOQOL Group, 1995) underscore the importance of patients' ratings of their own QOL as having the most clinical relevance to treatment outcome. Quality of life has been generally associated with a person's satisfaction with life and ability to complete valued life activities. Valued life activities often include occupations, social and intimate relationships, leisure activities, and spiritual activities. Life satisfaction is often derived from financial conditions, health status, living conditions, family involvement, and a sense of control over one's life and future.

In 1995, the World Health Organization (WHO) published a position paper that outlined its development of the World Health Organization Quality of Life Assessment (WHOQOL). The WHO designed the WHOQOL as an instrument that could be used for research in different cultural settings. When designing their instrument, the WHO identified six domains that are important in determining a patient's QOL. The domains identified by the WHO include (a) a physical domain, (b) a psychological domain, (c) the patient's level of independence, (d) social relationships, (e) the environment, and (f) spirituality, religion, and personal beliefs. The WHO (1995) defined QOL as "individuals' perception of their position in life in the context of culture and value systems in which they live and in relation to their goals, expectations, standards and concerns" (p. 1405).

When patients suffer from a chronic medical illness, they often feel a loss of control over their lives. Patient reactions to their initial diagnosis often include denial, depression, and withdrawal. It is not uncommon for patients either to embrace religious and spiritual beliefs to derive strength, or to feel as if a higher power is punishing them unfairly. Patients also encounter significant changes in their physical abilities; for example, patients with chronic back pain have difficulty standing up or sitting down for long periods of time, and patients with rheumatoid arthritis may no longer be capable of tying their own shoes. Declines in patients' levels of independence and changes in patients' social relationships reduce their QOL. Patients who were highly independent prior to the onset of their illness may resent having to rely on others to complete tasks for them that they once could complete on their own. Social relationships change following the onset of chronic medical illness due to several factors: (a) friends and family members may avoid these patients, because seeing them suffer is too difficult emotionally; (b) patients may be focused on their symptoms, and friends and family may interpret this as constant complaining; and/or (c) patients may not be physically able to go to the places that they used to go to socialize with friends and family members. Each of these factors impacts specifically on patients' life satisfaction and their ability to complete valued life activities; however, they are not mutually exclusive. Many, if not all, of the factors that are used to determine a patient's QOL have significant interrelationships.

Wenger et al. (1984) identified three major domains of QOL in patients diagnosed with medical conditions. The first domain is a patient's functional capacity or ability to perform activities of daily living, and the patient's level of social, intellectual, emotional, and economic functioning. The second domain includes a patient's satisfaction with life and perceptions of well-being. The final domain encompasses the physical sequelae of the disease such as disease specific symptomatology and related areas and levels of impairment.

QOL ISSUES IN SPECIFIC MEDICAL ILLNESSES

Cancer

Early diagnosis, corresponding early intervention, and advancements in treatments have led to a greater number of patients surviving cancer, or living a longer period postdiagnosis (Moinpour et al., 1995). Cancer patients face many negative treatment-related events that compound the already negative symptoms of their disease. Moinpour et al. (1995) report that beyond the pain associated with tumors, cancer patients must also deal with nausea and vomiting caused by chemotherapy as well as fatigue, loss of hair, and other side effects associated with radiation therapy. The authors point out that cancer patients often experience a decline in their QOL as a result of both the disease process and treatment of the disease.

Padilla et al. (1990) investigated the QOL of a sample of cancer patients with varying diagnoses who reported experiencing chronic pain related to their disease and treatment. In their conceptualization of QOL, the authors distinguish between the QOL factors that can be associated with physical well-being and those associated with psychological well-being. The patients in their sample reported a decrease in QOL due to aspects of impaired physical well-being, including feelings of not having a normal life, a sense of dependence, and feeling sick (Padilla et al., 1990). These patients also identified physical weakness and not being able to work as being significant contributors to a decrease in QOL. The increase and decrease of pain sensation was also linked in this study to decreases and increases in QOL, respectively. A few patients in the sample undergoing chemotherapy or radiation also listed vomiting, nausea, and lack of sleep as significantly contributing to a poor or diminished QOL. Psychological well-being in this patient sample was related to both cognitive and affective factors of QOL. The most widely endorsed factor was whether the patient was enjoying life. Other factors the patients found important included the ability to concentrate, level of self-esteem, spiritual support, happiness, and a sense of inner peace (Padilla et al., 1990).

Patients diagnosed with lung cancer often see increased QOL as the most important treatment outcome, at times preferring improved QOL to an increase in length of survival (Montazeri et al., 2003). A preference for improved QOL is particularly salient in lung cancer patients because their treatment is more often palliative than curative (Montazeri et al., 2003). Silvestri, Pritchard, and Welch (1998) found that patients diagnosed with non-small cell lung cancer would choose chemotherapy if it were to improve their QOL but would not make the same choice if the outcome were a 3-month increase in survival. In their study, Montazeri et al. (2003) found that decreases in lung cancer patients' QOL was related to deterioration in physical mobility, energy level, and role functioning. The authors also point out that functional impairment is the most significant factor related to increased depression in lung cancer patients.

Cancer is nonselective in that it affects adults and children alike. However, it is possible that QOL considerations may differ for adults and children. Hinds et al. (2004) indicate that QOL for children and adolescents diagnosed with cancer can have significant ramifications on treatment outcome. Hinds et al. found that QOL in children and adolescents can be negatively impacted by the inability to engage in activities such as going to school and completing homework. The ability to spend time outside of the hospital, and to spend time with friends and relatives, was associated with an increase in QOL. Nausea, fatigue, and pain were all associated with decreases in QOL. Hinds et al. also provide evidence for the prediction that QOL definitions and considerations may differ between adults and children. The children in their study did not explicitly relate QOL to perceived satisfaction with their current circumstances, a sense of control over their lives, a perceived disability, or the meaning of their illness experience. Each of these factors is predicted to affect QOL, and all or most of these factors are included in definitions of QOL, such as the WHO Group's definition presented earlier. Hinds and colleagues did find that children's ideas of QOL also included factors similar to those predicted by QOL definitions including an overall sense of well-being, the ability to participate in relationships with others and common activities, and the impact of the disease.

HIV/AIDS

At the time Acquired Immune Deficiency Syndrome (AIDS) was first diagnosed in the United States, patients did not learn of their Human Immunodeficiency Virus positive (HIV+) status until they had developed symptoms associated with advanced stages of the disease (Lutgendorf et al., 1995). Due to the relatively late diagnosis of the disease, the period between diagnosis and death was so brief that issues of QOL were not addressed in treatment (Lutgendorf et al., 1995). Today, advances in HIV antibody testing have led to significant increases in the period of life between diagnosis and mortality. Lutgendorf et al. report that due to the changes brought about by earlier detection, HIV infection now is seen as a chronic, degenerative disease with serious implications for QOL.

Lutgendorf and her colleagues have separated HIV infection into three distinct stages with separate QOL issues for each of the stages. These distinct stages coincide with a patient's CD4+ T lymphocyte count. CD4+ cell counts are an excellent marker of disease progression because the HIV virus infects and destroys cells expressing the CD4 surface protein. Therefore, the lower the CD4+ cell count the more advanced the HIV disease. The first stage is asymptomatic HIV infection, defined by CD4 cell counts at 500 or greater (normal cell count is between 500 and 1600). At this stage of the disease patients may express a decrease in QOL due to depression, anxiety, or anger after they learn of the diagnosis. Patients' social functioning may impact QOL due to self- or other-imposed isolation, stigmatization, withdrawal, and difficulties trusting in relationships. Physical and work functioning are usually intact at this stage of illness and do not negatively and may even positively impact QOL.

The second stage of disease progression, described as symptomatic HIV infection, is defined as a CD4 cell count between 200 and 499. During this stage of the illness patients' depression, anxiety, and anger continue to have negative impacts on their QOL. Symptoms may begin to interfere with a patient's ability to work at this stage, although many patients are still capable of working. QOL may be decreased during this stage due to a patient's reduced energy, possible emergence of cognitive deficits, and the experience of pain related to symptomatology. The final stage, as described by the authors, is AIDS, defined as a CD4 cell count less than 200 or less than 14% of T-lymphocytes present. During this final stage patients' QOL may improve with a relief from depression, anxiety, and anger related to a facing and/or acceptance of death. However, QOL is likely to be negatively impacted by the patient no longer being able to work, as well as by impairments in self-care and in cognitive deficits.

Carballo et al. (2004) have shown that QOL factors can have significant effects on antiretroviral therapy adherence in patients diagnosed with HIV/AIDS. Specifically, these researchers have demonstrated that impaired cognitive functioning, low financial status, and little access to or poor medical care were factors associated with reduced adherence to antiretroviral therapy. Younger patients and those without a stable home were also shown to have lower adherence rates. Remple et al. (2004) reported that antiretroviral treatments often improve QOL; however, side effects, toxicities, and pill-intensive regimens are often responsible for decreases in patients' QOL. In their study, Carballo et al. found that adherence to antiretroviral therapy was diminished when patients were maintained on a pill regimen of 14 or more pills a day.

Diabetes

Studies of Type I and Type II diabetes have not incorporated QOL assessments until rather recently (Jacobson, de Groot, & Samson, 1995). Studies show some overlap in effects on QOL between Type I and Type II diabetes, but there are also many type-specific effects. Jacobson, de Groot, and Samson (1994) found that patients with either Type I or Type II diabetes had decreases in their QOL which correlated highly with increases in disease-related complications. Wells, Golding, and Burnam (1988) found rates of depression for patients with either type of diabetes to be higher than that of healthy controls but lower than that for patients with other chronic diseases (i.e., chronic obstructive lung disease and coronary vascular disease). Relatively higher rates of QOL due to psychological well-being may be linked to the finding that patients with either type of diabetes seem to have a greater sense of control over their disease and treatment than do patients with other chronic medical illnesses (Jacobson et al., 1995).

In their work on developing a measure of diabetes dietary satisfaction, Ahlgren et al. (2004) reported that the QOL domain most affected by Type II diabetes was enjoyment of food. Dietary issues are often of great concern for patients with diabetes. They are required to eliminate fat and sugar from their diets. The foods they are required to purchase to comply with their new diets are often more expensive than those they bought prior to diagnosis. Social support for a new diet is often absent from family members and friends, who fear that the patient's new diet will also negatively impact their own eating habits.

Hart et al. (2003) conducted research on the QOL of patients with Type I diabetes. The authors point out that micro- and macrovascular complications associated with the disease impact patients' psychological and physical functioning on a daily basis. They found that QOL was most impacted by macrovascular complications, including (a) transient ischemic attack (blockage of blood flow in secondary vessels in the brain that can lead to temporary blurring of vision, slurring of speech, numbness, or paralysis), (b) cerebrovascular incident (stroke), (c) angina pectoris (brief attacks of chest pain associated with decreased oxygen supply to the heart muscles), and (d) myocardial infarction (heart attack). Hyperglycemia was also found to cause decreases in QOL due in large part to the negative physical symptoms that accompany it, including (a) polyphagia (frequent hunger), (b) polyuria (frequent urination), (c) polydipsia (frequent thirst), (d) impotence, and (e) recurrent infections such as vaginal yeast infections, groin rash, or external ear infections.

Cardiac Conditions

There are a vast number of cardiac conditions including arythmia (irregular heartbeat), coronary artery disease, congestive heart failure, hypertension (high blood pressure), dyslipidemia (a defect in lipid metabolism), myocardial infarction (heart attack), and so on, that can affect a patient's QOL. Although an exhaustive coverage is beyond the scope of this contribution, an overview of QOL issues associated with a small number of these conditions will be presented.

Müller-Nordhorn et al. (2004) investigated QOL issues in patients undergoing coronary artery bypass grafting (rerouting blood flow around blocked arteries in the heart [CABG]). They report that QOL, measured preoperatively, is a predictor of mortality 6 months postoperative. A decrease in pain following surgery was responsible for the largest relevant positive change in QOL. Apart from the CABG itself, higher income and higher exercise ability were associated with positive improvements in physical domains of QOL. Mental domains of QOL improved with an increase in patient age. These authors hypothesize that high QOL mental domains in older patients may be a result of patients' viewing diseases as more common or expected in older age (age > 65 years). Wray et al. (2004) investigated QOL outcomes for patients undergoing minimally invasive direct coronary artery bypass (MIDCAB; similar to CABG but does not require the stoppage of the heart or the use of a heart and lung machine during surgery). MIDCAB is a newer procedure that is frequently being recommended for patients who, in the past, would have undergone CABG. They report that following MIDCAB patients report their QOL as being excellent. The authors also report that MIDCAB has a lower prevalence of postoperative QOL decreases as a result of depression and anxiety than conventional CABG.

Congestive heart failure (a condition where at least one chamber of the heart is not pumping efficiently, which may lead to congestion in the lungs and the pulmonary blood vessels as well as possible swelling of the lungs, legs, and ankles [CHF]) contributes to significant declines in QOL by negatively impacting work, social, and physical functioning and leading to increased psychological symptomatology (Carels, 2004). In his study of 58 patients diagnosed with CHF, Carels found that depressive symptoms had a greater negative impact on patients' ratings of QOL than did functional impairment or the degree of cardiac dysfunction. Indeed, symptoms of depression were found to directly decrease physical and emotional quality of life in CHF patients. Carels also found that for CHF patients, the greater number of depressive symptoms they experienced, the greater the likelihood of their reporting CHF-related physical symptoms.

Hypertension in cardiac patients has been shown to negatively impact their QOL (Lalonde et al., 2004). Hypertensive cardiac patients report an increase in psychological distress, lower subjective ratings of their health status, an increase in physical disabilities, and a decrease in the amount of time they spend engaging in social activities. The QOL of hypertensive patients has been shown to increase and decrease as a result of such factors as the intensity or type of care they receive (treatments that are not intensive are rated higher than intensive treatments on Time Trade-off [Stiggelbout et al., 1995], but lower on the Mental Health and Vitality scales of the SF-36 [Ware et al., 1993]) and their compliance with programs designed to lower their blood pressure (compliance with medication regimen, dietary modification, weight loss, and exercise led to higher QOL) (Lalonde et al., 2004). The Time Trade-off is a preference-based approach to QOL. It measures a patient's strength of preference for health conditions. Specifically, a patient is asked to make a choice between perfect health for a set period of time followed by death; and a less than perfect health state for a set period of time followed by death. The set period of time is adjusted for the perfect health state to find the point where the patient is indifferent to which of the two choices is preferable (Stiggelbout et al., 1995).

Table 1 presents the QOL domains to assess for each of the chronic medical illnesses discussed (Diabetes Types I and II, Cardiac Conditions, HIV/AIDS, and Cancer). Several of the domains overlap across the chronic medical illnesses. However, serveral of the illnesses have QOL domains that are unique.

TABLE 1: Summary of QOL Domains to Assess by Specific Chronic Medical Illnesses

Diabetes Types I and II	Cardiac Conditions	HIV/AIDS	Cancer
Mood	Pain	Isolation	Pain
Fatigue	Fatigue	Stigmatization	Nausea
Social support	Depression	Withdrawal	Vomiting
Family functioning	Anxiety	Work functioning	Fatigue
Physical functioning	Work functioning	Physical functioning	Loss of hair
Chronic pain	Physical functioning	Depression	Feelings of dependence
Sleep problems	Cognitive deficits	Anxiety	Physical weakness
Frequent infections	Social functioning	Anger	Concentration
Diet restrictions	Compliance with treatment	Fatigue	Self-esteem
	Exercise ability	Pain	Spiritual support
		Cognitive deficits	Inner peace
		Access to medical care	Social relationships

MEASURING AND INTERVENING WITH QOL

General Domains to be Evaluated in the Clinical Interview

A thorough clinical interview is the first step in diagnosing and developing treatment strategies for patients with chronic medical illnesses. However, slight variations or additions to a standard clinical interview may be needed to address specific QOL issues. Lehman (1983) developed the Lehman Quality of Life Interview (QOLI) as a structured self-report interview for use with severely mentally ill patients that yields a numeric rating of the patient's QOL. Although not applicable to the chronic medical illness population, Lehman (1983) emphasized two important aspects of interviewing for QOL that are relevant to all clinical interviews for QOL. The first important aspect is objective QOL, or patients' personal evaluation of what they do and experience. The other important aspect is subjective QOL, or the feelings patients associate with their experiences.

When conducting a clinical interview, practitioners usually follow a format that includes gathering information about a patient's family of origin and developmental history, educational history, relationship history, occupational history, legal history, medical and psychological history, and lifestyle and health behaviors. When conducting a QOL clinical interview, clinicians should also ask patients about how their chronic medical illness is interacting with their sexual functioning, ability to complete tasks of daily living, ability to enjoy recreational activities, the impact the illness has on family interaction and social support systems, and their level of vocational satisfaction. Of particular interest to clinicians assessing QOL issues is how differences between current and premorbid functioning have impacted the patient's life, how the patient understands these changes, and the emotions the patient associates with these differences. The patients who attempt to go back to work too soon after chemotherapy and find that they are too fatigued to be productive may feel like failures and become depressed. Clinicians who interview these types of patients need to realize the negative effect the patients' fatigue and expectations together have on their QOL and can suggest appropriate interventions that may include starting with an hour or two of work and slowly progressing back to full-time.

The purpose of the clinical interview may change based on whether the patient is being seen prior to a specific medical treatment or procedure, after diagnosis of a chronic medical illness, or when palliative interventions are the only treatment options available. The patient who is being seen prior to a specific medical procedure can be interviewed and given one or more QOL measures to establish a baseline that can be compared to postprocedure QOL functioning. The QOL interview for those patients already diagnosed with a chronic medical illness will most likely focus on identifying the areas of their life that specific medical treatments have not improved, but may be improved by psychological or other allied health interventions. QOL clinical interviews for those patients whose only treatment options are palliative interventions will likely focus on the patients' expectations and desires for minimizing discomfort and maximizing social and family functioning.

The assessment of QOL is not limited to the clinical interview or the administration of one or more instruments at the beginning of treatment. For most patients, their QOL will be as fluid as their disease symptoms. Therefore, the most effective use of QOL instruments will be to administer them at the outset of treatment along with a clinical interview focused on aspects of the patient's QOL, and then at several points along the way. Many QOL measures are sensitive to both subtle and major changes, which make them ideal for measuring treatment effectiveness and outcome. The next two sections of this contribution are devoted to brief overviews of selected general QOL measures and selected illness-specific measures respectively. See page 18 for particular domains of QOL to include in addition to those covered in a standard clinical interview.

General QOL Measures

Quality of Life Rating (QOLR)

The QOLR is a 20-item self-report instrument developed by Gust (1982) for use in rehabilitation populations. Huebner et al. (1998) assessed the psychometric properties of the instrument. The instrument uses a 5-point scale for each item to measure a patient's perceived quality of life, where 5 means *quality is excellent: no improvement necessary* and 1 means *quality is extremely poor: I need to make changes as soon as possible* (Huebner et al., 1998). The questions of the QOLR have been shown through factor analysis to load on five domains: Self-Esteem and Well-Being, Interpersonal Attachment, Economics or Basic Needs, Avocational, and Spiritual. Scoring and interpretation of the QOLR is relatively simple, with total scores ranging from 20 to 100 points. Among 384 undergraduate students, the total score on the QOLR was determined to have a mean of 73.99 and a standard deviation of 10.11 (Huebner et al., 1998). The QOLR can be used at the beginning of treatment, and may aid the tracking of progress if readministered at critical intervals throughout treatment.

The QOLR demonstrated good reliability with a Cronbach alpha of 0.87, the test-retest coefficient of stability was 0.74, and adequate concurrent validity was established with a correlation coefficient between the total score of the QOLR and the Satisfaction With Life Survey (SWLS) at 0.69 (Huebner et al., 1998). Although generalizability of the results of the Huebner et al. study may be reduced due to the homogeneity of their sample, the QOLR is a good generic measure of QOL, sensitive to change, and practical to use. The QOLR is reproduced on pages 203 to 204.

Short Form-36 Health Status Survey (SF-36)

The SF-36 is a self-report questionnaire, originally designed by Ware and colleagues (Ware et al., 1993) at the New England Medical Center, which can be administered as an interview schedule, in a computer-administered version, and in a paper-and-pencil version. A 5-point scale is used for each item. The SF-36 provides eight scales for interpretation, including physical functioning, role-physical, bodily pain, general health, vitality, social functioning, role-emotional, and mental health.

Tsai, Bayliss, and Ware (1997) have reported that the published reliability statistics in more than 25 studies looking at internal consistency and test-retest methods have exceeded the minimum standard of 0.70 recommended for measures used in group comparisons, while convergent validity has been shown between the Mental Health Subscale and other measures including the Physical Performance Test (Reuben & Siu, 1990), the Quality of Well-Being Scale (Fryback et al., 1993), and the General Health Rating Index (Read, Quin, & Hoefer, 1987).

The SF-36 offers a short administration time, computer-assisted scoring, and an impressive list of conditions that have been studied in over 50 publications. Some of the conditions that have been extensively researched using the SF-36 include cancer, cardiovascular disease, chronic obstructive pulmonary disease, diabetes, HIV/AIDS, hypertension, irritable bowel syndrome, multiple sclerosis, stroke, and transplantation (Turner-Bowker, Bartley, & Ware, 2002).

World Health Organization Quality of Life-100 (WHOQOL-100)

The WHOQOL-100 is a 100-item cross-cultural, general use, self-report measure of QOL. It has been developed by an international collaboration of 15 countries for use with both non-ill and ill populations. Reminiscent of the previous discussion of the WHO's definition of QOL, the items of the WHOQOL-100 are organized into six domains: physical, psychological, independence, social, environment, and spirituality, religion, and personal beliefs, and the items cover 24 important factors, four items on a factor, and four general items that measure overall QOL and health (WHOQOL Group, 1995). Each item is scored on a 5-point Likert scale. Although the WHOQOL-100 uses a self-administered format, if the patient is likely to have difficulty completing the instrument, it can be modified to an interview format (WHOQOL Group, 1998a).

Psychometric properties for the WHOQOL-100 have been developed from data collected with large samples of both well and sick people across the 15 countries taking part in the instrument's development. Internal consistency has been demonstrated to be good with a range of 0.66 to 0.93 across studies. Discriminate validity has been demonstrated by various studies that examined the differences in scores between well and sick sample populations. Highly valuable as well for treatment monitoring and outcomes data, the WHOQOL-100 has been shown to be sensitive to clinical change (Skevington, Bradshaw, & Saxena, 1999).

The WHOQOL-100 has recently been modified into a brief instrument, the WHOQOL-BREF. The WHOQOL-BREF is a short form made up of 26 items taken from the WHOQOL-100 and is scored in four instead of six domains. The psychometric properties of the short form are consistent with the long form (WHOQOL Group, 1998b).

The Nottingham Health Profile (NHP)

The NHP was developed by McKenna et al. as a measure of general quality of life (Hunt, McEwen, & McKenna, 1985). The NHP is a 38-item questionnaire designed to measure a patient's perceived physical, emotional, social, and health problems. The instrument has been separated into two sections. The first section has questions measuring a patient's energy, pain, emotional reactions, sleep, social isolation, and physical mobility. The second section is considered to be optional, and has seven items that measure the effects that a patient's health problems are having on his or her work; activities of daily living; social, family, and sexual functioning; and hobbies and holidays. Although the second section is optional, it offers a great deal of information that relates directly to a patient's QOL and may be pertinent to treatment planning and outcome evaluation.

The test-retest reliability for the NHP has been found to range from 0.75 to 0.88, while content validity has been reported as very high. Of further importance, the NHP has been shown to discriminate between different types of patients and has been correlated with other questionnaires (Sajatovic & Ramirez, 2001).

Disease-Specific QOL Measures

Functional Assessment of Cancer Therapy-General (FACT)

The FACT-G is a 28-item self-report instrument designed to measure QOL in cancer patients who are receiving radiation or chemotherapy (Cella et al., 1993). Each item of this measure is scored on a 5-point (0-4) Likert-type format. Raw scores are transformed into scale scores ranging from 0 to 112. Five subscales are derived from the 28 items; these subscales include physical, functional, social, and emotional well-being as well as the patient-physician relationship.

Validity of the five subscales of the FACT-G was demonstrated using factor analysis. Convergent and discriminant validity have been demonstrated by the FACT-G's correlation with other instruments. The physical and functional subscales and the total scale have further confirmed the validity of the measure by their ability to differentiate among groups of patients by stage of disease (Cella et al., 1993).

The reliability of the FACT-G has been demonstrated with test-retest correlations between .82 and .88 for the subscales and total score correlation of .92. Internal consistency assessed with Cronbach's alpha yielded an overall alpha of .89 (Cella et al., 1993).

Perhaps the most important factor for clinical use of the FACT is that several modifications have been undertaken to make the instrument more relevant to specific types of cancer. With this goal in mind, the FACT-B for use with breast cancer, the FACT-L for use with lung cancer, and the FACT-H&N for use with head and neck cancer have all been developed to assess the QOL of patients with specific forms of cancer (Brady et al., 1997; Cella et al., 1995; List et al., 1996).

The Multidimensional Quality of Life Questionnaire For Persons With HIV/AIDS (MQOL-HIV)

The MQOL-HIV is a 40-item measure of 10 separate domains of QOL in persons with HIV (New England Research Institute [NERI], 1997). The 10 domains include sexual functioning, medical care, partner intimacy, financial status, cognitive functioning, social functioning, social support, physical health, physical functioning, and mental health (NERI, 1997). Each domain is measured by scoring the responses to four items. Responses are coded on a 7-point Likert scale where 1 is never and 7 is always. Each statement is preceded by the statement "How often have each of these statements been true for you in the past 2 weeks" (NERI, 1997). Both domain scores and an overall QOL index can be computed. Domain scores range from 4 to 28. The overall QOL index is computed by using the mental health and physical functioning domain scores. When scoring the instrument, a lower domain score represents poor QOL and higher scores indicate improving or good QOL (NERI, 1997).

The authors (NERI, 1997) report that psychometric testing has found the MQOL-HIV to be both reliable and internally consistent. They also indicate that the measure is sensitive to changes in symptomatology. Benefits of the MQOL-HIV include the 10 minutes or less time to complete, the flexibility in form of administration (in-person interview, self-report, by telephone, or by mail), and existing Spanish, German, and Japanese translations of the instrument.

The Diabetes Quality of Life Measure (DQOL)

The Diabetes Quality of Life Measure (DQOL) is a 46-item self-report measure originally designed for use with patients with Type I diabetes (Jacobson, 1994). The scale consists of four major dimensions: treatment satisfaction, treatment impact, worry about long-term complications, and worry about social/vocational issues. Each item is scored by responses to a 5-point Likert scale where 1 indicates *no impact, no worries, or always satisfied*, and a score of 5 represents *always affected, always worried, or never satisfied* (Jacobson, 1994).

The DQOL is the most widely used instrument for use with diabetes patients, and validity has been demonstrated in studies that demonstrate associations between lower scores and more frequent and severe long-term complications as well as glycemic control (Polonsky, 2000). Polonsky (2000) provides an excellent overview of several diabetes-specific QOL measures.

The Seattle Angina Questionnaire (SAQ)

The Seattle Angina Questionnaire (SAQ) was developed by Spertus and colleagues (1995) for use with coronary artery disease patients. The SAQ is a 19-item self-administered instrument measuring five dimensions of coronary artery disease. The five dimensions are physical limitation, anginal stability, anginal frequency, treatment satisfaction, and disease perception (Spertus et al., 1995). The SAQ was found to correlate significantly with other measures of patient functioning and diagnosis, with correlation coefficients ranging from 0.31 to 0.70. Spertus and colleagues also report that the SAQ is a valid and reliable instrument, sensitive to dramatic as well as subtle clinical changes.

Tactics for Improving QOL

Much of the research reviewed in this contribution thus far has specifically focused on how to measure QOL in patients with chronic medical illnesses. In this section, we provide suggestions for interventions to improve patients' QOL. Again, interventions designed to improve the quality and satisfaction of the patients' valued life activities are of particular relevance to patients with chronic medical illnesses.

Several of the studies reviewed in the earlier sections of this contribution indicate that improving a patient's level of social support and family involvement will dramatically improve a patient's QOL. For patients who must spend several weeks or months in the hospital due to their treatment demands, a weekend vacation home or a day trip from the hospital can be organized. Such a vacation can give the patient a valuable opportunity to interact with friends and family members. Time away from the hospital may also give the patient a brief escape from the feeling that his or her identity is solely that of a patient or a person with a disease.

A second area of intervention that can improve patients' QOL is promoting a sense of control over their life. Interventions include allowing patients to make decisions about their treatment. A patient who undergoes chemotherapy in the morning, but whose family members are unable to visit until the afternoon, may not be able to enjoy the time with the family. The patient may be tired or experiencing negative physical symptoms related to the chemotherapy when the family members are visiting. Allowing the patient to choose to undergo chemotherapy after his or her family members have visited may increase the patient's enjoyment of the time spent with them. In the case of patients with HIV/AIDS, their sense of control may be improved by an increased involvement in activities promoting awareness of the disease to others, as well as political activism to increase funding for HIV/AIDS research. Therapists working with these patients should be aware of the opportunities and organizations in their community that patients could become active in. Increased involvement in such efforts will likely also result in increased social support for the patient.

Restricted diets are often associated with patients who have been diagnosed with both diabetes and cardiac conditions. These diets can often be upsetting for patients and their family members alike. In particular, if the patient is responsible for buying groceries, other family members may resent the drastic change in foods purchased. Therapists may suggest that both the patient and the patient's family members, who are going to be impacted by the dietary changes, meet with the dietician so that all can be well informed about what foods are appropriate. Once educated about the restrictions of the patient's diet, the family members may be able to find many meals that they would enjoy and would be appropriate for the patient. Family members will also be important in reinforcing the patient to remain on a diet. The therapist can work with the family members to develop ways in which they can be more supportive of the patient and his or her adjustment to the new diet.

Flexibility is a key term for health professionals to keep in mind when trying to improve a patient's QOL. Often treatments and procedures are followed in the same manner for all patients with a particular disease. Keeping in mind that the patient will have an individualized symptom presentation and experience of a chronic medical illness, health professionals will have a greater ability to create innovative treatments to improve the patient's QOL.

Specific psychological interventions may vary by patient and presenting illness just as theoretical orientation may vary by clinician. Research has indicated that particular orientations or techniques associated with particular orientations are effective for improving the QOL in patients with various chronic medical illnesses. Lutgendorf et al. (1995) reported that cognitive-behavioral strategies to modify patients' beliefs about their stressors, improve their sense of control, and teach adaptive coping strategies may improve their QOL. Behavior modification and cognitive-behavioral strategies are also helpful for diabetes patients who must incorporate regular checking of glucose levels and insulin injections into their daily routines. Techniques such as charting weight loss or diet compliance can be beneficial to patients adjusting to a new dietary regimen. Cancer and HIV/AIDS patients may also benefit from behavioral and cognitive-behavioral interventions. However, when medical treatment becomes palliative, psychological treatment may need to shift focus to more humanistic/existential orientations and techniques. Topics of death and isolation are likely themes for therapy with patients diagnosed with terminal illnesses. Interventions that allow patients to plan their own death and funeral, write their own obituary, and "make peace" with those they feel they have wronged may improve their QOL by giving them a greater sense of control over their own death.

CASE EXAMPLES*

Case 1

Mr. H was a 52-year-old married white man who had been diagnosed with coronary artery disease and was scheduled to undergo cardiac bypass surgery. He presented for treatment of symptoms related to anxiety and depression. Mr. H was administered the Nottingham Health Profile and the Seattle Angina Questionnaire. On the NHP his responses indicated that he was experiencing reduced energy, frequent pain, problems sleeping, and decreased mobility. Mr. H's QOL related to sexual functioning, work, and social and family relationships were also impaired. Mr. H reported that while he was frequently tired, he had difficulty getting to sleep due to frequent experiences of pain. He indicated that his depression stemmed from his inability to work and his decreased sexual functioning. His responses to the SAQ indicated that his QOL was being most influenced by his physical limitations. Mr. H reported that his major social outlet had been participating in a work-sponsored bowling league. However, his doctor had advised him to avoid the physical exertion and the cigarette smoke associated with bowling. Mr. H was employed in a warehouse, and his job required some heavy lifting. He had always prided himself on being able to keep up the same rigorous pace at work as his coworkers in their early 20s. Mr. H's anxiety was related both to his upcoming bypass surgery and his fears of not being able to return to the physical demands of his job.

---

* Names and identifying characteristics have been changed to protect confidentiality.

Mr. H entered into individual therapy for issues related to his anxiety and depression. His anxiety surrounding the surgery was greatly reduced, but the depression seemed refractory to therapy. After 4 weeks of individual therapy Mr. H still reported significant problems in his social and family relationship as well as problems with sexual functioning. Mr. H then underwent the cardiac bypass surgery. Two weeks after surgery he reported that he was no longer experiencing anxiety. He reported that he was going to return to work in 4 more weeks in a new position as a supervisor that would not require as many physical demands. He also indicated that he was experiencing a great deal less pain and was able to sleep through the night. Mr. H was administered both the NHP and the SAQ again at 4 weeks postoperative. His quality of life scores were dramatically improved except in family functioning and sexual functioning. It was recommended that Mr. H be seen with his wife for couples therapy. During the couples sessions Mr. H was able to report to his wife that she had been "doing everything" for him and that he felt like she was treating him like an "invalid." Mrs. H. reported that she was concerned about how Mr. H's anxiety and depression were "affecting his heart" and was trying to "ease his burden." They both agreed to communicate more openly, which they both reported had been difficult prior to the surgery because Mr. H had seemed withdrawn. Apart from the idea that he may never be able to return to work, Mr. H reported that his problems with sexual functioning had caused him the greatest distress. During the couples sessions Mr. and Mrs. H both reported concerns about the possible consequences of sexual activity on Mr. H's heart. The therapist suggested that Mr. and Mrs. H consult with Mr. H's physician to see if regaining sexual activity would be problematic. They were informed by the physician that there was no reason they could not resume a "normal" sex life. However, 2 weeks after meeting with the physician, Mr. and Mrs. H. reported that they were still experiencing problems with Mr. H's sexual functioning. The therapist prescribed a week of sexual expression without intercourse. On night one the couple was to get into bed naked and kiss, caress, and touch without any breast/genital stimulation. Night two allowed for genital stimulation, but again intercourse was forbidden. By the end of night two Mr. and Mrs. H had violated the no intercourse rule, and Mr. H's sexual functioning was restored.

Case 2

Ms. Y was an 18-year-old, African-American female who was diagnosed with breast cancer. The cancer was diagnosed early and the doctors were able to remove the tumor before it had a chance to spread. Following the removal of the tumor, Ms. Y began a course of chemotherapy. It was during the course of the chemotherapy that the therapist was called in to consult with the patient. Ms. Y was experiencing several negative reactions to the chemotherapy including nausea, fatigue, and pain. Apart from these physical symptoms she also seemed to be evidencing a great many symptoms of depression including crying spells, loss of pleasure, low frustration tolerance, and withdrawal. At the time of the clinical interview Ms. Y was asked to complete the SF-36 and the FACT-B. Her responses to the SF-36 indicated that her QOL was being dramatically impacted by bodily pain and poor social functioning. Her responses to the FACT-B also indicated that physical and social well-being were her most impaired domains of QOL. Ms. Y reported decreases in her negative physical symptoms between chemotherapy treatments, but her depressive symptoms remained stable. Her problems with social functioning were explored in depth. She reported that prior to her diagnosis and treatment she had been in the first semester of her senior year of high school. She stated that she had been an active member of several student organizations and was a cheerleader. Unfortunately, the chemotherapy left her too exhausted to attend school. Ms. Y admitted that she was concerned that her illness was going to have a negative impact on her ability to get into a "good school." She also had fears about whether she would be able to graduate or not. Perhaps the most distressing thought that Ms. Y had was that she would not be able to attend her senior prom.

Ms. Y was able to identify goals that she believed would help relieve her depressive symptoms. These goals included increased social activity and decreased physical symptoms. Some physical symptom reduction was achieved through the use of relaxation training and distracting techniques that she could use when feeling pain or discomfort. However, the biggest change in the number and severity of reported negative symptoms came when Ms. Y, with the help of the therapist, asked her school's principal if she could participate as a member of the prom planning committee. She was granted permission and began attending the committee meetings. Attending the meetings allowed her to have increased social interaction with her friends and made her worry less about whether she would be able to attend the prom itself. As Ms. Y's depressive symptoms decreased so did her negative physical symptoms.

Both case examples illustrate the need to assess for both disease-specific and general QOL factors. If the therapists had focused only on the success of the patients' medical treatments, they would have ignored the most significant factors affecting the patients' QOL. In the case of Ms. Y, we can see the dynamic interaction of psychological variables on the patient's physical symptoms. Had the therapist not intervened to treat her depression, it is likely that she would have continued to experience much more discomfort as a result of her chemotherapy. Mr. H provides a contrasting example where it was a fear of exacerbating his physical condition that led to his symptoms of anxiety and depression.

SUMMARY

In this contribution we have provided a definition of quality of life as well as an overview of several chronic medical illnesses that impact QOL. Our aim has not been an exhaustive review of the literature; rather it has been to provide a starting point for health professionals who are interested in improving the QOL of their patients. The QOL measures reviewed are merely a small sample of the hundreds of measures that exist, but each one has been used extensively in the research of QOL issues. Clinicians should explore the different measures to determine which seem best suited to the patients they are working with. However, it is our recommendation that a general instrument be combined with an illness-specific instrument to get maximum coverage of the domains of QOL. Flexibility is the key when intervening to improve patient's QOL, and no two patients' symptom presentations will be the same or have an effect on the same domains of quality of life.

Additional Domains to Include During a QOL-Specific Clinical Interview

Psychosocial Changes

<u>Instructions</u>: Check all that apply.

Affective:

❏ Changes in mood	❏ Depression	❏ Anxiety	❏ Stress level
❏ Irritability	❏ Energy level	❏ Obsessing/Worrying	❏ Anger

❏ Other (describe): _____

Behavioral:

❏ Sleep habits	❏ Sexual functioning	❏ Eating	❏ Movement

❏ Other (describe): _____

Social:

❏ Relationship with spouse/partner	❏ Relationship with parents
❏ Relationship with children	❏ Relationship with significant other
❏ Social activities ❏ Work relationships	❏ Activities at home

❏ Other (describe): _____

Physical Symptoms

_____ Pain (rating on a 1 to 10 scale; 10 being the worst pain, 1 being no discomfort)

❏ Nausea	❏ Vomiting	❏ Fatigue	❏ Muscle weakness
❏ Frequency of infections	❏ Thirst	❏ Hunger	❏ Vision problems

❏ Bladder function

❏ Other (describe): _____

Spiritual Considerations

❏ Spiritual support	❏ Sense of inner peace	❏ Belief in meaning of life

❏ Other (describe): _____

CONTRIBUTORS

Jeremy M. Bottoms, MA, is currently a doctoral candidate in clinical psychology at the School of Professional Psychology, Wright State University, Dayton, Ohio. He received his Masters degree in counseling from Ball State University. His research interests include quality of life issues, and memory impairment in Multiple Sclerosis. Mr. Bottoms may be contacted at 1821 Monroe-Concord Road, Troy, OH 45373. E-Mail: bottoms.2@wright.edu

Jeffery B. Allen, PhD, ABPP-CN, is board certified in Clinical Neuropsychology by the American Board of Professional Psychology. He is currently a Professor in the School of Professional Psychology at Wright State University and teaches courses in physiological psychology and clinical neuropsychology. Dr Allen completed a postdoctoral fellowship at the Rehabilitation Institute of Michigan in Detroit. He is widely published in the areas of neuropsychology, head injuries, and memory and recently completed the text, *A General Practitioner's Guide to Neuropsychological Assessment* (American Psychological Association, in press). Dr. Allen's interests include neurobehavioral disorders, quality of life in medical populations, cognitive and neuropsychological assessment, and outcome measurement in rehabilitation. Dr. Allen can be reached at SOPP, Wright State University, 3640 Colonel Glenn Highway, Dayton, OH 45435-0001. E-mail: jeffery.allen@wright.edu

RESOURCES

Ahlgren, S. S., Shultz, J. A., Massey, L. K., Hicks, B. C., & Wysham, C. (2004). Development of a preliminary diabetes dietary satisfaction and outcomes measures for patients with type 2 diabetes. *Quality of Life Research, 13*, 819-832.

Brady, M. J., Cella D. F., Mo, F., Bonomi, A. E., Tulsky, D. S., Lloyd, S. R., Deasy, S., Cobleigh, M., & Shiomoto, G. (1997). Reliability and validity of the Functional Assessment of Cancer Therapy-Breast (FACT-B) quality of life instrument. *Journal of Clinical Oncology, 15*, 974-986.

Carballo, E., Cadarso-Suarez, C., Carrera, I., Fraga, J., de la Fuente, J., Ocampo, A., Ojea, R., & Prieto, A. (2004). Assessing relationships between health-related quality of life and adherence to antiretroviral therapy. *Quality of Life Research, 13*, 587-599.

Carels, R. A. (2004). The association between disease severity, functional status, depression and daily quality of life in congestive heart failure patients. *Quality of Life Research, 13*, 63-72.

Cella, D. F., Bonomi, A. E., Lloyd, S. R., Tulsky, D. S., Kaplan, E., & Bonomi, P. (1995). Reliability and validity of the Functional Assessment of Cancer Therapy-Lung (FACT-L) quality of life instrument. *Lung Cancer, 12*, 199-220.

Cella, D. F., Tulsky, D. S., Gray, G., Sarafian, B., Linn, E., Bonomi, A., Silberman, M., Yellen, S. B., Winicour, P., & Brannon, J. (1993). The Functional Assessment of Cancer Therapy Scale: Development and validation of the general measure. *Journal of Clinical Oncology, 11*, 570-579.

Fryback, D. G., Dosbach, E. J., Klein, R., Klein, B., Dorn, N., Peterson, K., & Martin, A. M. (1993). The Beaver Dam Health Outcomes Study. Initial catalog of health state quality factors. *Medical Decision Making, 13*, 89-102.

Gust, T. (1982). *Quality of Life Rating.* Unpublished instrument.

Hart, H. E., Bilo, H. J. G., Redekop, W. K., Stolk, R. P., Assink, J. H., & Meyboom-de Jong, B. (2003). Quality of life of patients with type I diabetes mellitus. *Quality of Life Research, 12*, 1089-1097.

Hinds, P. S., Gattuso, J. S., Fletcher, A., Baker, E., Coleman, B., Jackson, T., Jacobs-Levine, A., June, D., Rai, S. N., Lensing, S., & Pui, C.-H. (2004). Quality of life as conveyed by pediatric patients with cancer. *Quality of Life Research, 13*, 761-772.

Huebner, R. A., Allen, J. B., Inman, T. H., Gust, R., & Turpin, S. G. (1998). Quality of life rating: Psychometric properties and theoretical comparisons. *Journal of Rehabilitation Outcomes Measurement, 2*(5), 8-16.

Hunt, S. M., McEwen, J., & McKenna, S. P. (1985). Measuring health status: A new tool for clinicians and epidemiologists. *Journal of the Royal College of General Practitioners, 35*(273), 185-188.

Jacobson, A. M. (1994). The DCCT Research: The Diabetes Quality of Life Measure. In C. Bradley (Ed.), *Handbook of Psychology and Diabetes* (pp. 65-87). Switzerland: Harwood Academic Publishers.

Jacobson, A. M., de Groot, M., & Samson, J. (1994). Quality of life in patients with type I and type II diabetes mellitus. *Diabetes Care, 17*, 167-274.

Jacobson, A. M., de Groot, M., & Samson, J. (1995). Quality of life research in patients with diabetes mellitus. In J. E. Dimsdale & A. Baum (Eds.), *Quality of Life in Behavioral Medicine Research* (pp. 241-262). Hillsdale, NJ: Lawrence Erlbaum Associates.

Lalonde, L., O'Conner, A., Joseph, L., Grover, S. A., & The Canadian Collaborative Cardiac Assessment Group. (2004). Health-related quality of life in cardiac patients with dyslipidemia and hypertension. *Quality of Life Research, 13*, 793-804.

Lehman, A. F. (1983). The well-being of chronic mental patients. *Archives of General Psychiatry, 40*, 369-373.

List, M. A., D'Antonio, L. L., Cella, D. F., Siston, A., Mumby, P., Haraf, D., & Vokes, E. (1996). The Performance Status Scale for head and neck cancer patients and the Functional Assessment of Cancer Therapy-Head and Neck (FACT-H&N) scale: A study of utility and validity. *Cancer, 77*, 2294-2301.

Lutgendorf, S., Antoni, M. H., Schneiderman, N., Ironson, G., & Fletcher, M. A. (1995). Psychosocial interventions and quality of life changes across the HIV spectrum. In J. E. Dimsdale & A. Baum (Eds.), *Quality of Life in Behavioral Medicine Research* (pp. 205-239). Hillsdale, NJ: Lawrence Erlbaum Associates.

Moinpour, C. M., Savage, M., Hayden, K. A., Sawyers, J., & Upchurch, C. (1995). Quality of life assessment in cancer clinical trials. In J. E. Dimsdale & A. Baum (Eds.), *Quality of Life in Behavioral Medicine Research* (pp. 79-95). Hillsdale, NJ: Lawrence Erlbaum Associates.

Montazeri, A., Milroy, R., Hole, D., McEwen, J., & Gillis, C. R. (2003). How quality of life data contribute to our understanding of cancer patients' experiences: A study of patients with lung cancer. *Quality of Life Research, 12*, 157-166.

Müller-Nordhorn, J., Kulig, M., Binting, S., Völler, H., Gohlke, H., Linde, K., & Willich, S. N. (2004). Change in quality of life in the year following cardiac rehabilitation. *Quality of Life Research, 13*, 399-410.

New England Research Institute (NERI). (1997). *Multidimensional Quality of Life Questionnaire for Persons With HIV/ AIDS (MQOL-HIV) Administration and Scoring Manual.* Watertown, MA: Author.

Padilla, G. V., Ferrell, B., Grant, M. M., & Rhiner, M. (1990). Defining the content domain of quality of life for cancer patients with pain. *Cancer Nursing, 13*(2), 108-115.

Polonsky, W. H. (2000). Understanding and assessing diabetes-specific quality of life. *Diabetes Spectrum, 13*, 36-41.

Read, J. L., Quin, R. J., & Hoefer, M. A. (1987). Measuring overall health: An evaluation of three important approaches. *Journal of Chronic Disease, 40*(Supp.), 75-215.

Remple, V. P., Hilton, B. A., Ratner, P. A., & Burdge, D. R. (2004). Psychometric assessment of the Multidimensional Quality of Life Questionnaire for Persons With HIV/AIDS (MQOL-HIV) in a sample of HIV-infected women. *Quality of Life Research, 13*, 947-957.

Reuben, D. B., & Siu, A. L. (1990). An objective measure of physical function of elderly outpatients: The Physical Performance Test. *Journal of the American Geriatric Society, 38*, 1105-1112.

Sajatovic, M., & Ramirez, L. F. (2001). *Rating Scales in Mental Health.* Hudson, OH: Lexi-Comp.

Silvestri, G., Pritchard, R., & Welch, H. G. (1998). Preferences for chemotherapy in patients with advanced non-small cell lung cancer: Descriptive study based on scripted interviews. *British Medical Journal, 317*, 771-775.

Skevington, S. M., Bradshaw, J., & Saxena, S. (1999). Selecting national items for the WHOQOL: Conceptual and psychometric considerations. *Social Science and Medicine, 48*, 473-487.

Spertus, J. A., Winder, J. A., Dewhurst, T. A., Deyo, R. A., Prodzinski, J., McDonnell, M., & Fihn, S. D. (1995). Development and evaluation of the Seattle Angina Questionnaire: A new functional status measure of coronary artery disease. *Journal of the American College of Cardiology, 25*(2), 333-341.

Stiggelbout, A. M., Kiebert, G. M., Kievit, J., Leer, J. W., Habbema, J. D., & DeHaes, J. C. (1995). The "utility" of the time trade-off method in cancer patients: Feasibility and proportional trade-off. *Journal of Clinical Epidemiology, 48*(10), 1207-1214.

Tsai, C., Bayliss, M. S., & Ware, J. E. (1997). *SF-36® Health Survey Annotated Bibliography: Second Edition (1988-1996).* Boston, MA: Health Assessment Lab, New England Medical Center.

Turner-Bowker, D. M., Bartley, P. J., & Ware, J. E. (2002). *SF-36® Health Survey & "SF" Bibliography: Third Edition (1988-2000).* Lincoln, RI: QualityMetric Incorporated.

Ware, J. E., Snow, K. K., Kosinski, M., & Gandek, B. (1993). *SF-36 Health Survey Manual and Interpretation Guide.* Boston: Medical Outcomes Trust.

Wells, K. B., Golding, J. M., & Burnam, M. A. (1988). Psychiatric disorders in a sample of the general population with and without chronic medical conditions. *American Journal of Psychiatry, 145*, 976-981.

Wenger, N. K., Mattson, M. E., Furberg, C. D., & Elinson, J. (1984). Assessment of quality of life in clinical trials of cardiovascular therapies. *American Journal of Cardiology, 54*, 908-913.

World Health Organization Quality of Life Group. (1995). The World Health Organization Quality of Life Assessment (WHOQOL): Position paper from the World Health Organization. *Social Science and Medicine, 41*, 1403-1409.

World Health Organization Quality of Life Group. (1998a). The World Health Organization Quality of Life Assessment (WHOQOL): Development and general psychometric properties. *Social Science and Medicine, 46*(12), 1569-1585.

World Health Organization Quality of Life Group. (1998b). Development of the World Health Organization WHOQOL-BREF quality of life assessment. *Psychological Medicine, 28*, 551-558.

Wray, J., Al-Ruzzeh, S., Mazrani, W., Kanamura, K., George, C., Ilsley, C., & Amrani, M. (2004). Quality of life and coping following minimally invasive direct coronary artery bypass (MIDCAB) surgery. *Quality of Life Research, 13*, 915-924.

Understanding and Assessing Cognitive and Psychological Deficits Accompanying Chronic Medical Disease

Tricia M. Giessler and Jeffery B. Allen

When the general clinician encounters a client who has impaired cognitive or psychological functioning, it is important to know that such impairment may or may not be the result of actual functional psychiatric conditions. Chronic medical factors and psychological factors and conditions are interrelated with overall functioning and the manner in which psychotherapeutic, case management, rehabilitation, and family assistance services are delivered. Developmental and psychological conditions, such as learning disability (LD) and depression, often result in neuropsychological impairment; likewise, neurological and other medical conditions can produce psychological symptoms that in turn affect neuropsychological performance. Accordingly, if a client exhibits deficits in neuropsychological functioning, those deficits could be the result of a developmental or psychological condition, a psychological condition that occurs in response to medical illness, or a chronic medical condition itself.

Obviously, differential diagnosis is challenging when the influences of developmental, psychological, or psychosocial factors become entangled with the effects of medical illness. In such cases, the general clinician can benefit from referring the client for a neuropsychological consultation to clarify the extent of neuropsychological involvement rather than simplistically placing the client in either the "organic" (biological) or "functional" (behavioral) diagnostic group.

Moreover, cognizance of the etiology and nature of the developmental, psychological, and psychosocial consequences generated by medical conditions is necessary in the long-term management and treatment of such conditions. The psychological and psychosocial aspects of head injury, for example, are critical in predicting which individuals will successfully return to various social and occupational roles. Additionally, patients who experience physiological conditions with accompanying psychological and behavioral repercussions may recover from the physiological symptoms but retain psychological and behavioral changes that need to be addressed by the mental health clinician.

When making an appropriate referral and integrating the findings of subsequent cognitive and neuropsychological evaluation into the general assessment and treatment plan, it is crucial to understand the relationship between nonneurological elements and neuropsychological impairment. These constructs should be viewed as overlapping or additive, rather than mutually exclusive. A richer comprehension of the relationship may be facilitated by placing the complex nonneurological factors that influence neuropsychological performance along a continuum rather than into restrictive categories such as organic or functional. The following discussion will provide examples of a number of specific medical conditions that are both relatively frequent in the general public and accompanied by reasonably consistent patterns of psychological and cognitive symptom pictures. Following this summary, information will be provided to assist the mental health clinician in conducting effective interviews and formal testing to assist in the differential diagnostic process. The contribution will conclude with practical information concerning psychological interventions with clients who are dealing with chronic medical/health conditions.

MEDICAL CONDITIONS WITH PSYCHOLOGICAL AND NEUROPSYCHOLOGICAL MANIFESTATIONS

Multiple Sclerosis

Appearing in adults as young as 20 years old, multiple sclerosis can have lifelong debilitating effects. Multiple sclerosis is characterized by destruction of myelin sheaths surrounding central nervous system axons. This demyelination results in slowed or blocked nerve impulses and often in vision impairments, loss of sensation, coordination difficulties, bladder disturbances, sexual dysfunction, weakness, and fatigue (Cairns, 2004; Devins & Shnek, 2000). The disease may take various progressive courses. The majority of multiple sclerosis patients (65%-70%) experience a relapsing-remitting course, characterized by periods of increased symptomatology followed by periods of symptom relief. A second course, experienced by 15%-20% of the patient population, is characterized by continuous, progressive symptomatology, without periods of symptom remission. A third course, considered a benign course, is experienced by the remaining patients. This course involves little to no progression and few symptoms for several years after onset (Devins & Shnek, 2000).

Throughout the illness, many patients experience several cognitive, affective, and psychological consequences. Cognitive effects include impaired attention, memory, concentration, verbal fluency, and word finding; problem-solving and reasoning difficulties; and decreased processing speed (Cairns, 2004; Demaree et al., 1999; Devins & Shnek, 2000; Mohr & Cox, 2001).

Affective changes include increased depression and/or anxiety, anger, and euphoria (Mohr & Cox, 2001). Psychological effects include difficulty managing stress related to the illness, uncertainty related to when the next period of increased symptoms will occur, hopelessness related to living with a chronic illness, and reduced self-efficacy (Devins & Shnek, 2000). Additionally, patients experience significant lifestyle changes due to the effects of the disease. Many patients are unable to continue working and must change their daily activities due to fatigue, coordination problems, and cognitive deficits. Patients also experience difficulties with interpersonal relationships due to sexual dysfunction, care requirements, cognitive difficulties, and increased affective changes (Devins & Shnek, 2000; Mohr et al., 1999).

Metabolic Conditions or Endocrine Disorders

Many potentially reversible metabolic conditions or endocrine disorders can lead to acute or gradual mental status changes and neurobehavioral symptoms. Symptom patterns of these disorders are discussed below.

The endocrine disorders hyperthyroidism and hypothyroidism (overactivity and underactivity of the thyroid gland, respectively) can produce dramatic affective, cognitive, and behavioral alterations. Some hyperthyroid patients display a characteristic hyperactivity or agitation; others exhibit affective elements that are more typical of depressive illness. Individuals who have hypothyroidism often demonstrate decreased intellectual functioning and elements of cognitive and/or motor slowing. This symptom picture can emerge gradually and at times resemble the progressive decline often associated with dementia. The distinction is critical, however, as thyroid conditions are often treatable once they are diagnosed. Dysfunction of the pituitary or adrenal system also can produce acute or gradual mental status deficits and psychological symptoms.

Metabolic deficiencies or disorders of specific bodily organs also can result in direct or indirect neuropathologic changes that may lead to cognitive and intellectual dysfunction. One such condition is Wilson's disease, in which a rare disorder of copper metabolism causes copper ions to remain in the liver and in some subcortical regions of the brain. Due to the subcortical pathology of the disorder, many of the early neurological symptoms are motoric and often include tremor, rigidity, and dysarthria (motor speech impairment). When a behavioral or psychological component exists with the condition, it often includes emotional lability; silly, immature, or impulsive behavior; and sexual promiscuity (Strub & Black, 1988). Many patients also demonstrate decreased memory and attentional and higher order cognitive difficulties (e.g., judgment, reasoning).

Hypoxia, or the reduced availability of oxygen to the brain, is a broad neuropathologic category that may be brought on by different traumatic or medical circumstances. Cardiac failure, restricted circulatory functioning, and respiratory arrest can produce hypoxia, or even anoxia – a complete loss of oxygen to the brain. Situations that can lead to hypoxic states include carbon monoxide poisoning, smoke inhalation, electrocution, and strangulation. Given the neuron's inability to store oxygen for later use, brain cells are destroyed within approximately 5 minutes when anoxia is complete, resulting in permanent injury or brain death. Hypoxia may produce deficits of attention, memory, or judgment.

Another endocrine condition that may present with largely behavioral or psychiatric disturbance is hypoglycemia (low blood sugar). Because glucose is a nutritional staple of the central nervous system, even temporary deficiencies in the brain's available supply of glucose may result in neurological complications. Hypoglycemia is not a specific disease process; it results from situations that lead to reduced blood sugar. When these situations occur, the sympathetic nervous system responds with symptoms of hypertension, tachycardia, sweating, and malaise. Cognitive or emotional features may include only irritability or anxiety or more dramatic symptoms such as disorientation, confusion, suspiciousness, and hallucinatory experiences. In the most severe cases, individuals experience loss of consciousness or coma. The reversibility of an acute hypoglycemic episode is startling once correctly identified and appropriately treated with intravenous glucose. Cases have been reported in which individuals who were incoherent and confused and exhibiting psychotic characteristics became cogent and manageable within minutes following the administration of glucose.

Cardiac Conditions

Several cardiac conditions have significant neuropsychological, affective, and psychological implications. Often characterized as an early cardiovascular disease, hypertension can lead to several other cardiac conditions. Hypertension is typified by high blood pressure levels and includes two subtypes, essential hypertension and secondary hypertension. Essential hypertension entails sustained blood pressure elevation with no known etiology. Secondary hypertension involves heightened blood pressure with a known cause such as renal pathology or a hormonal disorder (Waldstein et al., 2001).

Characterized by several neuropsychological deficits, hypertension can lead to impairments in learning, memory, attention, psychomotor abilities, abstract reasoning, and visuospatial, visuoperceptual, and visuoconstructional abilities (Waldstein & Katzel, 2001; Waldstein et al., 2001). The deficits are related to age and education levels. The age effect indicates that a more significant difference in performance levels exists between hypertensive young adults and healthy young adults than between hypertensive middle-aged adults and healthy middle-aged adults. The education effect indicates that lower education is related to poorer cognitive function in hypertension patients (Waldstein et al., 2001).

Atherosclerosis is a cardiac disorder characterized by plaque formations in artery walls that diminish blood supply to the heart and decrease the heart's ability to efficiently pump blood throughout the body. Atherosclerosis may lead to angina pectoris, myocardial infarction, and stroke. Cognitive effects of atherosclerosis are measured by the disease's severity level. Greater severity levels are associated with more impaired verbal and nonverbal memory, mental status, verbal fluency, cognitive flexibility, and perceptuomotor speed (Everson et al., 2001; Waldstein et al., 2001).

Angina pectoris is a cardiac condition that involves chest pain due to decreased oxygen in the cardiac muscle. The condition has several possible etiologies, including atherosclerosis, imbalance in cardiac demand and supply, vascular heart disease, cardiomyopathy, and left ventricular outflow (Waldstein et al., 2001).

Myocardial infarction involves death of a region of heart muscle known as the myocardium. Transmural myocardial infarction is characterized by death across layers of heart muscle. Nontransmural myocardial infarction does not involve all layers of the heart. Several etiologies may explain myocardial infarction, including coronary emboli, atherosclerosis within the coronary artery, coronary vasospasm, thrombotic disease, vasculitis, and trauma (Waldstein et al., 2001). Cognitive deficits related to myocardial infarction include dementia symptomatology, difficulties with fine motor skills, disorientation, and impaired memory, verbal fluency, verbal learning, and psychomotor speed. Affective changes include comorbid depression (Vingerhoets, 2001).

Cardiac arrhythmias (abnormal heartbeats) are caused by irregularities in the initiation of the heartbeat and/or in the conduction of the heartbeat. Ventricular fibrillation, the most severe form of cardiac arrhythmia, can lead to cardiac arrest. Cardiac arrhythmias are characterized by several cognitive deficits, including impaired attention, learning, memory, verbal fluency, and executive function and declines in mental status functioning. Cardiac arrests present with more profound deficits, including amnesia, memory problems, and visuoconstructive deficits (Vingerhoets, 2001; Waldstein et al., 2001).

Chronic Obstructive Pulmonary Disease

Characterized by a group of diseases including emphysema and chronic bronchitis, chronic obstructive pulmonary disease (COPD) involves obstruction of the patient's airflow. This obstruction results in lung hyperinflation, impaired gas exchange, shortness of breath, dyspnea (patient's experience of labored breathing), coughing, hypoxemia (displacement of oxygen from the hemoglobin molecule), and wheezing (Hopkins & Bigler, 2001). This symptomatology places increased stress on the patient's respiratory muscles, making it increasingly harder to breathe. COPD is often caused by cigarette smoking, which accounts for 80% to 90% of COPD development (Boyle & Locke, 2004). However, inhalation of other toxic substances also may lead to this disease. COPD often involves significant psychological, cognitive/neuropsychological, affective, and psychosocial consequences. The severity of neuropsychological impairments is often related to the impact of hypoxemia on neural tissue. Consistent with the diffuse nature of hypoxemia, the cognitive impairments seen in COPD are also variable and diffuse and may include impaired memory, attention, and psychomotor speed and decreased abstract reasoning skills (Hopkins & Bigler, 2001). End-stage COPD patients experience additional neuropsychological impairments. They experience deficits in immediate free recall and long-term retrieval, set-shifting, cognitive processing speed, and visuomotor scanning (Crews et al., 2001).

In addition to experiencing cognitive difficulties, many COPD patients also experience affective changes. Depression, anxiety, and hypochondriasis are common comorbid conditions with COPD. Although the affective changes may be related to chemical imbalances resulting from the effects of hypoxemia, they are also as likely due to the lifestyle changes that COPD patients are expected to undergo (Hopkins & Bigler, 2001). COPD patients often experience new limits placed on their daily activities due to difficulty breathing after periods of exertion. Psychological responses also may include grief, loneliness, and powerlessness (Boyle & Locke, 2004). Due to the significant cognitive, affective, and psychological consequences of COPD, patients often experience reduced quality of life. Recently, several researchers have examined quality-of-life issues related to COPD patients (Nicolson & Anderson, 2003; Van der Molen et al., 2003; Van Stel et al., 2003). In a focus group of COPD patients, emotional distress, reliance on medication, disruption of interpersonal relationships, and negative self-esteem emerged as themes related to decreased quality of life (Nicolson & Anderson, 2003). Additionally, ability to manage daily activities, physical and social functioning, levels of pain and difficulty breathing as well as experience of depression and/or anxiety relate to COPD patients' quality of life (Van Stel et al., 2003). Further variables implicated in quality of life include preventing disease progression, decreasing symptoms, and improving functional abilities (Van der Molen et al., 2003).

ASSESSMENT OF NEUROPSYCHOLOGICAL AND PSYCHOLOGICAL FACTORS IN PATIENTS WITH CHRONIC MEDICAL ILLNESSES

Behavioral Observations

Conducting a thorough assessment for psychological and neuropsychological factors with a medically ill patient includes behavioral observation. Before beginning behavioral observation, it is important to be aware of cultural variations in behaviors (e.g., eye contact). Five components of nonverbal behavior are important to note when conducting an assessment. The first variable, kinesics, includes body gestures, eye contact, facial expressions, and body movements. Paralinguistics include characteristics of the patient's speech, such as loudness, pitch, rate of speech, and verbal fluency. A third variable, proxemics, refers to physical distance between the patient and others (including the assessor). A fourth variable is related to how the client responds to the environment in which the assessment is occurring. A final variable related to nonverbal behavior is time, particularly the patient's values regarding time and use of time during the evaluation (S. Cormier & B. Cormier, 1998).

Other important considerations regarding behavioral observations include the patient's affect, congruence of affect with discussion material, and attention to and interest in the evaluation. During evaluations with medically ill clients, it is important to observe health-related behaviors and be aware of how the client deals with pain or discomfort during the evaluation.

Formal Testing

Formal testing with medically ill patients can be conducted within two categories, general assessments and disease-specific assessments. Several assessment instruments used for general mental health population clients have been used widely with medically ill patients as well, to assess mood, personality, and neuropsychological functioning. One instrument used widely in medical settings to measure mood is the Beck Depression Inventory-II (BDI-2; Beck, Steer, & Brown, 1996). The BDI has shown strong reliability and validity in recognizing depressive symptomatology; however, this instrument should be used with caution as medical patients may have elevated depression levels due to experiencing several somatic symptoms. An instrument used widely to measure personality characteristics is the Minnesota Multiphasic Personality Inventory-II (MMPI-2; Butcher et al., 1989). The MMPI-2 has been used with multiple sclerosis patients (Nelson et al., 2003); however, use of this scale in medical populations should follow the same cautionary note as the BDI. Patients may elevate on somatic scales due to physical illness symptoms; therefore, patient profiles should be examined regarding endorsement of somatic symptomatology to determine if it is disease related or personality related. Alternatively, the Millon Behavioral Health Inventory (MBHI) may allow the clinician to gather information on a broader array of patient attitudes toward health and health professionals. Importantly, there is some evidence that the MBHI may overly pathologize some patients seen in a medical context (Elliott & Umlauf, 1995).

Assessment of neuropsychological functioning in medical patients often involves the use of standard neuropsychological instruments. Studies of neuropsychological function in multiple sclerosis patients have included standard tests such as the Wechsler Adult Intelligence Scale-Third Edition (WAIS-III; Wechsler, 1997a), which assesses intellectual ability; the Wechsler Memory Scale-Third Edition (WMS-III; Wechsler, 1997b); the California Verbal Learning Test-2nd Edition (CVLT-2; Delis et al., 2000), which measures memory and learning; and the Wisconsin Card Sorting Test (WCST; Heaton et al., 1993), which measures executive function (Mohr & Cox, 2001). Additionally, several studies have used neuropsychological tests within the Halstead-Reitan battery (Reitan & Wolfson, 1985) to measure neuropsychological deficits within medical illnesses.

When using tests intended for the general population, the practitioner must consider the patient's medical limitations when selecting proper tests. A patient with left-side paralysis, for example, would have difficulty with a test requiring use of the left hand. Likewise, many patients with the medical conditions discussed in this contribution experience attention and concentration difficulties as well as impaired psychomotor speed and visuoperceptual skills. These clients may have particular difficulty with timed tests. Although it will be necessary to complete the test in a standardized fashion, after completion of the test, the examiner may opt to revisit a failed task to evaluate whether the patient is able to succeed without time constraints.

Several instruments have been created to address specific medical populations. These instruments may provide a unique perspective on a patient's experience with his or her medical condition; however, the tests should be used with caution as they may be less psychometrically sound. Disease-specific instruments include the Clinical Chronic Obstructive Pulmonary Disease Questionnaire (CCQ), which examines functional status, symptomatology, and quality of life for COPD patients (Van der Molen et al., 2003); the Quality of Life for Respiratory Illness Questionnaire (QoLRIQ), which examines life satisfaction and functional status in pulmonary rehabilitation patients (Van Stel et al., 2003); and the Guy's Neurological Disability Scale (GNDS), a measure of physiological and cognitive symptomatology in multiple sclerosis patients (Sharrack & Hughes, 1999).

Please find a neuropsychological history form and referral worksheet that can be used in clinical interviews on pages 27 to 30.

CONCLUSION

Issues related to initial diagnosis of neurological impairment may be handled by treating physicians, neurologists, and neuropsychologists, but management and treatment of behavioral symptoms is often left to the psychologist. Anticipating the broad array of emotional and psychosocial difficulties that often plague clients with neurological involvement may greatly enhance treatment planning and eventual outcome of psychotherapeutic interventions. Awareness of the specific cognitive deficits that accompany many neurobehavioral syndromes can assist in expediting and focusing the delivery of psychological services that are better tailored to the unique needs of the cognitively involved client. This last consideration is especially relevant given the increasing economical demands of a service delivery affected by the constraints of a managed care environment.

Cognitive/Neuropsychological History

Client Identification

Client Name: _____ Age: _____

Date of Birth: _____ Education: _____ Gender: _____ Race/Ethnicity: _____ Marital Status: ____

Client Address/Telephone:

_____

_____

Date of Evaluation: _____

Presenting Complaints

_____
_____
_____
_____

History of Specific Neurological Events

_____
_____
_____
_____

History of Symptoms With Potential Neurological Significance

_____
_____
_____

Previous Neurological Procedures and Findings

_____
_____
_____

Cognitive Changes (Check any that apply)

Language deficits:	❑ word finding	❑ verbal comprehension	
Attentional deficits:	❑ task maintenance	❑ distractibility	❑ impulse control
Memory deficits:	❑ name retrieval	❑ recall of recent personal events	
Visuospatial deficits:	❑ visual perception	❑ spatial orientation	
Cognitive speed deficits	❑		
Problem-solving and reasoning deficits	❑		

Description (describe the nature of any problem noted above):

_____
_____
_____
_____

Psychosocial Changes

Affective:

_____
_____
_____

Behavioral:

_____
_____
_____

Social:

_____
_____
_____

Description (describe the nature of any problem noted above):

_____
_____
_____

Significant Medical History

Previous surgeries/hospitalizations:

_____
_____
_____

Serious conditions/illnesses:

_____
_____
_____

Family medical history:

_____
_____
_____

Birth/Developmental History

_____
_____
_____

Educational and Social History

_____
_____
_____

Other

_____
_____
_____
_____

Neuropsychological Referral Worksheet

Client Name: _____ Identification Number: _____

Education: _____ Date of Birth: _____ Age: _____ Gender: _____

Marital Status: _____ Occupational Status: _____

Address/Telephone:

_____

_____

Referring Clinician/Telephone:

_____

Loss of consciousness (circle): Yes / No

Cause: _____

_____

_____

REASON FOR REFERRAL FOR NEUROPSYCHOLOGICAL SERVICES

Diagnostic Questions to be Addressed

_____

_____

_____

_____

Questions Regarding Client's Functional Status and Potential

_____

_____

_____

_____

_____

Recommendations for Providing Psychological Intervention to the Client

_____

_____

_____

_____

Client's Current Psychological and Cognitive Symptoms

_____

_____

_____

_____

Recent Psychological Test Scores

Full Scale IQ: _____ Verbal IQ: _____ Performance IQ: _____

Test Administered: _____

Date: _____

Achievement Test Results (standard scores)

Reading: _____ Math: _____ Written Expression: _____

Other: _____

Conclusions Regarding Objective or Projective Personality Testing

_____

_____

_____

_____

_____

Comments

_____

_____

_____

_____

_____

CONTRIBUTORS

Tricia M. Giessler, BS, is currently completing a predoctoral internship with the Veterans Affairs North Texas Health Care System, in Dallas, Texas. She is a doctoral student at Wright State University, School of Professional Psychology. Prior to attending Wright State University, she received a Bachelor of Science degree in Psychology from Xavier University. Her interests include intervention and assessment in medical populations. Ms. Giessler may be contacted at 2531 Falconbridge Drive, Cincinnati, OH 45238. E-mail: tmgiessler@hotmail.com

Jeffery B. Allen, PhD, ABPP-CN, is board certified in Clinical Neuropsychology by the American Board of Professional Psychology. He is currently a Professor in the School of Professional Psychology at Wright State University and teaches courses in physiological psychology and clinical neuropsychology. Dr Allen completed a postdoctoral fellowship at the Rehabilitation Institute of Michigan in Detroit. He is widely published in the areas of neuropsychology, head injuries, and memory and recently completed the text, *A General Practitioner's Guide to Neuropsychological Assessment* (American Psychological Association, in press). Dr. Allen's interests include neurobehavioral disorders, quality of life in medical populations, cognitive and neuropsychological assessment, and outcome measurement in rehabilitation. Dr. Allen can be reached at SOPP, Wright State University, 3640 Colonel Glenn Highway, Dayton, OH 45435-0001. E-mail: jeffery.allen@wright.edu

RESOURCES

Beck, A. T., Steer, R. A., & Brown, G. K. (1996). *The Beck Depression Inventory-II*. San Antonio: The Psychological Corporation.

Boyle, A. H., & Locke, D. L. (2004). Update on chronic obstructive pulmonary disease. *Nursing, 13*(1), 42-48.

Butcher, J. N., Dahlstrom, W. G., Graham, J. R., Tellegen, A., & Kaemmer, B. (1989). *MMPI-2: Manual for Administration and Scoring*. Minneapolis: University of Minnesota Press.

Cairns, N. J. (2004). Neuroanatomy and neuropathology. In L. H. Goldstein & J. E. McNeil (Eds.), *Clinical Neuropsychology: A Practical Guide to Assessment and Management for Clinicians* (pp. 23-55). West Sussex, England: John Wiley and Sons.

Cormier, S., & Cormier, B. (1998). Nonverbal behavior. *Interviewing Strategies for Helpers* (pp. 78-95). Pacific Grove: Brooks/Cole.

Crews, W. D., Jefferson, A. L., Bolduc, T., Elliott, J. B., Ferro, N. M., Broshek, D. K., Barth, J. T., & Robbins, M. K. (2001). Neuropsychological dysfunction in patients suffering from end-stage chronic obstructive pulmonary disease. *Archives of Clinical Neuropsychology, 16*, 643-652.

Delis, D. C., Kramer, J. H., Kaplan, E., & Ober, B. (2000). *California Verbal Learning Test Manual* (2nd ed.). San Antonio, TX: The Psychological Corporation.

Demaree, H. A., DeLuca, J., Gaudino, E. A., & Diamond, B. J. (1999). Speed of information processing as a key deficit in multiple sclerosis: Implications for rehabilitation. *Journal of Neurology, Neurosurgery, and Psychiatry, 67*, 661-663.

Devins, G. M., & Shnek, Z. M. (2000). Multiple sclerosis. In R. G. Frank & T. R. Elliot (Eds.), *Handbook of Rehabilitation Psychology* (pp. 163-184). Washington, DC: American Psychological Association.

Elliott, T. R., & Umlauf, R. L. (1995). Measurement of personality and psychopathology following acquired physical disability. In L. A. Cushman & M. J. Scherer (Eds.), *Psychological Assessment in Medical Rehabilitation* (pp. 325-358). Washington, DC: American Psychological Association.

Everson, S. A., Helkala, E., Kaplan, G. A., & Salonen, J. T. (2001). Atherosclerosis and cognitive functioning. In S. R. Waldstein (Ed.), *Neuropsychology of Cardiovascular Disease* (pp. 105-120). Mahwah, NJ: Lawrence Erlbaum.

Heaton, R. K., Chelune, G. J., Talley, J. L., Kay, G. G., & Curtiss, G. (1993). *Wisconsin Card Sorting Test Manual: Revised and Expanded*. Odessa, FL: Psychological Assessment Resources.

Hopkins, R. O., & Bigler, E. D. (2001). Pulmonary disorders. In R. E. Tarter, M. Butters, & S. R. Beers (Eds.), *Medical Neuropsychology* (pp. 25-50). New York: Kluwer Academic/Plenum Publishers.

Mohr, D. C., & Cox, D. (2001). Multiple sclerosis: Empirical literature for the clinical health psychologist. *Journal of Clinical Psychology, 57*(4), 479-499.

Mohr, D. C., Dick, L. P., Russo, D., Pinn, J., Boudewyn, A. C., Likosky, W., & Goodkin, D. E. (1999). The psychosocial impact of multiple sclerosis: Exploring the patient's perspective. *Health Psychology, 18*(4), 376-382.

Nelson, L. D., Elder, J. T., Tehrani, P., & Groot, J. (2003). Measuring personality and emotional functioning in multiple sclerosis: A cautionary note. *Archives of Clinical Neuropsychology, 18*, 419-429.

Nicolson, P., & Anderson, P. (2003). Quality of life, distress, and self-esteem: A focus group study of people with chronic bronchitis. *British Journal of Health Psychology, 8*, 251-270.

Reitan, R. M., & Wolfson, D. (1985). *The Halstead-Reitan Neuropsychological Test Battery: Theory and Clinical Interpretation*. Tucson, AZ: Neuropsychology Press.

Sharrack, B., & Hughes, R. C. (1999). The Guy's Neurological Disability Scale (GNDS): A new disability measure for multiple sclerosis. *Multiple Sclerosis, 5,* 223-233.

Strub, R. L., & Black, F. W. (1988). *Neurobehavorial Disorders: A Clinical Approach.* Philadelphia: F. A. Davis.

Van der Molen, T., Willemse, B. W. M., Schokker, S., Hacken, N. H. T. T., Postma, D. S., & Juniper, E. F. (2003). Development, validity, and responsiveness of the Clinical COPD Questionnaire. *Health and Quality of Life Outcomes, 1*(13). Retrieved July 28, 2004, from http://www.hqlo.com/content/1/1/13

Van Stel, H. F., Maille, A. R., Colland, V. T., & Everaerd, W. (2003). Interpretation of change and longitudinal validity of the Quality of Life for Respiratory Illness Questionnaire (QoLRIQ) in inpatient pulmonary rehabilitation. *Quality of Life Research, 12,* 133-145.

Vingerhoets, G. (2001). Cognitive consequences of myocardial infarction, cardiac arrhythmias, and cardiac arrest. In S. R. Waldstein & M. R. Elias (Eds.), *Neuropsychology of Cardiovascular Disease* (pp. 143-163). Mahwah, NJ: Lawrence Erlbaum.

Waldstein, S. R., & Katzel, L. I. (2001). Hypertension and cognitive function. In S. R. Waldstein & M. R. Elias (Eds.), *Neuropsychology of Cardiovascular Disease* (pp. 15-36). Mahwah, NJ: Lawrence Erlbaum.

Waldstein, S. R., Snow, J., Muldoon, M. F., & Katzel, L. I. (2001). Neuropsychological consequences of cardiovascular disease. In R. E. Tarter, M. Butters, & S. R. Beers (Eds.), *Medical Neuropsychology* (pp. 51-83). New York: Kluwer Academic/ Plenum Publishers.

Wechsler, D. (1997a). *Wechsler Adult Intelligence Scale-Third Edition.* San Antonio, TX: The Psychological Corporation.

Wechsler, D. (1997b). *Wechsler Memory Scale-Third Edition. Administration and Scoring Manual.* San Antonio, TX: The Psychological Corporation.

Assessment and Treatment Of the Psychosocial Aspects Of Breast Cancer

Nicole L. Glick and Maurice F. Prout

In this contribution, the authors wish to offer the reader a current overview of the physiological and psychosocial impact of breast cancer throughout its progression from initial diagnosis to recovery and recurrence. A summary of the risk factors, the types of breast cancer, screening procedures, staging, and treatment provide the reader with the background to understand the emotional sequelae that occur in response to this disease. Breast cancer must be conceptualized not only from the perspectives of the patients but also from those of family members, friends, and caregivers. As clinicians providing support to these individuals, we must be cognizant of the ways in which individuals affected by this disease attempt to cope and adapt. It is also essential to recognize that efforts to adjust to breast cancer may not always prove successful, leading to symptoms of depression and anxiety that require intervention. Psychosocial treatment may be presented in a variety of modalities from psychoeducation to supportive-expressive and cognitive-behavioral therapies. Mental health professionals carefully assess the needs of the patients and the severity of the symptoms in order to provide the appropriate level of care.

An extensive exploration of the vast psychosocial impact of breast cancer and its corresponding interventions is warranted because it is the most common cancer in women and it threatens an organ that is intimately associated with self-esteem, sexuality, and femininity (Rowland & Holland, 1989). Breast cancer is also the most widely studied cancer with respect to its psychological impact. Although researchers have identified common themes with regard to psychological responses in individuals with breast cancer, Rowland and Holland indicate that women differ extensively in their reactions to diagnosis, treatment, survival, recurrence, and fatality.

According to the American Cancer Society (2005), one out of seven women are diagnosed with breast cancer, classifying it as the most commonly occurring cancer among women. Over 211,000 women in the United States are expected to develop breast cancer in 2005, while nearly 1,700 cases in men are also anticipated. Over the past 2 decades, the largest increase in breast cancer rates has occurred in women age 50 or older, with 70% of all cases occurring among this age group. Breast cancer is second to lung cancer as the principal cause of mortality in women; however, mortality rates have been declining, most likely due to earlier detection and improved treatment. More than two million cancer survivors live in the United States (Elk & Morrow, 2003).

PRIMARY RISK FACTORS

Although less than 25% of women in the United States possess recognized risk factors, several features have been identified that increase women's vulnerability to developing breast cancer. Primary risk factors include being age 50 or older, being North American or Northern

European, experiencing a personal history of breast cancer, having two or more first-degree relatives (mother, sister, daughter) with breast cancer, the presence of bilateral or premenopausal breast cancer in a first-degree relative, identification of atypical hyperplasia (excessive cell growth), and occurrence of ductal carcinoma in situ (precancerous cells in the lining of the milk ducts) and lobular carcinoma in situ (cell changes in the lining of the lobes of the breast).

The risk of cancer is related to a positive family history and is strongly correlated with the number and ages of affected relatives. Familial breast cancer refers to a family history of one or more first-degree relatives with breast cancer. The genes associated with this type seem to be tumor suppressor genes that undergo mutations, allowing for malignant cell growth. Hereditary breast cancer represents positive family history of related cancers (i.e., ovarian), early onset, bilateral breast involvement, and other multiple cancers.

Genetic Predisposition

Two autosomal gene mutations that increase vulnerability have been isolated, one on chromosome 17 called BRCA1 and one on chromosome 13 called BRCA2. Susceptibility genes are associated with a strong likelihood that the effect of the mutation will result in disease for families with multiple breast and ovarian cancers. Cancersource (2000) documents that BRCA1 and BRCA2 mutations may be passed from either parent to a child, and each child, regardless of gender, has a 50% likelihood of inheritance. Women who have inherited a mutation on BRCA1 or BRCA2 generally have an 85% risk of developing breast cancer by age 70. BRCA2 seems to be associated with male breast cancer and early-onset female breast cancer.

TYPES OF BREAST CANCER

According to Cancersource (2000), carcinoma in situ is a precancerous condition within cells that are still contained within the site of origin. A carcinoma in situ in the breast has the ability to convert into an invasive cancer but does not necessarily do so. Ductal carcinoma in situ (DCIS) is the most common form of noninvasive breast cancer in women and occurs in approximately 5% of male breast cancer. Invasive or infiltrating ductal carcinoma, the most frequently occurring type of breast cancer, originates in the ducts and invades the surrounding breast tissue (Elk & Morrow, 2003). Cancersource (2000) cites that lobular carcinoma in situ (LCIS) functions as an indicator of elevated risk for developing an invasive ductal or lobular cancer. LCIS may be associated with increased risk within both breasts and occurs predominantly in postmenopausal women. Palpation or mammography does not typically detect LCIS. Instead, it is most frequently identified microscopically when breast tissue is removed for another reason.

SCREENING PROCEDURES

Breast cancer may be detected by noninvasive and interventional methods. A mammogram is conducted as both a screening device and a diagnostic tool. This X-ray of the breasts allows radiologists to identify characteristic benign masses with defined borders and malignant lesions with speculated or imprecise masses, asymmetric densities, and microcalcifications. Interventional procedures may be used to provide more thorough assessment for potential malignancy. Fine-needle aspiration is utilized when an abnormality is known to be solid or to determine if the lump is a cyst. A lump that is actually a cyst should disappear after the aspiration is completed, while a solid lump will require further examination. According to

Cancersource (2000), core needle biopsy is generally used for solid, palpable masses that have some suspicion of cancer. Stereotactic Needle-Guided Biopsy is mainly employed to identify nonpalpable lesions in the breast that were detected by mammography. Wire localization biopsy is utilized to assist the surgeon in locating the nonpalpable lesion for excisional biopsy and to minimize the volume of tissue removed to avoid unnecessary deformity. Open biopsy or excisional biopsy is the most invasive diagnostic procedure and is performed when a sonogram displays the lesion as solid and nonspecific, cytology and histology results are inadequate, clinical or mammographic findings are suspicious, or when patients with low-risk lesions request biopsies to alleviate anxiety.

BREAST CANCER STAGING

Following screening and biopsy, the tissue sample is examined thoroughly and considered along with findings from a physical examination, mammogram, and medical history. The information collected from these assessments is utilized to confirm the diagnosis and determine treatment options and prognosis. The patient is clinically staged on the basis of the characteristics of the primary tumor, the physical examination of the axillary lymph nodes, and the presence of distant metastases (Cancersource, 2000). Stage 0 is also known as carcinoma in situ and manifests as localized abnormal cell growth in the lining of the ducts (DCIS) or in the lobes of the breast (LCIS). Stage I represents a tumor that is 0 to 2 cm, negative lymph nodes, and lack of evidence of metastasis. Stage II breast cancer refers to a small tumor with positive lymph nodes or a larger tumor with negative lymph nodes. Stage III is diagnosed for more advanced regional disease with suspected but undetectable metastases. Finally, Stage IV signifies the presence of distant metastases.

Stage, Treatment, and Prognosis

The level of disease of the tumor cells and lymph nodes plays a significant role in determination of treatment and prognosis. Cancersource (2000) asserts that the more differentiated the tumor cells, the better the prognosis and response to treatment. Additionally, there is a clear positive correlation between systemic risk of recurrence and tumor size. The involvement of axillary nodes is recognized as a key feature in establishing prognosis in breast cancer, in that the prognosis worsens as the number of positive lymph nodes increases. Additionally, recurrence is seen in approximately 75% of women with many positive nodes. When breast cancer metastasizes, the first site is usually local or regional. Thereafter, according to Cancersource (2000), it spreads widely and to nearly all organs of the body, but primarily to the bone, lungs, nodes, liver, and brain.

METHODS OF TREATMENT

Methods of treatment include local therapy and systemic treatment. Local therapy is selected when the goal is to remove or destroy breast cancer in specific areas. Examples of local therapy are surgery and radiation therapy. Systemic treatment aims to destroy or control cancer throughout the body and is conducted via chemotherapy, hormonal therapy, or biological therapy. Selecting an appropriate treatment option depends on several factors including age and menopausal status, general health, size and location of the tumor, stage of cancer, results of laboratory tests, size of breasts, and tumor cell features such as whether they depend on hormones to grow.

Surgery

Surgery is the most common treatment for breast cancer and can incorporate removal of specific cancer sites, parts of the breast, lymph nodes, the entire breast, or both breasts. A lumpectomy is performed to remove the cancerous cells but not the breast, though some normal surrounding tissue may be removed during this procedure. A segmental mastectomy involves removal of the cancerous area, a larger area of normal breast tissue, and frequently the axillary lymph nodes under the arm as well. Axillary lymph node dissection entails removal of the lymph nodes under the arm to determine whether the cancer cells have entered the lymphatic system. A mastectomy involves removal of the whole breast in addition to the axillary nodes. Removal of the whole breast, most of the lymph nodes under the arm, and the lining over the chest muscles refers to a modified radical mastectomy. Finally, a radical mastectomy is an infrequently occurring procedure in which the breasts, both chest muscles, all lymph nodes under the arm, and additional fat and skin are removed.

Surgical Side Effects

There are many potential side effects associated with the various types of surgical treatments. Short-term pain and tenderness in the area of operation occurs frequently. Women who undergo these procedures may be at risk for infection, poor wound healing, bleeding, and reaction to anesthesia. Removal of a large breast can cause a weight imbalance, leading to neck and back discomfort. Following surgery, the skin around the incision may be tight and the muscles of the arm and shoulder may feel stiff. Some women have permanent loss of strength in the muscles following mastectomy. Another potential side effect may be numbness and tingling in the chest, underarm, shoulder, and upper arm if nerves were injured or cut. Lymphedema, a build-up of lymph fluid due to a slower flow, often leads to swelling in the hand and arm.

Surgery and Psychological Response

Women who undergo surgical treatment of their breast cancer may encounter emotional difficulties that are specific to this intervention. Jacobson and Holland (1989) indicate that "the universal reaction to an anticipated surgical procedure is fear and anxiety" (p. 119). These worries manifest as fears about separating from home and family, fears of loss of control or death under anesthesia, fears of being partially awake during surgery, and fears of damage to body parts during the procedure. According to Jacobson and Holland, fears tend to be greatest in individuals who have chronically high levels of anxiety. Individuals often have concerns about entrusting their lives to strangers performing the surgery. Self-image and appraisal of attractiveness frequently shift, leading to body image disturbance, diminished sense of femininity, and sexual and marital disruptions (A. M. Nezu, C. M. Nezu, & Geller, 2003). All of these psychological effects represent threats to women's sense of personal invulnerability.

Rose and Perotti (2003) recommend that women create a presurgical ritual to give themselves a sense of protection during surgery, to say goodbye to their breast or breasts, or prepare for other changes in their bodies. Jacobson and Holland (1989) suggest additional methods of creating psychological preparation for surgery. They emphasize the importance of preoperative education in order to increase women's sense of control. These authors also suggest participation in brief psychotherapy to allow patients to express concerns and fears and to provide reassurance and support. Behavioral interventions may be useful for coping with the effects of surgery both in anticipation of the procedure and during recovery. Relaxation training, progressive muscle relaxation, and imagery with calming self-statements all contribute to reduction of the fears associated with surgery. Women may also benefit from stress inoculation training, which includes self-monitoring for cognitive and physiological signs of stress, deep breathing, muscle relaxation, pleasant imagery, and substitution of coping self-statements for negative self-statements (Jacobson & Holland, 1989).

After surgery, women may feel as if their bodies have been damaged or assaulted by cancer and by treatment. Women may have difficulty reorienting their bodies to feel pleasure or to feel sexy after enduring physical discomfort or emotional distress. Some women opt to receive breast reconstruction, as they do not feel whole without their breast or breasts. Women who undergo this procedure tend to experience an increase in psychological, social, and sexual function (Rowland & Holland, 1989). Additionally, Moyer (1997) found that women who received breast-conserving surgical treatment exhibited improvements in psychological adjustment, marital-sexual adjustment, social adjustment, body image, and cancer-related fears and concerns.

Chemotherapy

Chemotherapy is a systemic treatment that involves the use of a combination of drugs to kill cancer cells. This form of treatment is administered either by pill or injection. Chemotherapy is typically provided on an outpatient basis, though inpatient treatment may be used depending on the type of drugs used and the general health of the patient. Chemotherapy often occurs in conjunction with radiation therapy or surgery.

Chemotherapy Side Effects

The side effects of chemotherapy are generally experienced for a brief duration and depend on the type and dosage of drugs used. Chemotherapy typically affects rapidly dividing cells such as blood cells, hair cells, and digestive tract cells. When blood cells are affected, women become vulnerable to infections, bruising, bleeding, and fatigue. Chemotherapy that impacts the hair cells in the roots leads to hair loss. When digestive tract cells are implicated, the result is likely to be poor appetite, nausea, vomiting, diarrhea, and mouth or lip sores. Many of the above side effects can be controlled by medication. More permanent adverse effects include the cessation of hormone production, leading to menopausal symptoms such as hot flashes, vaginal dryness, irregular or stopped menstruation, and infertility. Hormone production does not typically return for women over age 35. Other long-term effects of a weakened heart and leukemia rarely occur but are quite serious.

Chemotherapy and Psychological Response

When chemotherapy is prescribed to treat breast cancer, many women experience emotional distress prior to initiating treatment and as a side effect of the systemic therapy. Rose and Perotti (2003) note that it is common for women to feel anticipatory anxiety before the first treatment. Common effects of the treatment include nausea, vomiting, weakness and fatigue, and weight loss, which may invite reactions from others that the individuals appear sick. Anticipatory nausea and vomiting occur when cues present during chemotherapy become associated with the experience of nausea and vomiting. Many women find these symptoms embarrassing, as these symptoms can persist after treatment and may generalize to other situations. For some, the symptoms are so aversive that they lead to discontinuation of treatment. Weight gain may also occur, especially when chemotherapy is administered with other medication (Holland & Lesko, 1989). Many women who lose their hair believe that this effect is the most traumatic aspect of treatment (Rose & Perotti, 2003). Some women have trouble sleeping during periods of chemotherapy, which can intensify feelings of exhaustion, frustration, or depression. Additionally, women may experience a change or disruption in their sexual desire, arousal, or ability to achieve orgasm during or after chemotherapy, due to the suppression of estrogen and the interruption of the body's normal reproductive and sexual functions. Holland and Lesko (1989) suggest that, upon completing chemotheraphy, some women experience a paradoxical anxiety in that they are afraid to stop due to concern that the treatment benefit will end.

Relaxation techniques, guided visualization, meditation, and hypnosis especially prove effective for the anticipatory anxiety and anxiety symptoms that may occur during the treatment (Holland & Lesko, 1989). Establishing a routine of something to look forward to at the end of each treatment can also alleviate psychological distress. It is especially important for women undergoing systemic treatment to maintain involvement with people and projects to boost mood and self-confidence. Rose and Perotti (2003) emphasize the importance of being assertive throughout the course of treatment so that unpleasant effects can be addressed promptly.

Radiation

Radiation therapy is the use of high energy rays to kill cancer cells and occurs within two modalities: external radiation and implant radiation. External radiation is conducted on an outpatient basis and uses a machine to direct the rays at the breast. Implant radiation involves radioactive material in thin plastic tubes implanted directly into the breast. This treatment requires an inpatient stay, and the implants are not removed until discharge from the hospital several days later. Some women receive both external and implant radiation treatment. Additionally, radiation therapy is often used in conjunction with surgery or chemotherapy and can be implemented either before or after these procedures.

Radiation Side Effects

The side effects of radiation treatment are generally temporary. Women undergoing this type of therapy tend to feel significant fatigue, especially following several treatments. Subsequent to repeated radiation therapy, the breast may feel heavy and hard. Skin in the treated area may become red, dry, tender, or itchy. However, toward the end of treatment, skin often becomes moist and weepy.

Radiation and Psychological Response

Radiation therapy may elicit psychological reactions that make the treatment more distressing and difficult to tolerate. Holland (1989b) noted that individuals may experience fear of painful radiation burns as well as fear that radiation will not help. Like chemotherapy, anticipatory anxiety is common especially before the first treatment. Fear of harmful effects of radiation often occurs because many people associate radiation with atomic bombs, nuclear accidents, radiation sickness, and ionizing radiation in the atmosphere. The closed space in the treatment room may also aggravate claustrophobia. Additionally, Holland notes that depression may occur due to misinterpretation that the side effects represent irreparable damage. Individuals who have preexisting agoraphobia are particularly vulnerable to poor tolerance for separation from familiar others while in the treatment room. To alleviate anticipatory fears, some women arrange to see the room for radiation treatment ahead of time to increase familiarity with the setting. Cognitive-behavioral techniques prove effective in reducing physiological anxiety and challenging cognitive distortions or irrational beliefs about the procedure.

Hormonal Therapy

Hormonal therapy is utilized to prevent the cancer cells from access to the hormones that they need to grow. According to Cancersource (2000), tumors with identifiable receptor activity respond to the stimulatory effects of estrogen and progesterone and are thus influenced by hormone therapy. This type of treatment may include use of medication to change the way hormones work or surgery to remove the ovaries, inducing severe menopause. Tamoxifen, used for early stages of breast cancer since FDA approval in 1998, is the most common hormonal treatment known to mimic the effects of estrogen in selected tissues and act as estrogen antagonists in other tissues. Tamoxifen is also utilized as a form of chemoprevention, which is proposed to alter the course of disease for those with known risk factors (Cancersource, 2000).

Newer hormone treatments include aromatase inhibitors and antiestrogens. Aromatase inhibitors (AIs) inhibit an enzyme that converts androgen to estrogen, thus lowering the levels of estrogen that are available to cancer cells (Elk & Morrow, 2003). Arimidex, Femara, and Aromasin are three new generation AIs that have been proven effective in treating postmenopausal women with metastatic breast cancer while producing fewer side effects. Elk and Morrow report that recent testing on pure antiestrogens such as Faslodex, which destroy estrogen receptors, have been shown effective in treating women with metastatic breast cancer.

Biological Therapy

Biological therapy is utilized to enhance the body's natural defenses against cancer. Herceptin is an example of a biological treatment that blocks human epidermal growth factor receptor-2 (HER-2), a protein that causes breast cancer cells to grow. Herceptin functions by slowing or stopping the growth of breast cancer cells. This biological treatment may be given by itself or with chemotherapy.

Biological Therapy Side Effects

Rashes or swelling at the injection site and flu-like symptoms, the side effects of biological therapy, typically become less severe after the first treatment. However, Herceptin may cause damage to the heart leading to heart failure. Thus, women receiving this treatment are examined for heart and lung problems carefully.

COMPLETION OF TREATMENT

During treatment, adjustment is focused primarily on coping with apprehensions about painful procedures, unwanted side effects, disruption in daily functioning, and changes in life roles (National Cancer Institute, 2004). The completion of active treatment can be a time of celebration and relief. It may also yield heightened distress due to a sense of vulnerability from the cessation of active medical efforts and less frequent physician contact. Individuals may experience disappointment about intermittent periods of anxiety and depression that persist following active treatment. During this posttreatment period, women feel significant uncertainty about the future. As a consequence, some feel that they must maintain an emotional vigilance due to concern that cancer may surprise them again if they begin to move forward and enjoy life. It is important for women to be aware of their ambivalence and to articulate these feelings to others for greater understanding and support.

Positive Response to Treatment

Women whose breast cancer responds positively and comprehensively to treatment must undergo the transition from patient to healthy status. Women experiencing this change must also anticipate and adjust to reduction of the special support and concern they received throughout the treatment phase. These individuals also face reentry into their social and employment circles, where they may be regarded by others as different, experience job insecurity or discrimination, encounter negative employer and peer attitudes, and receive health and life insurance difficulties. Tross and Holland (1989) cite several interventions that facilitate adjustment to this stage. They recommend that professionals focus on helping patients to anticipate fears of recurrence, exploring adjustment to living with compromises, providing education about anger, anxiety, and depression, and emphasizing the importance of becoming part of a community of survivors. These women also benefit from preparation in dealing with expectations of others and helping the family to prevent overprotection.

Recurrence

When women experience a recurrence of breast cancer, the initial elation ends and the painful uncertainty of the future becomes magnified. Women are faced with the notion that the treatment that offered the greatest hope has failed (Holland, 1989a). During this time, women tend to experience intensified existential concerns, sadness, depression, insomnia, restlessness, and anxiety. Some individuals undergoing a recurrence of breast cancer search for a cause for the recurrence by blaming themselves or their doctors. The fear of dying becomes particularly salient, as there is much apprehension about the potential of a painful death. Suicidal thoughts are common, and some individuals develop plans for a worst-case scenario. Many women fear abandonment by the doctor and by their families, leading them to feel very alone. This period especially engenders a desire for assurance that there will be an aggressive approach to the control of cancer to ensure that the disease will never return (Holland, 1989a).

ADJUSTMENT

From the period of assessment and diagnosis, the process continues to be dynamic and unpredictable, placing significant demands on the individuals affected. The challenges that the women encounter throughout the course of the illness require significant strength and flexibility. Ability to adjust and cope with these distressing experiences markedly impacts the level of distress that occurs as a result. The National Cancer Institute (2004) highlights Brennan's (2001) definition of adjustment or psychosocial adaptation "as an ongoing process in which the individual patient tries to manage emotional distress, solve specific cancer-related problems, and gain mastery or control over cancer-related life events" (p. 2). From this view, adjustment is a series of coping responses to multiple tasks associated with living with cancer. The responsibilities related to living with cancer yield different demands during major stages of the disease. Diagnosis, treatment, posttreatment and remission, recurrence and palliative care, and survivorship represent common periods that create significant challenge to coping among the individuals and their loved ones. Each period has certain coping tasks, particular existential questions, common emotional responses, and specific problems.

Normal or successful adjustment can be conceptualized as the ability to minimize disruptions to life roles, regulate emotional distress, and remain actively involved in aspects of life that continue to hold meaning and importance. According to the National Cancer Institute (2004), there are several important factors that influence women's adjustment to breast cancer. These factors are distinguished by the demands that the situation places upon the individuals and the resources that the individuals possess to cope with these stressors. Situational demands may incorporate the type of cancer, its stage, its prognosis, and where the patient falls in the process of diagnosis, treatment, and recurrence. The developmental stage of life of women with breast cancer and the availability and quality of social support also impact adaptation to cancer. Society-derived factors such as general views of cancer, access to treatment, level of openness about discussing the illness, and popular beliefs about causes of cancer can further influence adjustment.

COPING

An essential aspect of emotional adjustment to cancer regards the manner in which individuals attempt to cope with the difficulties. As conceptualized by Lazarus and Folkman's (1984) Transactional Stress and Coping Paradigm, coping represents the cognitive and behavioral endeavors that individuals employ to manage distressing events (A. M. Nezu et al., 2003).

Coping responses are a dynamic succession of interactions between individuals and their environments in order to regulate affective states and modify the interactions. Nezu et al. indicate that another important aspect of coping involves the cognitions associated with the way individuals appraise or perceive their relationships with the environment. Appraisals of the harm or loss posed by the stressor, belief in the degree of controllability of the stressor, evaluation of the outcome of their coping efforts, and their expectations for future success are determinants of the coping strategies selected.

Types of Coping

Coping strategies are situation specific and are categorized into three dimensions: problem solving, emotion focused, and meaning focused. Problem-solving strategies are aimed at altering the problematic situation, such as information seeking and deliberate, thoughtful problem resolution. A. M. Nezu et al. (2003) assert that those who engage in a problem-solving strategy tend to increase their flexibility and perceived control with regard to approaching distressing situations. Emotion-focused coping targets the regulation of emotional responses to stressors. Cognitive reassessment of the stressor and minimization of the problem are examples of emotion-focused approaches. Coping strategies that are meaning focused facilitate understanding of why this has happened and what impact cancer will have.

Lazarus and Folkman (1984) proposed that the amount of distress experienced by patients is dependent on the balance between perception of the demands that a situation places upon them and perception of the resources they possess to effectively manage these demands (A. M. Nezu et al., 2003). Generally, individuals who adjust well typically remain committed and actively engaged in the process of coping with cancer and continue to find meaning in their lives. Those who do not adjust well often become disengaged, withdraw, and feel hopeless. Stanton and Snider (1993) suggest that avoidance coping may impede effective cognitive processing and problem solving that is essential for making rapid, life-altering decisions associated with cancer treatment. A. M. Nezu et al. (2003) report that individuals who engage in habitual avoidance and denial tend to feel helpless and subsequently experience increased levels of anxiety and depression.

Those who possess a fighting spirit and a strong sense of optimism are likely to adjust more positively and experience less distress (A. M. Nezu et al., 2003). Coping style has also been linked to cancer survival. Improved survival appears to be correlated with individuals who are emotionally expressive, demonstrate a fighting spirit, and possess an optimistic orientation. On the other hand, poor survival seems to be related to individuals who are unable to express negative affect, engage in suppression of hostility and anger, exhibit passive responses, display stoic acceptance, experience a sense of helplessness and hopelessness, and possess a pessimistic orientation.

COGNITIVE PROCESSING THEORY

Cognitive processing theory suggests that traumatic events can challenge individuals' core assumptions about themselves and their world. For example, a diagnosis of breast cancer can challenge women's assumptions about being personally invulnerable to illness. Individuals attempt to comprehend and revise these core beliefs by engaging in cognitive activities that help them view undesirable events in personally meaningful ways, find ways of understanding the negative aspects of the experience, and ultimately reach a state of acceptance. As a consequence, individuals may be better able to cope with the losses they experience. Another benefit of cognitive processing may be that individuals find a new appreciation for life or place a greater value on relationships. Further, cognitive processing allows for development of a more benign explanation for the illness by using existing views of the world, such as attributing it to God's will or assuming responsibility for the illness because of a lifestyle. Sears, Stanton, and Danoff-Burg (2003) term this positive reappraisal as benefit finding, a method of identifying positive aspects from adversity.

SOCIAL SUPPORT AND ADAPTATION

Social support has been one of the most studied predictors of psychological adaptation to health problems (A. M. Nezu et al., 2003). Bloom (1982) proposed that perception of social support is measured by family cohesiveness and the frequency of social contact. It represents the strongest predictor of health coping responses and may even contribute to immunological defense (A. M. Nezu et al., 2003). Communication with significant others and shared decision making have especially positive effects on adjustment and coping. Advice and guidance from others may alter the threatening appraisal of a difficult situation to a more benign assessment of a situation. Social support can function as a coping aide, by identifying adaptive coping strategies and providing assistance in implementing these strategies. Some research suggests that perception of social support and coping is stronger for good cancer prognosis.

INITIAL EMOTIONAL RESPONSE

After being diagnosed with breast cancer, many women describe feeling vulnerable and alone, which may be especially acute for women whose partners are unable to provide adequate support, women without partners, or women who live alone (Rose & Perotti, 2003). It is also common for women to minimize the frightening nature of the facts as temporary protection against overwhelming anxiety. "One of the cardinal issues that confronts every cancer patient is the constant uncertainty about the future" (Holland, 1989a, p. 78). Women are especially vulnerable to experiencing high levels of stress at several key points of the illness progression. These moments occur at diagnosis or disease recurrence, when facing the prospect of having surgery, during adjuvant therapy, at the time of a medical examination, and when living with advanced breast cancer (National Breast Cancer Centre, 2000). Psychological variables also influence the amount and impact of distress throughout the process. The level of women's emotional discomfort and the changes in life patterns that occur consequent to the illness are particularly salient. The extent of the fears and concerns regarding treatment outcome is another mediating factor in ongoing distress. Changes in life patterns are related to physical discomfort, marital or sexual disruption, and altered activity level. Intensity of anguish may also be determined by the point in the life cycle at which the breast cancer occurs and the subsequent social tasks that are threatened or interrupted (Rowland & Holland, 1989). Prior association with breast cancer, response from other significant people, and support from women who have been through the experience also have a bearing on the development of distress throughout the progression of the illness.

IDENTIFYING PSYCHOLOGICAL DISTRESS

The National Comprehensive Cancer Network aims to establish standards of care so that all patients experiencing psychosocial distress will be accurately and routinely identified, recognized, and treated (National Cancer Institute, 2004). These guidelines include recommendations for screening, triage, and initial evaluation, as well as referral and treatment guidelines for participating professions (mental health, social work, palliative care, and pastoral care). Screening is a rapid method of identifying patients with psychosocial distress, typically via brief self-report questionnaires.

Measures of Psychological Distress

Several facilities renowned for their excellence in cancer research and treatment utilize standardized screening methods to identify individuals who are experiencing significant distress and who require additional support (National Cancer Institute, 2004). Memorial Sloan-Kettering Center uses a distress thermometer modeled after those used to measure pain in which the patients rate their distress that particular day on a scale of zero to 10, with 10 representing extreme distress. This facility also includes a problem list to identify which potential sources of stress are relevant. The Johns Hopkins Cancer Center gives all new patients an 18-item version of the Brief Symptom Inventory, which lists 18 problems people sometimes experience (e.g., dizziness, lack of interest in things, loneliness, nausea). The patients are asked how much they are distressed by each of the problems during the past 7 days, including the day of assessment. The Oncology Symptom Control Research Group at Community Cancer Care typically screens all incoming patients with the Zung Self-Rating Depression Scale (ZSDS). The ZSDS is a 20-item self-report depression screen that has been used to detect depression and more general distress. Additionally, single items on the questionnaire are also used to screen for conditions such as fatigue.

Screening and Referral

When identifying individuals who are experiencing marked distress, most patients will respond to the recommendations of health care professionals who exhibit trust, expertise, warmth, care, and concern (National Cancer Institute, 2004). It is especially important to normalize the procedure of screening and referral by avoiding words that suggest the stigma of serious mental illness in favor of words that focus on distress or concerns related to the illness or treatment. After initial screening and referral, psychosocial assessment typically follows as a semistructured interview during which the professional evaluates adjustment to the current demands of the illness among the patients, the patients' families, and other significant people in the patients' lives.

CHARACTERISTICS OF WOMEN WITH POOR ADJUSTMENT

The National Breast Cancer Centre (2000) identified common characteristics of women with breast cancer that are associated with poor adjustment and increased risk of psychosocial problems. Younger women who are single, separated, divorced, or widowed are especially vulnerable due to reduced availability of social supports. Women who have children under the age of 21 and have experienced cumulative stressful life events tend to have a higher risk of distress, due to encountering many demands. Economic difficulties, perceived inadequate social support, and poor marital or family functioning place additional stress on women with breast cancer. Finally, those who have a history of psychiatric problems or a past history of alcohol or other substance abuse are particularly vulnerable to psychosocial problems.

DEPRESSION

The severity of depressive symptoms varies according to several factors, including individuals' coping abilities, access to support and resources, and degree of illness advancement. For example, women whose malignancies are discovered in the early stages of cancer development experience distress in response to the threat of diagnosis, treatment, and the subsequent changes in individual and relational functioning. Additionally, the severity of distress may be mediated by the potential responsivity to treatment. Women who are in the advanced stages of their breast cancer and who experience poorly controlled pain are at risk for experiencing depression. Additionally, certain treatments with medication and concurrent illnesses that produce depressive symptoms can induce severe mood changes and may lead to suicidal ideation (Massie, 1989b). Vulnerability to depression is high among those with a history of an affective disorder or alcoholism.

Assessment of Depressive Symptoms

According to A. M. Nezu et al. (2003), depressive symptoms are present in approximately 20% to 60% of cancer patients and are responsible for the largest percentage of psychiatric consultations among cancer patients. In order to determine the level of acuteness, a thorough clinical evaluation should be conducted, incorporating a careful assessment of symptoms, mental status, physical status, treatment effects, laboratory data, previous depressive episodes, family history of depression or suicide, concurrent life stressors, and availability of social support. Although diagnosis of depression in physically healthy individuals relies significantly on the presence of symptoms of appetite and sleep disruption, lack of energy, fatigue, psychomotor slowing, and decreased libido, these indicators have less diagnostic value in cancer patients because they are common in both cancer and depression. Massie (1989b) indicates that "depression in cancer patients is best evaluated by the severity of dysphoric mood, the degree of the feelings of hopelessness, guilt, and worthlessness, and the presence of suicidal thoughts" (p. 287).

Treatment of Depressive Symptoms

Psychiatric consultation is indicated when depressive symptoms persist for more than 1 week, worsen over time, and interfere with individuals' abilities to function or cooperate with treatment. Patients who meet these criteria are typically referred for short-term supportive psychotherapy, an approach based on a crisis-intervention model. The goal of this intervention is to assist patients in regaining a sense of self-worth, correct misconceptions about the past and present, and integrate the present illness into a continuum of life experiences. Supportive psychotherapy also functions to emphasize past strengths, encourage formerly successful ways of coping, and mobilize internal resources (Massie, 1989b). Adjustment to illness appears to be mediated by individuals' abilities to remain engaged in previous activities after diagnosis and treatment (Carver, Lehman, & Antoni, 2003). Family involvement is particularly important to challenge families' perceptions that depressive symptoms indicate that patients have resigned themselves to their cancer. Patients are also frequently referred for participation in a support group.

ANXIETY DISORDERS

Anxiety disorders appear to be more common in people with cancer than in controls or individuals with other chronic illnesses in the general population (A. M. Nezu et al., 2003). For some individuals, the anxiety can be so severe that they may be unable to adhere adequately to their medical treatment and seek to avoid fear-provoking procedures. Nezu et al.

cite research conducted by Dow (1991) and Henderson (1997) suggesting that people with cancer may respond to the psychological distress and uncertainty about the future by displaying posttraumatic stress disorder with symptoms similar to those experienced by victims of war or environmental disasters. Posttraumatic stress symptoms may manifest as somatic vigilance, recurrent recollections of illness-related events, and emergence of symptomatology around anniversary dates. Over time, these symptoms appear to dissipate as the fear of recurrence lessens.

Assessment of Anxiety

When assessing for the presence of anxiety, clinicians should look for the following symptoms: fear that encompasses dread and apprehension; fear of death and body dysfunction; respiratory and cardiovascular symptoms; gastrointestinal disturbance such as reduced appetite, diarrhea, heartburn, and constipation; gynecological and genitourinary symptoms, including impotence, painful intercourse, urinary urgency and frequency, and reduced libido or ability to achieve orgasm (Massie, 1989a).

Types of Anxiety

Common types of anxiety exist which reflect a variety of contributing factors and levels of severity. Massie (1989a) asserts that reactive or situational anxiety is related to crisis or transitional points including (a) anticipation of test results, diagnosis, new procedures, treatment, and surgery; (b) termination of long-term treatment; and (c) the advanced and terminal stages of the illness. Anxiety associated with medical influences may be caused by pain, abnormal metabolic states, hormone-producing tumors, and anxiety-producing medication, especially corticosteroids that frequently produce anxiety, motor restlessness, and agitation. According to Massie (1989a), this type of anxiety cannot be adequately assessed until the pain and physical distress have been controlled. Preexisting anxiety disorders such as phobias, panic, and Generalized Anxiety Disorder may also be exacerbated by medical illness. Anxiety related to termination of treatment, participating in clinical trials, and anticipatory nausea and vomiting also represent specific circumstances that may evoke anxiety symptoms.

Treatment of Anxiety Symptoms

Reactive anxiety may be managed by providing adequate information and support, preparation about what to expect, and assisting individuals in mentally "walking through" events. If these interventions do not adequately diminish the reactive anxiety, psychopharmacological treatment may be utilized (Massie, 1989a). Preexisting anxiety may be treated by teaching behavioral techniques such as relaxation, distraction, and mental rehearsal of anticipated frightening events. Relaxation modalities may include progressive muscle relaxation and breathing exercises that are prescribed for daily practice. Many of the symptoms of posttraumatic stress disorder such as pervasive anxiety, intrusive thoughts, and avoidant behaviors occur among breast cancer survivors (Andrykowski et al., 1998). When the anxiety manifests itself as posttraumatic stress disorder, mental health professionals aim to provide support, encourage exploration of the traumatic event in order to reduce the physiological, cognitive, and emotional responses associated with the event, and employ medication when needed.

PSYCHOSOCIAL INTERVENTIONS

"Psychosocial interventions for cancer patients are systematic efforts applied to influence coping behavior through educational or psychotherapeutic means" (Massie, Holland, & Straker,

1989, p. 459). Mental health professionals provide psychosocial interventions through psychoeducation, supportive psychotherapy, and cognitive-behavioral therapy. Massie et al. (1989) add that these interventions serve a variety of functions including augmenting knowledge of the disease and its associated features; increasing sense of control; improving coping ability, self-esteem, and resolution of problems; and reducing emotional distress. Clinicians typically implement these interventions within a supportive, short-term psycho-therapy model. On average, visits occur once or twice per week for 4 to 6 weeks of the initial crisis phase. Professionals need to maintain flexibility with scheduling and are encouraged to provide phone calls or visits if patients are hospitalized for medical reasons. Massie et al. (1989) suggest that when psychological responses or concurrent stressors reach a level of severity greater than that of typical emotional reactions, clinicians may need to shift their treatment from a supportive, short-term modality to exploratory psychotherapy. Medication may also serve as an adjunct to therapy if symptoms are extensive and do not abate. A combi-nation of individual and group therapy often proves most effective (Chang & Haber, 1997).

Psychoeducation

Clinicians can play an educational role by serving as an extension to patients' social environments – family, treating doctor and staff, employer, and school. An important function of psychoeducational interventions is to impart information regarding the technical aspects of the disease and its treatment, potential side effects, possible emotional impact, and issues around coping and adjustment. It is especially important for mental health professionals to clarify information that was not fully understood due to anxiety and correct any misinformation. Written permission must be obtained in order for clinicians to function as a liaison between patients and their physicians.

Patients benefit greatly from reassurance about the situation and explanations of common emotional reactions to cancer, including why they occur, why they are normal, and why they are not cause for alarm. Professionals may also provide interpretation and clarification of psychological mechanisms as a means to encourage more effective ways of coping (Massie et al., 1989). Psychoeducational information can assist individuals in anticipating problems likely to be encountered on return to home, school, or work. This modality of support also enhances patients' knowledge regarding navigating the medical system, maximizing physician-patient relationships, and accessing community resources. Information may be shared by providing written and audio materials and offering opportunities to attend lectures. The goal of educa-tional interventions is to reduce distress and improve individuals' sense of control that may appear undermined by lack of knowledge and feelings of uncertainty (A. M. Nezu et al., 2003).

Supportive Psychotherapy

Supportive psychotherapy promotes expression of emotions about the illness and its outcome and provides assistance through empathic listening and encouragement (National Breast Cancer Centre, 2000). These functions help to provide a sense of security that the therapist and the medical staff are reliable and accessible. Clinicians clarify and interpret feelings, behaviors, and defenses to facilitate increased awareness and understanding. Supportive inter-ventions also explore the impact that previous experiences, such as death in the family by cancer, have on present emotional responses. This approach additionally serves to explore areas of concurrent stress that may exacerbate a negative psychological response. Supportive psychotherapy provides opportunities to examine existential concern and ways of coping with uncertainty about the future (Massie et al., 1989). In fact, Giese-Davis et al. (2002) found that expressing painful emotions in response to existential concerns contributed to positive change in affect regulation.

Cognitive-Behavioral Therapy

Cognitive-behavioral interventions serve to identify and change behavioral, cognitive, and affective variables that mediate the deleterious effects of cancer and its treatment. The methods through which this objective is achieved include contingency management, biofeedback, relaxation training, and systematic desensitization. Cognitive distraction, cognitive restructuring, guided imagery, and problem-solving techniques may also be utilized to alter the perceptions that contribute to adverse impact of the illness. Mental health professionals may assist women in reducing emotional distress by encouraging development of problem-solving and assertive communication skills, teaching cognitive reframing and management of emotions, and promoting the scheduling of pleasurable activities. Problem-solving training involves guiding individuals to become more effective problem solvers, thus improving their abilities to manage stressful life situations and gradually adapt to fears (National Breast Cancer Centre, 2000). These cognitive-behavioral interventions function to promote empowerment and effective coping.

Negative thoughts may be controlled by utilizing several cognitive techniques. One method of thought stopping involves teaching individuals to yell "STOP" really loudly in their minds and visualize a big red STOP sign. Clinicians may also advise patients to slap themselves on the wrist with a rubber band, splash water on their faces, get up and move to a different spot, or initiate a pleasant, engaging activity (Houts & Bucher, 2000). Instructing individuals to arrange a time and place for negative thinking may also minimize negative cognitions. Distraction techniques involve suggesting that patients take a vacation in their minds or perform mental time travel into the future, such as to an event they are eagerly anticipating. Individuals may also argue against their negative thoughts by providing evidence for both sides of the issue, distinguishing facts from assumptions, identifying gray areas, recognizing when taking things out of context, and attempting to find flaws with the negative side (Houts & Bucher, 2000).

Behavioral techniques are especially productive in managing special problems in patient care that are often resistant to conventional treatment alone. These difficulties include chemotherapy-induced anticipatory nausea and vomiting, anxiety, eating and sleep disorders, control of pain, and enhancement of sense of self-control and well-being (Mastrovito, 1989). Mastrovito adds that hypnosis may be implemented as an adjunct in the management of cancer pain in order to enhance individuals' control over the pain. Progressive muscle relaxation combined with guided imagery is frequently utilized to reduce the nausea and vomiting often associated with chemotherapy.

Group Therapy

Group therapy provides a milieu for people with similar experiences to impart emotional support (A. M. Nezu et al., 2003). Group support should be made up of women at comparable stages of the disease and provides emotional support and allows for opportunities to learn from experiences of others. Professionals facilitate these groups for patients and their families by using educational, psychotherapeutic, or cognitive-behavioral methods. This modality offers the advantage of being cost-effective for patients and time-efficient for mental health professionals. A supportive-expressive group approach provides supportive interaction among participants, encouragement to express emotions, and discussion of cancer-related problems. A. M. Nezu et al. (2003) cite the assertion of Spiegel, Bloom, and Yalom (1981) that this modality especially leads to reduced anxiety, depression, confusion, and fatigue for women with metastatic breast cancer. Self-help or mutual support groups are often composed of patients with the same tumor site or treatment and maintain a focus on education, practical advice, modeling, coping, and advocacy (Massie et al., 1989).

COUPLES ISSUES

When breast cancer occurs within newly married couples, it may shatter the union and shift women toward dependency with their parents and siblings while excluding their spouses (Rait & Lederberg, 1989). Parents who have young children and are affected by illness have reduced available energy for childrearing duties, marital needs, and negotiating boundaries with families of origin, friends, and the larger community. When breast cancer occurs among families with adolescents and young adults, it may disrupt adolescents' process of separation and intimacy with peers. As a consequence, regression may occur, creating severe conflicts in dependence and autonomy. Rait and Lederberg note that the older family is likely to experience role reversals as a consequence of the illness, requiring a refocus on personal and interpersonal goals.

For some couples, adapting to changes in the intimate areas of their relationship causes significant strain. Sometimes, problems that were not addressed in earlier stages of marriage or partnership will increase with the stress of dealing with breast cancer.

The major goals of couples' treatment involve alleviating anxiety and restoring hope. Anxiety stems from a variety of sources, including misinformation, the fear of pain and rejection, altered appearances, financial concerns, and the impact of illness on relationships, partners, children, or parents. Women with breast cancer particularly fear estrangement, abandonment, being burdensome to their partners, and infidelity (Auchincloss, 1989).

Sexual Difficulties

Body image problems are very common, especially among women who undergo breast surgery. These women tend to experience distress over their scars, leading to feelings of decreased sexual attractiveness and restricted use of certain items of clothing.

It is beneficial for clinicians working with women who experience difficulty with arousal and sexual desire to provide reassurance that this difficulty is normal. In fact, these sexual issues can continue 1 to 2 years posttreatment, impacting quality of life (A. M. Nezu et al., 2003). Nezu et al. also offer that women with negative self-schema are less likely to resume sex or have pleasurable sexual functioning after treatment. Loss of sexual desire and inability to achieve orgasm may be due to fatigue, pain, weakness secondary to cancer treatment, opiate and pain medications, and antidepressant or antipsychotic medications. These difficulties may also be associated with depression, body image concerns, feelings of guilt, or misbeliefs about the development and spread of cancer.

Sex Therapy

It may be helpful to distinguish primarily physical changes in sexual response from emotional alterations, such as self-consciousness or anger about body changes. Mental health professionals can support couples in accepting physical changes without ignoring or obsessing about them (Auchincloss, 1989). When women find that the loss of a breast or breasts diminishes their sexual arousal, they may benefit from exploration of new techniques to enhance sexual pleasure. Masters and Johnson's (1970) technique of sensate focus encourages mutual exploration without touching the genitals or breasts in order to locate other areas of the body that provide sensual pleasure. Rose and Perotti (2003) also recommend gradual exposure as a gentle way to adjust to changes in women's breasts.

Professionals working with couples recommend increased time on foreplay, communication when there is discomfort or pain, and adjustment of sexual activities. Other techniques that may be of benefit include relaxation and Kegel exercises and sequenced vaginal penetration either digitally or using vaginal dilators (Auchincloss, 1989). These difficulties may improve by increasing the amount of time planned for the couple, using sexual fantasies, and challenging anxious or negative distracting thoughts such as concern that partners are focusing on the altered breasts (Auchincloss, 1989).

It is also helpful for women to explore other ways to become comfortable with their bodies, especially if they do not have steady partners. One way to increase women's comfort is to engage in massage. It is important that couples express their feelings or fears about sex, as establishing open communication will help avoid misunderstandings and enable them to address concerns as soon as they arise.

FAMILY RESPONSE

Breast cancer impacts family members differently throughout the progression of the illness. Rait and Lederberg (1989) suggest that some family members may be more acutely distressed than the patient. The acute phase of the illness is a time of rallying and mobilization among family members. Relatives may also reduce their communication and create a "conspiracy of silence" in an effort to avoid upsetting the individuals with cancer (Rait & Lederberg, 1989, p. 587). During the chronic phase, family members attempt to juggle the needs of the patients with the needs of other family members. Although this period focuses significantly on illness, it also requires a resumption of normal developmental tasks. Rait and Lederberg state that relatives may express disagreement on goals and important decisions leading to anger, jealousy, and neediness among other family members. Family members may experience a sense of isolation due to decreased support from family, friends, or coworkers. Coping must be carried out on a day-to-day basis.

Children

Children of women with breast cancer face particular challenges associated with their mothers' illness. Children's sense of security develops from routines and stability. Therefore, changes over which children have no control often threaten this feeling of safety (Houts & Bucher, 2000). Numerous alterations in aspects of children's daily lives occur, including changes in routines, relationships, and experiences to which children are accustomed. Their mothers may undergo alterations in appearance and energy levels, leading to differences in the amount of attention children receive. The distribution of household duties as well as the individuals who are in the home may change.

Houts and Bucher (2000) assert that children benefit most when adults are honest with them, as children are observant and sensitive to changes in the people they love. Providing accurate information is especially important when children create their own interpretations of the information. For example, children may worry about getting cancer themselves, fear that no one will take care of them, or believe they did something to cause the illness (Houts & Bucher, 2000). Parents' avoidance of discussing the topic of cancer may intimate that it is too distressing to discuss, consequently increasing the children's fears of the disease. If children discover the truth from others, they will likely feel betrayed that their parents did not tell them. Fears may also exacerbate difficulties children may already be having due to changes in family life. Commonly occurring problems include sleep or appetite disruption, difficulties in school, withdrawal, irritability, and fighting. Parents should inform their children of the diagnosis, what treatments are expected, how they will affect the individuals with cancer, and how they might affect other family members. The prognosis may be shared in response to direct questions from children. However, Houts and Bucher warn that if the prognosis is less clear, parents should focus on reassuring children that someone will always be there to care for them.

To facilitate children's expression of their own feelings, parents should encourage them to explore a multitude of modalities. Art, role-playing, and storytelling are especially effective methods of communication of emotions (Houts & Bucher, 2000). It is important that parents make a conscious effort to be available to their children in order to foster opportunities for discussion. Women with cancer should develop a plan regarding how they will communicate with their children when they are not available at home. Parents should avoid trying to protect their children by withholding feelings such as anger, fear, or worries. However, children do not need to participate in discussions with their parents regarding aspects of treatment that would be especially scary. Using humor, allowing children to help, anticipating changes, and maintaining rules of discipline and rewards all facilitate children's adjustment and coping abilities (Houts & Bucher, 2000).

Adolescents

Adolescents sometimes feel more comfortable talking to others outside of their families. It is also important that parents routinely keep schools informed. Teenagers and young adults may want to discuss issues around religion, as questions are likely to surface. Maintaining hobbies, sports, and activities is important, though family and lifestyle changes may be unavoidable. Parents should be careful to avoid loading down adolescents with too much responsibility in order to maintain a sense of normalcy regarding family roles and routines. Adolescents are especially sensitive to deception by their parents, which will likely result in feelings of distrust. Given the importance of separation and individuation during this period, adolescents may experience guilt about wanting to exert their independence when they are needed at home. Embarrassment commonly emerges regarding being different from their peers or regarding their mothers' changes in physical appearance. Houts and Bucher (2000) assert that adolescents are also particularly vulnerable to confusion due to increased lack of control.

Special issues are likely to arise for adolescent daughters of mothers with breast cancer. Mothers may rely on their daughters for more assistance around the house. Daughters may be uncomfortable talking about issues related to breasts, as they are in the stage of undergoing breast development. These young women may also experience fears about their risk of developing breast cancer (Houts & Bucher, 2000). Overall, daughters of women with breast cancer exhibit greater fearfulness, withdrawal, and hostility, typically stemming from fears of developing the disease and greater demands placed upon them (Rowland & Holland, 1989).

CAREGIVERS

More care and recovery takes place at home due to earlier hospital discharges, greater reliance on outpatient care, and the increasing prevalence of chronic illness, thus generating a significant impact on caregivers. Most caregivers are laypersons and are often family members, which often leads to significant distress regarding the uncertainty of providing adequate support. According to Houts et al. (1996), "family members who are assuming these caregiving responsibilities are often uninformed about what to do and are emotionally involved as well" (p. 65).

Playing the role of a caregiver can prove markedly exhausting, both physically and emotionally. Many caregivers must give up many activities in order to provide 24-hour-per-day availability. The responsibility of caring for loved ones may affect family members' physical and emotional well-being. A. M. Nezu et al. (2003) report that caregivers with heightened stress experienced lowered self-esteem, less family support, more negative impact on schedules, and greater overall demands. Spouses who act as caregivers may experience elevated psychological distress and are vulnerable to developing eating disorders, sleep disturbances, anxiety, and depression, particularly when their own needs remain unsatisfied (A. M. Nezu et al., 2003).

Caregivers must be aware of important tasks in order to provide support and communicate effectively with the individuals with cancer (Houts & Bucher, 2000). Individuals with cancer require assistance with coping with the diagnosis emotionally and living their lives as normally as possible. Caregivers can support this goal by creating a climate that encourages sharing feelings and communicating their availability. The patients may not always elect to share by talking. Instead, they may feel more comfortable writing about their feelings or expressing them through an activity, gestures or expressions, or touching. Caregivers should also keep in mind that they don't always have to agree with their loved ones' thoughts or feelings.

Caregiver Emotional Responses

Many powerful emotions may arise among caregivers supporting individuals with cancer. When caregivers feel overwhelmed, it is helpful to avoid making important decisions while upset, instead electing to take time to sort things out. Caregivers also benefit from talking over important problems with others who have been helpful in the past. Caregivers are particularly vulnerable to experiencing anger that their lives have been disrupted due to taking on this stressful role. Caregivers may feel frustrated by the magnitude of responsibilities, especially when the individuals they are supporting may be demanding and irritable. Houts and Bucher (2000) indicate that caregivers who are used to fixing things must also learn to accept that they cannot fix cancer. To facilitate management of angry feelings, it is beneficial if caregivers can attempt to view situations from their loved ones' perspectives. Instead of withholding strong feelings, caregivers should express their anger in appropriate ways before becoming severe. When anger begins to cloud their abilities to support their loved ones, it is also helpful for caregivers to remove themselves from the situation temporarily.

Feelings of guilt also occur commonly among caretakers of individuals with cancer. Caregivers may believe that they did something to cause the illness or that they should have recognized it sooner. Caregivers may experience guilt due to their assertion that they are not adequately supporting their loved ones. Caregivers may blame themselves for not establishing time for their own needs. Guilt may occur in response to feeling angry with their loved ones for being ill when they are healthy (Houts & Bucher, 2000). Coping with feelings of guilt involves talking to other people who have gone through similar experiences. Caregivers should avoid dwelling on errors and placing demands on themselves to be perfect.

Caregivers may experience fear for what is to come and worry that they will not be able to manage what occurs in the future. Learning as much as possible about the potential impact of cancer on their loved ones can reduce this fear. Talking to others about the fears may also alleviate this feeling.

Caregiver Self-Care

Houts and Bucher (2000) warn that caregivers must be careful to avoid becoming so depleted that they cannot take care of themselves. As a consequence, caregivers must set limits on what tasks they can reasonably expect themselves to do and seek assistance from others. "Caregivers who have support from other people become less depressed and overwhelmed about the responsibilities of caregiving" (Houts & Bucher, 2000, p. 45). One way to maintain caregiver health is to schedule and focus on pleasurable experiences such as enjoyable activities with other people, activities that provide a sense of accomplishment, and activities that engender positive feelings. Problem-solving methods contribute to positive mental health by increasing caregivers' sense of mastery or control. This approach supports caregivers in identifying obstacles when they arise, defining the dilemmas, developing plans to overcome and prevent them, and learning when and how to obtain professional help.

COUNTERTRANSFERENCE

Mental health professionals must be aware of their own beliefs and countertransference issues when working with women with breast cancer. Clinicians must be cognizant of their personal views of death and their abilities to cope with losses. Massie et al. (1989) assert that "psychotherapeutic work in cancer demands a far more active stance and use of the self than is true of traditional psychotherapy, making the need for self-reflection more important" (p. 465). Clinicians must be willing to engage in introspection about their own vulnerabilities from prior losses. It is particularly important to be aware of a psychological need to try to "save" patients from their illness.

Therapists should seek out accurate information about their patients' diagnoses, treatments, and prognoses before undertaking psychotherapy. Working knowledge of treatment options and the capacity to adapt treatment to the patients' needs and illness changes are also essential functions. Mental health professionals must also be able to adjust interventions with physicians and nurses on behalf of the patients.

When clinicians struggle with their own emotional responses to their work, they often feel a sense of futility and discouragement, helplessness, and impotence (Massie et al., 1989). Therapists may experience low self-esteem, depression, and resentment toward their patients for creating these internal conflicts. Massie et al. warn that this resentment may cause therapists to encourage or expect inappropriate or impractical efforts on behalf of the patients that may contradict the reality of the circumstances. These feelings tend to occur more frequently when treatment goals shift to palliative care. Clinicians are also vulnerable to premature withdrawal from treatment due to frustration with their patients with advancing illness. Many therapists feel worried about causing their patients additional emotional distress by confronting them with evidence of maladaptive defenses. This concern may result in reluctance or refusal to broach painful topics for discussion in order to avoid additional discomfort.

CONCLUSION

Although breast cancer may manifest itself uniquely, the impact of the diagnosis often results in common responses such as sadness, low self-esteem, and fear. The influence of this disease goes beyond the direct effects on the women who are diagnosed; spouses, children, other family members, and friends also experience significant levels of distress. The breasts, typically symbols of femininity, sexuality, and attractiveness, come to represent physical discomfort, diminished self-concept, and a potential threat to women's lives.

The majority of women experience marked distress consequent to receiving this diagnosis, exhibiting symptoms of an Adjustment Disorder With Depressed or Anxious Mood. Common affective responses include low mood, fatigue, sense of hopelessness about the future, uncontrollable worry, and disruption in sleeping and eating patterns. Women frequently develop fears about side effects of treatment, potential changes in appearance, impact of the illness on daily functioning and relationships, and prognosis. Short-term interventions incorporating psychoeducation and supportive therapy are recommended to diminish distress and improve coping. Supportive therapy creates opportunities for expression and acceptance of emotions and often includes cognitive-behavioral techniques such as challenging negative thoughts and enhanced relaxation and stress management. When mood and anxiety symptoms persist in severity and duration beyond what would be expected, more intensive treatment may be required.

Mental health professionals must take into consideration that spouses and partners, children, friends, and caregivers also experience significant concerns. Clinicians may support couples by alleviating fears and encouraging communication and intimacy. Children's emotional responses and needs for support are dependent upon their developmental levels. Parents must look for opportunities for open discussion among family members. Due to their significant emotional and physical investment in their loved ones, caregivers must not ignore their own self-care and limitations. Like caregivers, therapists also become deeply invested in their patients with breast cancer. Personal issues regarding loss and fantasies of cure and rescue tend to surface while in this provider role. Therapists need to be cognizant of their emotional responses and of the value of self-care. Overall, support is most beneficial when established in a broader context, incorporating multiple areas of functioning and all individuals affected by the illness experience.

CONTRIBUTORS

Nicole L. Glick, PsyD, is currently a licensed psychologist for the Ashland School District in Ashland, Massachusetts. Her clinical interests include child and adolescent psychotherapy and the treatment of mood, anxiety, and eating disorders. Dr. Glick completed her training in clinical psychology at the Institute for Graduate Clinical Psychology at Widener University, where she specialized in School Psychology and Family Therapy. She presently holds certification in School Psychology in Massachusetts and Pennsylvania. Dr. Glick may be contacted at 395 Captain Eames Circle, Ashland, MA 01721. E-mail: NicoleGlick@aol.com

Maurice F. Prout, PhD, ABPP, is currently professor at the Institute for Graduate Clinical Psychology at Widener University, Chester, Pennsylvania. He also directs the respecialization program housed within the Institute. His clinical interests include the treatment of anxiety and mood disorders as well as topics related to behavioral medicine. He is a Diplomate in Clinical Psychology and a Founding Fellow of the Academy of Cognitive Therapy. Dr. Prout can be reached at Widener University, Chester, PA 19013. E-mail: Maurice.F.Prout@widener.edu

RESOURCES*

Cited Resources

American Cancer Society. (2005). All about breast cancer. Retrieved June 18, 2005, from http://www.cancer.org/docroot/CRI/CRI_2x.asp?sitearea=&dt=5

Andrykowski, M. A., Cordova, M. J., Studts, J. L., & Miller, T. W. (1998). Posttraumatic stress disorder after treatment for breast cancer: Prevalence of diagnosis and use of the PTSD Checklist – Civilian Version (PCL-C) as a screening instrument. *Journal of Consulting and Clinical Psychology, 66*(3), 586-590.

Auchincloss, S. S. (1989). Sexual dysfunction in cancer patients: Issues in evaluation and treatment. In J. C. Holland & J. H. Rowland (Eds.), *Handbook of Psychooncology: Psychological Care of the Patient With Cancer* (pp. 383-413). New York: Oxford University Press.

Bloom, J. R. (1982). Social support, accommodation to stress and adjustment to breast cancer. *Social Science and Medicine, 16*, 1329-1338.

Brennan, J. (2001). Adjustment to cancer—coping or personal transition? *Psychooncology, 10*(1), 1-18.

Cancersource. (2000). Breast cancer overview: Learn about cancer. Retrieved August 13, 2004, from http://www.cancersource.com/LearnAboutCancer/core

Carver, C. S., Lehman, J. M., & Antoni, M. H. (2003). Dispositional pessimism predicts illness-related disruption of social and recreational activities among breast cancer patients. *Journal of Personality and Social Psychology, 84*(4), 814-821.

Chang, A. F., & Haber, S. B. (1997). Breast cancer: How your mind can help your body. Retrieved August 13, 2004, from http://www.apahelpcenter.org/articles/article.php?id=47

Dow, K. H. (1991). The growing phenomenon of cancer survivorship. *Journal of Professional Nursing, 7*, 54-61.

Elk, R., & Morrow, M. (2003). *Breast Cancer for Dummies.* Hoboken, New Jersey: Wiley.

Giese-Davis, J., Koopman, C., Butler, L. D., Classen, C., Cordova, M., Fobiar, P., Benson, J., Kraemer, H. C., & Spiegel, D. (2002). Change in emotion-regulation strategy for women with metastatic breast cancer following supportive-expressive group therapy. *Journal of Consulting and Clinical Psychology, 70*(4), 916-925.

---

* Although all websites cited in this contribution were correct at the time of publication, they are subject to change at any time.

Henderson, P. (1997). Psychological adjustment of adult cancer survivors: Their needs and counselor interventions. *Journal of Counseling and Development, 75*, 188-194.

Holland, J. C. (1989a). Clinical course of cancer. In J. C. Holland & J. H. Rowland (Eds.), *Handbook of Psychooncology: Psychological Care of the Patient With Cancer* (pp. 75-100). New York: Oxford University Press.

Holland, J. C. (1989b). Radiotherapy. In J. C. Holland & J. H. Rowland (Eds.), *Handbook of Psychooncology: Psychological Care of the Patient With Cancer* (pp. 134-145). New York: Oxford University Press.

Holland, J. C., & Lesko, L. M. (1989). Chemotherapy, endocrine therapy, and immunotherapy. In J. C. Holland & J. H. Rowland (Eds.), *Handbook of Psychooncology: Psychological Care of the Patient With Cancer* (pp. 146-162). New York: Oxford University Press.

Houts, P. S., & Bucher, J. A. (Eds.). (2000). *Caregiving: A Step-By-Step Resource for Caring for the Person With Cancer at Home*. Atlanta, GA: American Cancer Society.

Houts, P. S., Nezu, A. M., Nezu, C. M., & Bucher, J. A. (1996). The prepared family caregiver: A problem-solving approach to family caregiver education. *Patient Education and Counseling, 27*, 63-73.

Jacobson, P., & Holland, J. C. (1989). Psychological reactions to cancer surgery. In J. C. Holland & J. H. Rowland (Eds.), *Handbook of Psychooncology: Psychological Care of the Patient With Cancer* (pp. 117-133). New York: Oxford University Press.

Lazarus, R., & Folkman, S. (1984). *Stress, Appraisal, and Coping*. New York: Springer.

Massie, M. J. (1989a). Anxiety, panic, and phobias. In J. C. Holland & J. H. Rowland (Eds.), *Handbook of Psychooncology: Psychological Care of the Patient With Cancer* (pp. 300-309). New York: Oxford University Press.

Massie, M. J. (1989b). Depression. In J. C. Holland & J. H. Rowland (Eds.), *Handbook of Psychooncology: Psychological Care of the Patient With Cancer* (pp. 283-290). New York: Oxford University Press.

Massie, M. J., Holland, J. C., & Straker, N. (1989). Psychotherapeutic interventions. In J. C. Holland & J. H. Rowland (Eds.), *Handbook of Psychooncology: Psychological Care of the Patient With Cancer* (pp. 455-469). New York: Oxford University Press.

Masters, W., & Johnson, V. (1970). *Human Sexual Inadequacy*. Boston: Little, Brown, & Co.

Mastrovito, R. (1989). Behavioral techniques: Progressive relaxation and self-regulatory therapies. In J. C. Holland & J. H. Rowland (Eds.), *Handbook of Psychooncology: Psychological Care of the Patient With Cancer* (pp. 492-501). New York: Oxford University Press.

Moyer, A. (1997). Psychosocial outcomes of breast-conserving surgery versus mastectomy: A meta-analytic review. *Health Psychology, 16*(3), 284-298.

National Breast Cancer Centre. (2000). A guide for women with early breast cancer. Retrieved August 12, 2004, from http://www.nbcc.org.au/resources/documents/EBC_earlyguide.pdf

National Cancer Institute. (2004, July). Normal adjustment, psychosocial distress, and the adjustment disorders: Health professional version. Retrieved August 9, 2004, from http://www.cancer.gov/cancertopics/pdq/supportivecare/adjustment/healthprofessional

Nezu, A. M., Nezu, C. M., & Geller, P. A. (Eds.). (2003). *Health Psychology: Vol. 9* in I. B. Weiner (Ed.), *Handbook of Psychology*. New York: Wiley.

Rait, D., & Lederberg, M. (1989). The family of the cancer patient. In J. C. Holland & J. H. Rowland (Eds.), *Handbook of Psychooncology: Psychological Care of the Patient With Cancer* (pp. 585-597). New York: Oxford University Press.

Rose, A. R., & Perotti, J. (2003). Every woman's guide to breast cancer. Y-ME National Breast Cancer Organization. Retrieved August 9, 2004, from http://www.y-me.org/resource_library/every_womans_guide.pdf

Rowland, J. H., & Holland, J. C. (1989). Breast cancer. In J. C. Holland & J. H. Rowland (Eds.), *Handbook of Psychooncology: Psychological Care of the Patient With Cancer* (pp. 188-207). New York: Oxford University Press.

Sears, S. R., Stanton, A. L., & Danoff-Burg, S. (2003). The yellow brick road and the emerald city: Benefit finding, positive reappraisal coping, and posttraumatic growth in women with early-stage breast cancer. *Health Psychology, 22*(5), 487-497.

Spiegel, D., Bloom, J. R., & Yalom, I. D. (1981). Group support for patients with metastatic cancer: A randomized prospective outcome study. *Archives of General Psychiatry, 38*, 527-533.

Stanton, A. L., & Snider, P. R. (1993). Coping with a breast cancer diagnosis: A prospective study. *Health Psychology, 12*(1), 16-23.

Tross, S., & Holland, J. C. (1989). Psychological sequelae in cancer survivors. In J. C. Holland & J. H. Rowland (Eds.), *Handbook of Psychooncology: Psychological Care of the Patient With Cancer* (pp. 101-116). New York: Oxford University Press.

Additional Resources

Allen, S. M., Shah, A. C., Nezu, A. M., Nezu, C. M., Ciambrone, D., Hogan, J., & Mor, V. (2002). A problem-solving approach to stress reduction among younger women with breast carcinoma. *Cancer, 94*(12), 3089-3100.

American College of Physicians. (1997). Home care guide for advanced cancer. Retrieved June 30, 2004, from www.acponline.org/public/h_care/preface.htm

Breitbart, W. (1989). Suicide. In J. C. Holland & J. H. Rowland (Eds.), *Handbook of Psychooncology: Psychological Care of the Patient With Cancer* (pp. 291-299). New York: Oxford University Press.

Burnham, T., & Wilcox, A. (2002). Effects of exercise on physiological and psychological variables in cancer survivors. *Medicine and Science in Sports and Exercise, 34*(12), 1863-1867.

Cassidy, S. (2000). How individual and group psychological support can help cancer patients. *Primary Care and Cancer, 20*(5). Retrieved June 21, 2004, from http:www.cancernetwork.com/journals/primary/p0005i.htm

Coyle, N., Loscalzo, M., & Bailey, L. (1989). Supportive home care for the advanced cancer patient and family. In J. C. Holland & J. H. Rowland (Eds.), *Handbook of Psychooncology: Psychological Care of the Patient With Cancer* (pp. 598-606). New York: Oxford University Press.

McDaniel, S. H., & Speice, J. (2001). What family psychology has to offer women's health: The examples of conversion, somatization, infertility treatment, and genetic testing. *Professional Psychology: Research and Practice, 32*(1), 44-51.

Payne, D., & Massie, M. J. (1995). Monitor patient's emotional adaptation to breast cancer. *Oncology News International, 4*(11). Retrieved June 21, 2004, from www.cancernetwork.com/journals/oncnews/n9511v.htm

Quesnel, C., Savard, J., Simard, S., Ivers, H., & Morin, M. (2003). Efficacy of cognitive-behavioral therapy for insomnia in women treated for nonmetastatic breast cancer. *Journal of Consulting and Clinical Psychology, 71*(1), 189-200.

RealAge Breast Cancer Screening Health Assessment. (2004). Retrieved August 8, 2004, from http://www.realage.com/health_guides/BreastCancer/introduction.asp?memberId=&cbr=

Spencer, S. M., Lehman, J. M., Wynings, C., Arena, P., Carver, C. S., Antoni, M. H., Derhagopian, R. P., Ironson, G., & Love, N. (1999). Concerns about breast cancer and relations to psychosocial well-being in a multiethnic sample of early-stage patients. *Health Psychology, 18*(2), 159-168.

Spiegel, D. (2002). Group psychosocial therapy improves mood and pain in metastatic breast cancer patients. *Oncology News International, 11*(1). Retrieved June 21, 2004, from www.cancernetwork.com/journals/oncnews/n0201xx.htm

Williams, T. R., O'Sullivan, M., Snodgrass, S. E., & Love, N. (1995). Psychosocial issues in breast cancer: Helping patients get the support they need. *Postgraduate Medicine, 98*(4), 97-110.

Williamson, G. (2000). Extending the activity restriction model of depressed affect: Evidence from a sample of breast cancer patients. *Health Psychology, 19*(4), 339-347.

Yahoo Health. (2004). Breast cancer health center. Retrieved August 9, 2004, from http://health.yahoo.com/health/centers/breast_cancer/

Psychosocial Aspects of Obstetrics, Gynecology, and Fertility

Ann Morrison and Brenda J. B. Roman

The health and wellness of women is intimately linked to reproduction. For some women, menstrual cycle disorders and menopause also can compromise mental well-being. Certain phases and events of women's reproductive lives, such as pregnancy and the postpartum period, represent times of increased vulnerability to mental illness, especially mood and anxiety disorders. Complications of conception and pregnancy, such as infertility, multiple births, abortion, miscarriage, and stillbirth, may have psychological consequences. Finally, it should be noted that gender differences in the frequency, onset, severity, course, and characteristics of many mental illnesses, including depression, bipolar disorder, panic disorder, obsessive compulsive disorder, schizophrenia, and posttraumatic stress disorder, are well known. This contribution will focus primarily on the interface between women's reproductive health and mental health rather than these gender differences.

PREMENSTRUAL DISORDERS

Premenstrual disorders include the less severe premenstrual syndrome (PMS), which includes physical and psychological symptoms, and the more severe premenstrual dysphoric disorder (PMDD), which, as the name implies, emphasizes psychological symptoms. Prevalence estimates vary, but for the more severe disorders, Steiner and Born (2002), reviewing multiple studies, estimated it to be 3% to 8% of menstruating women. The 2001 study by Soares et al. reported a 6.3% prevalence. Table 1 (p. 58) presents PMDD as defined in the American Psychiatric Association *Diagnostic and Statistical Manual of Mental Disorders* (*DSM-IV-TR;* 4th ed. text rev., 2000). Essential symptoms include one or more of the following: depressed mood, anxiety, lability, and anger or irritability. Exclusionary criteria include exacerbation of a more pervasive mood or anxiety disorder, such as major depression or panic disorder, and prospective rating in at least two consecutive cycles is required. Premenstrual symptoms are very common, and even the more significant disorders of premenstrual syndrome and PMDD are fairly common; however, care must be taken that primary psychiatric disorders are not overlooked. Indeed, Caligor and Ormont (1999) relate that 30% to 50% of women presenting with PMS are found to have a major psychiatric illness, usually depression or anxiety disorder. Premenstrual worsening of psychiatric illnesses should also be distinguished from PMDD. An asymptomatic week during the follicular phase of menstrual cycles is indicative of PMDD (Caligor & Ormont, 1999). In addition, medical conditions such as thyroid disease, endometriosis, and others may mimic symptoms of PMDD (Nonacs & Cohen, 2002).

TABLE 1: Research Criteria for Premenstrual Dysphoric Disorder*

A. In most menstrual cycles during the past year, five (or more) of the following symptoms were present for most of the time during the last week of the luteal phase,** began to remit within a few days after the onset of the follicular phase, and were absent in the week postmenses, with at least one of the symptoms being either (1), (2), (3), or (4):

    (1)   markedly depressed mood, feelings of hopelessness, or self-deprecating thoughts

    (2)   marked anxiety, tension, feelings of being "keyed up," or "on edge"

    (3)   marked affective lability (e.g., feeling suddenly sad or tearful or increased sensitivity to rejection)

    (4)   persistent and marked anger or irritability or increased interpersonal conflicts

    (5)   decreased interest in usual activities (e.g., work, school, friends, hobbies)

    (6)   subjective sense of difficulty in concentrating

    (7)   lethargy, easy fatigability, or marked lack of energy

    (8)   marked change in appetite, overeating, or specific food cravings

    (9)   hypersomnia or insomnia

   (10)   a subjective sense of being overwhelmed or out of control

   (11)   other physical symptoms, such as breast tenderness or swelling, headaches, joint or muscle pain, a sensation of "bloating," weight gain

B. The disturbance markedly interferes with work or school or with usual social activities and relationships with others (e.g., avoidance of social activities, decreased productivity and efficiency at work or school).

C. The disturbance is not merely an exacerbation of the symptoms of another disorder such as Major Depressive Disorder, Panic Disorder, Dysthymic Disorder, or a Personality Disorder (although it may be superimposed on any of these disorders).

D. Criteria A, B, and C must be confirmed by prospective daily ratings during at least two consecutive symptomatic cycles. (The diagnosis may be made provisionally prior to this confirmation.)

---

* Reprinted with permission from the *Diagnostic and Statistical Manual of Mental Disorders*, Copyright © 2000. American Psychiatric Association.

****Note:** In menstruating females, the luteal phase corresponds to the period between ovulation and the onset of menses, and the follicular phase begins with menses. In nonmenstruating females (e.g., those who have had a hysterectomy), the timing of luteal and follicular phases may require measurement of circulating reproductive hormones.

Treatment of PMDD includes both pharmacologic and nonpharmacologic approaches. Treatment with a selective serotonin reuptake inhibitor (SSRI) antidepressant has shown consistent benefit in both the psychological and somatic symptoms of PMDD. These are considered first-line treatments (Steiner & Born, 2002). Indeed, PMDD seems to be more responsive than depression to treatments with an SSRI, with both quicker improvement and evidence from studies such as those by Freeman et al. (2004) reporting benefit from even intermittent dosing, a treatment strategy not recommended for depression or anxiety disorders. Other psychotropic medications with support of some efficacy (but less effectiveness than the SSRIs) from randomized controlled trials are the anxiolytics alprazolam and buspirone (Steiner & Born, 2002). Hormonal treatments have included suppression of ovulation with gonadotropin-releasing hormone (GnRH) and oral contraception. The former has shown benefit in most but not all studies (Steiner & Born, 2002). Oral contraceptives, on the other hand, have had more mixed results (Rapkin, Mikacich, & Moatakef-Imani, 2003). Two controlled studies support a decrease in physical symptoms from triphasic oral contraceptives (Steiner & Born, 2002), and one newer progestin containing oral contraceptive has shown quality of life, well-being, and physical symptom improvement (Borenstein et al., 2003). Nutritional supplements like tryptophan, an amino acid which is a serotonin precursor, have been shown to be more effective than placebo in the control of psychological symptoms of PMDD (Steinberg et al., 1999). Steiner and Born (2002) summarize that calcium supplements (1,200 mg calcium carbonate daily) reduced symptoms in one study. There is some evidence that vitamin B6 (pyridoxine up to 100 mg daily) may decrease symptoms overall, including depression, and magnesium (200 mg daily) may be beneficial in reducing water retention.

Nonpharmacologic approaches to PMS and PMDD include recommendations for prudent diet and exercise regimens. These typically call for limiting fat, simple carbohydrates, and salt in the diet, and decreasing methylxanthine (i.e., caffeine) consumption in foods, beverages, and drugs. Individual and group psychotherapy may be helpful in managing symptoms of depression and anxiety. Cognitive behavioral techniques are recommended by many (Nonacs & Cohen, 1998; Steiner & Born, 2002). Steiner and Born (2002), citing studies by Parry's and Lam's groups (Lam et al., 1999; Parry et al., 1993), support the use of light therapy during the luteal phase to decrease symptoms.

PERIMENOPAUSE AND MENOPAUSE

Popular belief and portrayal of menopause as a time of emotional turmoil has persisted for decades. Witness the tonics offered by medicine men of the 19th century, up through Edith Bunker's televised ordeal in the second half of the 20th century. Indeed the medical literature reflected this view in Kraeplin's (1921) concept of "involutional melancholia" as a time of increased vulnerability experienced by women as they entered the end of their reproductive years. However, scientific studies of the prevalence of mood disorders do not consistently confirm an increase in the menopausal years. Additionally, as in the case of menstrually related mood disorders, there are significant differences in prevalence depending upon the sample population; the threshold for the type, number, and severity of symptoms; and even the definition and confirmation of menopause. Treatment of mood symptoms in the perimenopausal and menopausal years likewise has been a mixture of conflicting studies and recommendations. Added to the biological controversies are the even more varied social and cultural expectations and changes within which menopause occurs and which affect women's physical and psychological experience.

Menopause is generally defined as 12 months of amenorrhea. Perimenopause is the time before this in which menses are irregular. The postmenopausal period is beyond the first 12 months of amenorrhea. Hormonal levels vary considerably between these periods (Khine et al., 2003). Postmenopausal women have elevated gonadotropins (follicle-stimulating hormone and luteinizing hormone) and low ovarian steroids (estradiol and progesterone) and relatively low androgens. In the perimenopause, hormones are in flux, with episodic gonadotropin secretion, periods of both normal and low estradiol, declining androgens, and both ovulatory and anovulatory cycles.

As mentioned earlier, there is no consistent evidence of increased mood disorders with postmenopausal women; however, there is some evidence that there may be increased vulnerability in the perimenopausal population. Among the more recent of these is the Cross National Epidemiologic Study by Weissman et al. (1988) indicating increased risk of depression in the perimenopausal years (45-50).

Typical symptoms of the perimenopausal and menopausal period include not only depression but also insomnia, hot flashes, night sweats, cognitive disturbance, anxiety, and sexual dysfunction due to both peripheral (pelvic) and central (brain) problems (Alexander et al., 2003). They describe peripheral (pelvic) problems to include decreased lubrication, atrophy of internal and external genital tissues, and loss of pelvic musculature. Central (brain) factors include the effects of diminished estrogen and testosterone on neurotransmitters, which ultimately leads to decreased libido. The possible interaction and relatedness of these physiologic and psychological complaints is reviewed by Ayubi-Moak and Parry (2002). Of special interest is the interplay between vasomotor symptoms, insomnia, and depression. They describe studies in which the awakenings appear to precede hot flashes, and in which the degree of sleep disruption seems to predict the degree of depression.

Although there remains controversy regarding the relationship between mood and menopause, there is more agreement regarding treatment of depression when it does occur in the perimenopausal and menopausal period. The treatment of choice is the standard treatment of depression, namely antidepressant therapy, such as an SSRI, and psychotherapy. Although low levels of estrogen replacement therapy alone improve mood and well-being in nondepressed women, studies on the role of hormone replacement in the treatment of clinical depression have failed to show any significant role for their use (Ayubi-Moak & Parry, 2002). Some studies in which women received estrogen replacement therapy and an SSRI, but not a tricyclic antidepressant (TCA), appear to show an augmentation of antidepressant efficacy (Ayubi-Moak & Parry, 2002). As the risks and benefits of hormone replacement therapy continue to be debated and studied, it would seem prudent to use augmentation only for refractory depression, or when otherwise indicated for the short-term amelioration of clinically significant menopausal complaints. As always, the risks and benefits of hormone replacement therapy must be weighed in the context of the patients' individual and family medical history, symptom complex, and available alternative treatments.

PREGNANCY

Psychiatric illnesses, especially mood and anxiety disorders, often emerge during the childbearing years in women. Thus, women may consult their clinicians regarding psychiatric medications that they have been taking when planning to conceive, or when unexpectedly pregnant. Additionally, some women may experience psychiatric symptoms for the first time while pregnant. Because symptoms may be severe enough to impair functioning, thus potentially affecting the developing fetus, the potential benefits of medication must be considered. All psychotropic medication passes across the placenta; thus, clinicians must be aware of the risks of prenatal exposure. With potential risks to the developing fetus, women generally are advised to discontinue medication; however, relapse rates during pregnancy in women with recurrent mood disorders are high (Viguera et al., 2000). Thus, one must keep in mind the risks of untreated mental illness to the mother and developing fetus, making a careful risk/benefit assessment. This risk assessment includes risk of fetal exposure to the medication, risk of untreated psychiatric illness to the mother, and risk of relapse if medication is discontinued (Nonacs, Viguera, & Cohen, 2002). No psychotropic medication is approved by the U.S. Food and Drug Administration for use during pregnancy; thus, clinicians must rely on available clinical data to assist in the risk assessment discussion.

Untreated major depression in the mother likely adversely affects the developing fetus, with increased risks of preterm labor, lower birth weight, smaller head circumference, and lower Apgar scores (Nonacs et al., 2002). Additionally, pregnant women with depression are more likely to smoke, consume alcohol, or use illicit drugs, further increasing risk to the fetus (Zuckerman et al., 1989). Thus, these risks must be weighed against potential risks of antidepressant medication. In general, antidepressants, particularly the SSRIs and TCAs, do not cause any known congenital anomalies. Neonatal withdrawal syndromes have been described with TCAs, primarily jitteriness and irritability, and with the SSRIs, again noting jitteriness, feeding problems, and mild respiratory distress (Nonacs et al., 2002).

For bipolar disorder, lithium is the safest mood stabilizer available for use during pregnancy. Although concern about Epstein's anomaly (a cardiac deformation) remains, the relative risk is very low (Cohen et al., 1994). Anticonvulsants, particularly valproate (Omtzigt et al., 1992; Robert & Guibaud, 1982) and carbamazepine (Rosa, 1991), have a well-established risk of 1% to 6% for neural tube defects, including craniofacial abnormalities, hydrocephalus, and micro-cephalous. Other problems include cardiovascular malformation, limb defects, and genital anomalies (Nonacs et al., 2002). Therefore, anticonvulsants must be avoided during pregnancy. Due to the high prevalence of postpartum mood disorders, they will be covered in the next section.

Anxiety disorders in pregnancy and the postpartum have varied courses. Cohen, Nonacs, and Viguera (2004) summarize that although some articles have described decreased panic symptoms during pregnancy, others have described the development and worsening of panic disorder during pregnancy. Similarly, the development of obsessive compulsive disorder (OCD) in pregnancy and the postpartum has been reported (Arnold et al., 2002). Of particular interest is the study by Neziroglu, Anemone, and Yaryura-Tobias (1992) in which 39% of women with OCD reported onset during pregnancy. As in the treatment of depression, psychotherapeutic and psychopharmacologic treatments may be used during both pregnancy and the postpartum. Cognitive behavioral therapy (CBT) for anxiety disorders can be effective for panic disorder and OCD. The same risk/benefit issues regarding treating depression associated with pregnancy and the postpartum apply to the treatment of anxiety disorders. SSRIs or trycyclics are effective medication classes for panic disorder and SSRIs are effective in OCD. Exposure to benzodiazepines is unclear and controversial, although Altshuler et al. (1996) suggest an increased risk of oral cleft problems in infants with first trimester exposure. Several researchers have described a benzodiazepine withdrawal syndrome consisting of jitteriness, autonomic dysregulation, and even seizures in infants with in utero benzodiazepine exposure (Nonacs et al., 2002).

As is the case with depression, severe anxiety disorders can impair a woman's ability to care for herself and her child, and effective treatments should not be withheld from her due to pregnancy or breast-feeding once an appropriate review of the risks/benefits and alternative therapies has taken place and she consents. In general, the recommendation is to use agents that are older, for which more information is available, and to which the woman has previously responded. Women with schizophrenia and other psychotic disorders should not forego treat-ment of the psychiatric illness due to pregnancy. Older, "typical" high-potency neuroleptics are often recommended because more information is available about their safety in pregnancy (Altshuler et al., 1996; Cohen et al., 2004; Nonacs et al., 2002). Case reports have noted transient extrapyramidal symptoms in infants exposed to antipsychotics during pregnancy (Nonacs et al., 2002). However, as always, decisions need to be made in the context of the woman's history of illness, medication response, and her wishes. For instance, although little information is available to date regarding clozapine, if this is the only antipsychotic to which the woman has responded and abrupt withdrawal of clozapine is reported to precipitate psychosis, there may be little benefit in switching medication, especially later in pregnancy, a time at which, unfortunately for many women, pregnancy is first detected. Acute psychosis is not good for either mother or infant; therefore, weighing treatment options with the woman is critical.

POSTPARTUM PSYCHIATRIC ILLNESSES

The connection between childbirth and psychiatric illness has long been known, with Hippocrates describing "puerperal fever" in 460 B.C. (Thurtle, 1995). The 11th century gyne-cologist Trotula of Salerno wrote, "If the womb is too moist, the brain is filled with water, and the moisture running over to the eyes compels them to involuntarily shed tears" (Steiner, 1990). Marce, in the 18th century, wrote the *Treatise on Insanity in Pregnant and Lactating Women*, describing puerperal psychosis and depression (Steiner, 1990). Despite this long known association and the fact that postpartum depression is more common than gestational diabetes, preeclampsia, and preterm delivery, far less attention is given to this clinical condition that is potentially devastating.

Childbirth itself is a major risk factor in the development of mental illness for women, as shown by several studies. Kendell et al. (1976) followed 35,000 deliveries and found a seven-fold increase in the rate of psychiatric admissions during the first 3 months postpartum. Further, this study showed that the risk of psychosis was 22 times higher than the prepregnancy rate. Yet, over 87% of the admissions were for mood disorders, with the majority having major depression (Kendell et al., 1981).

The most common postpartum mood disturbance is known as postpartum blues or baby blues. It is a transient state of heightened emotional reactivity that occurs in 50% to 80% of new mothers (Kennerley & Gath, 1989; O'Hara, 1991). The most common symptoms are mood lability, irritability, feeling overwhelmed, weepiness, and feeling "low spirited." These symptoms peak 3 to 5 days postdelivery and generally resolve within 2 weeks. No clear links have been found to various factors, including breast- or bottle feeding, labor difficulties, marital status, or parity (Hapgood, Elkind, & Wright, 1988). However, others (Kennerley & Gath, 1989; O'Hara et al., 1991b) have found that risk factors may include ambivalent feelings toward the pregnancy, fear of labor, poor social adjustment, a history of severe premenstrual tension, and stressful life events.

The etiology is unknown, although the mood changes may stem from the abrupt hormonal withdrawal. Harris et al. (1994) found that absolute levels of estrogen and progesterone have no effect on the development of postpartum blues, but rather the greater the difference between pregnancy and postpartum levels, the greater the risk of developing postpartum blues. Treatment includes reassurance and support.

Postpartum depression occurs in approximately 10% to 20% of women in the U.S. within 6 months of delivery (Steiner & Tam, 1999) and in approximately 26% of adolescent deliveries (Troutman & Cutrona, 1990). Risk factors include a personal history of major depression, depression during pregnancy, a history of premenstrual dysphoric disorder, and poor social support (O'Hara et al., 1991a; Steiner & Tam, 1999).

Interestingly, cultures with strong social support for new mothers have lower rates of postpartum depression (Miller, 2002). The diagnostic criteria are the same as for a major depressive episode (*DSM-IV-TR*; American Psychiatric Association, 2000), with a postpartum onset qualifier to a major depressive disorder if onset is within 1 month. More liberally, one may consider the postpartum period to extend to 1 year following delivery. However, the symptoms may be more difficult to ascertain. For example, sleep disturbances are characterized by difficulty falling asleep even when the baby is sleeping. Other risk factors may include a history of postpartum blues, marital discord, infant medical problems, unwanted pregnancies, and stressful life events during pregnancy (Arnold et al., 2002). In fact, up to 20% of women experiencing postpartum blues will experience a major depressive episode in the first postnatal year (Campbell et al., 1992; O'Hara, 1991). A high percentage of depressed women experience thoughts of harming their infants (Jennings et al., 1999). Fortunately, the majority of these women describe these thoughts as ego-dystonic, realizing their thoughts are irrational and that they would never act on such feelings (Miller, 2002). In addition to obsessional thoughts, these mothers may have excessive guilt, especially about a sense of failure as a mother.

However, in severe cases of depression, a woman may experience psychotic symptoms manifested by delusions and/or hallucinations as well as greater disorientation, bizarre behavior, lack of insight, suspiciousness, grandiosity, persecution, cognitive impairment, and mood lability (Wisner, Parry, & Piontek, 2002). At these times, a woman may become suicidal and also homicidal toward the baby out of a desire to protect her child and not abandon the child. These cases constitute a medical emergency, generally resulting in psychiatric hospitalization for concerns about safety for the mother, infant, and any other children.

O'Hara et al. (1991a) found that women who developed postpartum depression had significantly lower estradiol levels at 2 days postpartum compared to women who did not develop depression. Bloch et al. (2000) concluded, after exogenously inducing states of hormonal levels as in pregnancy and postpartum states in nonpregnant women, with and without histories of depression, that women who develop postpartum depression are differentially sensitive to the mood destabilizing effects of withdrawal from gonadal steroids at childbirth.

For mild to moderate symptoms of depression, cognitive behavioral therapy and interpersonal therapy are effective and should be considered first-line (O'Hara et al., 2000). Supportive psychotherapy, family and marital therapy, and group therapy may also be useful (Misri & Kostaras, 2002). Additionally, self-help groups such as Depression After Delivery, Inc. (http://www.depressionafterdelivery.com) and Postpartum Support International (http://www.chss.iup.edu/postpartum) can be helpful in providing support and education.

Antidepressant medication is utilized in moderate to severe depression. Although there are no absolute contraindications to the use of antidepressants during pregnancy or lactation, SSRIs are most often used, although the TCAs can be used (Miller, 1998). The clinician must consider the potential risk of medication exposure to the nursing infant, although, if the mother is already maintained on medication during pregnancy, she can continue while breast-feeding. Estrogen therapy has also been found to be more effective than placebo for treating postpartum depression (Ahokas et al., 2001; Gregoire et al., 1996). Women with severe depression with suicidal ideation or psychosis should be considered for electroconvulsive therapy, as it is highly effective and the effects are often more immediate (Miller, 1994).

Postpartum psychosis is a rare event, occurring in 1 out of 1,000 births (Kendell, Chalmers, & Platz, 1987). The differential diagnosis includes major depression with psychotic features, bipolar disorder, schizoaffective disorder, schizophrenia, schizophreniform disorder, brief reactive psychosis, and certain medical conditions and substances.

Although it may be difficult to distinguish between an affective disorder with psychotic features, particularly bipolar disorder, and a schizophrenic illness, most research supports a higher percentage of women with bipolar disorder as developing postpartum psychosis (Chaudron & Pies, 2003). The rate of postpartum relapse in women with bipolar disorder is 30% to 50%, and women with bipolar disorder have a 100-fold risk of developing postpartum psychosis (Chaudron & Pies, 2003). For women with a history of schizophrenia, the risk of psychiatric admission following childbirth was 3.4%, and for those with a history of major depression, it was 1.9%, yet the rate was over 21% for those women with a history of bipolar disorder (Kendell et al., 1987).

Most women who develop postpartum psychosis are generally ill within 3 weeks of delivery. The women often present with confusion, insomnia, disorganized behavior, delusions, and/or auditory hallucinations. Compared to nonpostpartum psychotic mood episodes, there tends to be greater mood lability and disorientation. Women who experience severe postpartum psychosis are at greater risk for suicide, up to 5%, and up to 4% may commit infanticide, defined as the killing of a child in the first year of life (Knopps, 1993).

Postpartum psychosis, regardless of etiology, is a medical emergency. Up to 30% of women who are psychotic experience thoughts of suicide and homicide toward their children (Misri & Kostaras, 2002). In 68% of the cases reviewed by Resnick (1969), women killed their children prior to killing, or attempting to kill, themselves. Resnick also found that 75% of mothers who committed infanticide had psychiatric symptoms prior to the offense, and 40% had been seen just prior to the tragedy by a family physician or a psychiatrist. The majority of these women were married but felt overwhelmed by responsibilities with little support, and were generally described as "devoted" mothers. Most ultimately were found not guilty by reason of insanity. Alder and Baker (1997), in a review of filicide/suicide cases, found that the women were generally over the age of 30, with two or more children, and felt overwhelmed by stressors. Ironically, the mother's concern for her children is often reflected in detailed instructions in the suicide note for the children's burial.

Women with postpartum psychosis should be psychiatrically hospitalized. There are no studies regarding clinical treatment of postpartum psychosis; however, as in any other psychiatric illness, other general medical causes must be ruled out, such as thyroiditis, vitamin B12 deficiency, or substances. Antipsychotics would be indicated. Typically, atypical antipsychotics would be first-line, although typical antipsychotics can certainly be used. If the mother is nursing, infants should be monitored for sedation and other adverse effects. With the high probability of bipolar disorder as the cause of the psychosis, mood stabilizers as well as antipsychotics are recommended. If the mother is breast-feeding, lithium is generally contraindicated due to higher levels in the breast milk and the possibility of toxic side effects in the nursing baby. Valproate may also be used, once again monitoring the nursing infants for adverse effects. Antidepressants, most commonly the SSRIs, can be added for severe depressive symptoms. For refractory patients, electroconvulsive therapy is an excellent option.

Finally, with neonaticide, the killing of an infant within the first 24 hours of life, a psychotic episode is less likely to be the reason for such action. More often, there has been complete denial of the pregnancy. These are not premeditated murders, but rather the act is committed in the face of intense emotion such as shock, shame, guilt, or fear. Interestingly, the women who commit neonaticide generally do not experience the typical symptoms, such as nausea, associated with pregnancy, and some still experience irregular or even regular periods (Brezinka et al., 1994). These mothers tend to be young and unmarried with strict fundamentalist backgrounds. As Spinelli (1998) explains, because pregnancy is viewed as a danger, it is split off from conscious awareness; thus, shocked by the onset of labor, these mothers typically deliver their infants alone and without experiencing pain. This dissociative syndrome is so profound that the mothers either leave their babies to die, often hidden in the trash, or may actively strangulate the newborn.

INFERTILITY

Chantilis and Carr (2000) estimate that infertility, failure to conceive after 1 year of unprotected intercourse, affects approximately 15% of married couples. Crosignani and Rubin (1996) report a lower 5% to 6% rate using the extended European Society of Human Reproduction and Embryology (ESHRE) 2-year timeframe. In either case, it is a problem leading to psychological distress in large numbers of couples. In addition, reproductive technologies used to evaluate and treat infertility are associated with physical and psychological burdens. Although the causes of infertility may be related to either the male or female partner or both, the burden of evaluation and treatment tends to weigh more heavily on the woman. The nature of the physical evaluation of the female, which might include physical and gynecological exams, blood tests, temperature charts, hysterosalpingograms, laparoscopy, endometrial biopsy, ovarian ultrasounds, and postcoital exams (Chantilis & Carr, 2000), tends to be more invasive and time-consuming. Further, as Greil (1997) summarizes, women report higher degrees of psychological distress such as depression, lower self-esteem, lower life satisfaction, and self-blame, as well as avoidance of children and pregnant women.

Treatments for infertility may be experienced by both partners as decreasing the satisfaction and quality of their marital and sexual relationships. These treatments likewise place more physical and psychological weight on the female partner. Operative procedures, such as gamete intrafallopian transfer (GIFT), the higher likelihood of multiple pregnancies, and preparatory hormonal treatments to promote ovarian stimulation, all necessarily fall dispro-portionately on women. Interestingly, Peterson, Newton, and Rosen (2003) point out that congruence or agreement between partners' perceived stress predicted higher levels of marital adjustment. Incongruence in perceived stress was also a risk factor for depression in women, but not men.

Infertility can result in a wide array of psychological symptoms. In addition, historically the literature also discussed psychogenic causes of infertility. Although the focus of the causes of infertility has shifted toward organic (physical) problems in recent years, there has been some renewed attention to the impact of stress management and other psychological interventions. Not only may psychotherapy alleviate the distress caused by infertility, but it also might improve pregnancy rates (Domar et al., 2000). Domar (2004) summarized the recent studies of the effect of distress on the success of in vitro fertilization (IVF): 10 studies support that distress is associated with lower pregnancies, two small studies show trends in this direction, and three show no relationship. In this same article, she points out that one determi-nant of success is the treatment dropout rate, which is also increased when people experience a higher emotional burden. Relatively brief, less intensive, and more cost-effective approaches, such as group therapy one to two times per week over a 3- to 5-week span using cognitive behavioral techniques described by McNaughton-Cassill and colleagues (2000), may be used to decrease stress.

The role of stress on male fertility likewise remains controversial. Lenzi et al. (2003) review that although some studies report decreased semen quality due to stress, others do not. They summarize the psychoanalytical causes of stress-induced male infertility as conflict about the pregnancy and fatherhood, rejection of the male role, suppressed aggression, and fear of the pregnancy. They also point out that males, as well as females, suffer from psychological sequelae caused by the experience of infertility and the evaluation and treatments directed at it. These include feelings of personal and sexual inadequacy, depression, anxiety, guilt, hostility, marital conflict, and sexual dysfunction.

Recognizing and treating these psychological sequelae of infertility capture the larger amount of attention. Although it is important not to ignore the suffering of men experiencing infertility, as noted earlier, the greater psychological and physical burden appears to fall on women. However, Greil, in a 1997 review, contends that this finding of severe psychological distress is more common in descriptive literature than it is in studies of psychological conse-quences. He concludes that studies looking for underlying psychopathology, such as personality disorders, have not found significant differences between fertile and infertile groups. He does report some evidence of differences in depression, anxiety, and self-esteem. Interestingly, in the area of mental adjustment and stress, he notes that although the descriptive literature reports infertility as a great stress for couples, studies actually show high or higher rates of marital satisfaction among infertile couples compared to fertile couples. In earlier interviews of infertile couples, Greil notes many found that infertility brought them closer together. This foreshadows the more recent work of Peterson et al. (2003) in which this congruence between couples' stress and need for parenthood was correlated with marital satisfaction for men and women, and incongruence was related to depression in women but not men. Although shared goals and needs seem to ameliorate infertility-induced stress, some continued discrepancy in the way men and women experience infertility is described in the work of Monga et al. (2004). They confirm the trend in the literature for women to experience poorer quality of well-being and mental adjustment and men to report less satisfaction with intercourse.

Even though there are discrepancies in the literature regarding the frequency and severity of psychological sequelae due to infertility, there is agreement that when individuals and couples do experience symptoms of stress, grief, depression, and anxiety that interfere with function, these problems should be treated. Nonacs and Cohen (1998) recommend supportive, insight-oriented, and cognitive behavioral psychotherapies. Other treatments described are cognitive behavioral therapy groups (Domar et al., 2000; McNaughton-Cassill et al., 2000) and standard support groups (Domar et al., 2000; Stewart, 1992). Given the possible importance of congruence of the couple on infertility-related stress (Peterson et al., 2003), one also suspects that interpersonal therapy for depressive symptoms would be effective, as it is for postpartum depression and depression in general. Finally, for more severe depression and anxiety symptoms, pharmacologic treatment with antidepressants or anxiolytics should be considered. However, as Nonacs and Cohen (1998) note, sexual side effects such as decreased libido, anorgasmia, and delayed ejaculation may occur in 30% to 50% of individuals taking the common antidepressants — SSRIs such as citalopram, fluoxetine, fluvoxamine, paroxetine, and sertraline — and thus may further complicate treatment and evaluation of infertility. Other psychotropic medications including tricyclic antidepressants, monoamine oxidase inhibitors, and antipsychotics may also lead to sexual side effects (Nonacs & Cohen, 1998).

Psychological interventions for infertility-related stress not only provide relief of symptoms of depression and anxiety, but also may have a direct impact on fertility and fertility treatments with an increased pregnancy rate (Domar et al., 2000). Treating the depression and anxiety also decreases the dropout rates from treatment, because the psychological burden is the most common reason for terminating infertility treatment (Domar, 2004).

Reproductive Technologies

As cited in the general discussion of infertility, the evaluation and treatment of infertility has physical and psychological costs. The rise and fall of hope with each treatment cycle, the financial burden, and the difficult decision regarding when to terminate treatment are all stressful for couples. Even successful treatment can frequently bring the additional complication of multiple births, which brings unique decisions and stressors. To begin, a simple summary of common reproductive treatments and technologies follows (Forti & Krausz, 1998; Nonacs & Cohen, 1998):

1. Intrauterine insemination (IUI): sperm are introduced into the uterus through the vagina.
2. In vitro fertilization (IVF) and embryo transfer (ET): ova and sperm are first harvested, then incubated together in culture; after 2 days the embryos (usually two or three) are transferred into the uterus.
3. Gamete intrafallopian transfer (GIFT): unfertilized ova and sperm are placed in the fallopian tube.
4. Zygote intrafallopian transfer (ZIFT): a zygote (a fertilized egg obtained through IVF) is placed in the fallopian tube.
5. Intracytoplasmic sperm injection (ICSI): sperm is directly injected into the cytoplasm of an ovum.

The risk for multiple births with many of these techniques exceeds the incidence in spontaneously conceived pregnancies. All multiple births carry greater risk for preterm labor and delivery and low or very low birth weight resulting in higher infant morbidity and mortality (DiRenzo et al., 2001). Ellison and Hall, in a 2003 study, note that twin rates have increased 55% and multiple births 423% since the 1970s. They also report studies that show not only increased physical risks to mother and babies associated with multiple births, but also increased psychosocial risks associated with IVF itself and multiple births. Reviewing earlier studies, they report that IVF parents were noted to be more emotionally invested or overly involved with children, were less sensitive to adolescent children, perceived their children as more vulnerable, were more child focused, had lower parental self-esteem, and had less sense of maternal competence. On the positive side, IVF parents had increased parental warmth, involvement, and satisfaction with the parental role. Ellison and Hall (2003) note that the literature supports multiple births itself as an independent stressor, as twin births are associated with more maternal depression than close singleton births, and triplet mothers experience high rates of persistent depression. In their study they examined the psychosocial issues related to multiple births. Analyzing the comments of focus groups that included high-risk multiple-birth mothers, low-risk multiple-birth mothers, and singleton mothers, they reported that multiple-birth mothers reported social stigma related to fertility treatments, high rates of pregnancy or neonatal loss (including loss due to selective reduction), varied impacts on marital satisfaction, stresses in dealing with children's health problems (from minor to severe), and an exponential increase in family needs (baby supplies, childcare, shelter). Additionally, these mothers identified magnified parenting stress with the attendant conflict of feeling that they ought not complain about the stress, intensified postnatal depression, and lingering dissatisfaction with some elements of infertility treatments, much of it centering on communication with and information sharing by physicians. Selective reduction came up as a particularly difficult issue, especially for younger women and those with higher religiosity or those who grew up in or desired a larger family. However, selective reduction, like elective abortion, is said for most to have transient effects (Schreiner-Engel et al., 1995). Clinicians need to be aware of the stress and vulnerability that may follow women and couples even after successful treatment of infertility with assisted reproductive technologies.

ABORTION AND SELECTIVE REDUCTION

Although abortion generates heated debates in this country, and many telephone lines and counseling centers exist to ostensibly help women deal with "crisis" pregnancies, there is little evidence that abortion frequently results in serious psychological sequelae. Major et al. (2000), in a study at three sites following women for 2 years, reported that 78% of women were satisfied with their decision at 2 years, and 69% would have the abortion again. Additionally, depression scores were lower postabortion than preabortion. Over 2 years, 20% reported depression after abortion, a rate equal to the national rate of depression for women in this age group. Those at increased risk for depression were those with prior clinical depression, 26% of the sample. Self-esteem postabortion was also higher than preabortion. Posttraumatic stress disorder associated with abortion was experienced by 1% of the women.

Selective reduction, as mentioned in the previous discussion of infertility, is the elective termination of one or more fetuses, usually as a result of multiple pregnancies created by artificial reproductive technologies. This is recommended to decrease the risk to maternal health and life as well as to improve the viability of and decrease the risk to the other fetuses. Selective reduction, like elective abortion, appears to carry little serious long-term psychological sequelae, although women and couples do anecdotally describe some emotional turmoil and conflict at the time of the decision (Ellison & Hall, 2003).

MISCARRIAGE AND STILLBIRTH

Approximately 20% of recognized pregnancies are spontaneously miscarried early in pregnancy (Dell, 2002). Although nearly all couples experience grief, it may be intensified when the pregnancy is planned; when there is a history of infertility, elective abortion, or prior pregnancy loss; when miscarriage occurs without warning or later in pregnancy; when there are no living children; or when problems of social isolation, relationship problems, prior history of depression, and poor coping exist (Brier, 1999). Following a pregnancy loss, the

American College of Obstetricians and Gynecologists (ACOG, 1985) outlines several stages including denial or disbelief, a searching stage in which a reason is sought, acceptance which may be accompanied by disorientation or depression, and finally reorganization. Time to be with a stillborn infant or to view the products of conception, allowing choices regarding obstetrical procedures when possible, and encouraging the use of natural support systems and support groups is recommended (ACOG, 1985). For those more severely affected, psychotherapy and antidepressants should be recommended.

Grief reactions, although most common after miscarriage and stillbirth, may also accompany any obstetrical event that falls short of the woman's and couple's expectations. These include complicated or operative deliveries, children born with congenital defects or disease, and the development of pregnancy-related or chronic disease, such as diabetes or depression during gestation or postpartum (Stotland, 1999). Stotland recommends availability, but not intrusive behavior, on the part of physicians and other health care providers to help parents manage grief reactions. She also encourages the use of other support systems such as family and clergy.

SUMMARY

For women, reproductive health and mental health have a strong alliance. Reproductive problems such as infertility, miscarriage, and stillbirth may produce a continuum of symptoms and distress from normal grief to clinical depression and may also affect the couple's relationship. Additionally, reproductive phases such as premenstrual days and perimenopause bring increased mood or anxiety problems for some women. Pregnancy and the postpartum period are a time of increased risk for some major psychiatric illnesses, especially depression and bipolar disorder. These can represent life-threatening disorders for both mother and child, and need to be identified and treated vigorously. Similarly, psychiatric illnesses present prior to a pregnancy, such as schizophrenia, depression, panic disorder, or OCD, cannot be ignored, or undertreated during the pregnancy if a positive outcome is to be obtained. The overall guiding principle for successful treatment of psychiatric problems that arise in the context of an obstetrical or gynecological problem or event is to address both conditions in an integrated manner. Standard treatment for psychiatric illnesses, albeit with some special considerations such as medication choice during pregnancy, are the mainstay of effective treatment of these disorders even when they occur in the context of an obstetrical or gynecological condition.

CONTRIBUTORS

Ann Morrison, MD, is the director of the Community Psychiatry Division of the Department of Psychiatry at Wright State University, Dayton, Ohio. Her clinical work is primarily with individuals with severe mental disorders and most recently with the homeless mentally ill. She also has special interests in women's mental health and cognitive behaviorial therapy. In 2004 she received the Exemplary Psychiatrist award from the National Alliance for the Mentally Ill (NAMI) for her work in developing a training program in public sector psychiatry. Dr. Morrison may be contacted at Wright State University, Department of Psychiatry, P.O. Box 927, Dayton, OH 45401-0927. E-mail: ann.morrison@wright.edu

Brenda J. B. Roman, MD, is an Associate Professor of Psychiatry at Wright State University School of Medicine in Dayton, Ohio. She serves as Director of Medical Student Education in Psychiatry, and is Director of the Resident Psychotherapy Clinic. Clinical interests include psychotherapy, medical student mental health, and women's issues, as well as serving the homeless mentally ill population. Dr. Roman can be reached at Wright State University School of Medicine, Department of Psychiatry, P.O. Box 927, Dayton, OH 45401-0927. E-mail: brenda.roman@wright.edu

RESOURCES

Ahokas, A., Kaukoranta, J., Wahlbeck, K., & Aito, M. (2001). Estrogen deficiency in severe post-partum depression. *Journal of Clinical Psychiatry, 62*, 332-336.

Alder, C. M., & Baker, J. (1997). Maternal filicide: More than one story be told. *Women and Criminal Justice 2*, 15-39.

Alexander, J. L., Kotz, K., Dennerstein, L., & Davis, S. R. (2003). The systemic nature of sexual functioning in the postmenopausal woman: Crossroads of psychiatry and gynecology. *Primary Psychiatry, 10*(12), 53-57.

Altshuler, L., Cohen, L. S., Szuba, M. P., Burt, V. K., Gitlin, M., & Mintz, J. (1996). Pharmacologic management of psychiatric illness during pregnancy: Dilemmas and guidelines. *American Journal of Psychiatry, 153*, 592-606.

American College of Obstetricians and Gynecologists. (1985). *Grief Related to Perinatal Death* (ACOG Technical Bulletin No 86). Washington, DC: Author.

American Psychiatric Association. (2000). *Diagnostic and Statistical Manual of Mental Disorders* (4th ed. text rev.; Appendix B; pp. 71-74). Washington, DC: Author.

Arnold, A. F., Baugh, C., Fisher, A., Brown, J., & Stowe, Z. N. (2002) Psychiatric aspects of the postpartum period. In S. G. Kornstein & A. H. Clayton (Eds.), *Women's Mental Health, A Comprehensive Textbook* (pp. 91-113). New York: Guilford.

Ayubi-Moak, I., & Parry, B. L. (2002). Psychiatric aspects of menopause. In S. G. Kornstein & A. H. Clayton (Eds.), *Women's Mental Health, A Comprehensive Textbook* (pp. 132-145). New York: Guilford.

Bloch, M., Schmidt, P. J., Danaceau, M., Murphy, J., Nieman, L., & Rubinow, D. R. (2000). Effects of gonadal steroids in women with a history of postpartum depression. *American Journal of Psychiatry 157*, 924-930.

Borenstein, J., Yu, H. T., Wade, S., Chiou, C. F., & Rapkin, A. (2003). The effect of an oral contraceptive containing ethinyl estradiol and drospirenone (Yasmin) on premenstrual symptomatology and health related quality of life. *Journal of Reproductive Medicine, 2*, 79-85.

Brezinka, C., Huter, O., Biebl, W., & Kinzl, J. (1994). Denial of pregnancy: Obstetrical aspects. *Journal of Psychosomatic Obstetrics and Gynecology, 15*, 1-8.

Brier, N. (1999). Understanding and managing the emotional reactions to miscarriage. *Obstetrics and Gynecology, 93*, 151-155.

Caligor, E., & Ormont, M. (1999). Women's health through the reproductive cycle: Premenstrual syndrome, postpartum disorders, and menopause. In R. E. Feinstein & A. A. Brewer (Eds.), *Primary Care Psychiatry and Behavioral Medicine: Brief Office Treatment and Management Pathways*. New York: Springer.

Campbell, S. B., Cohn, J. F., Flanagan, C., Popper, S., & Meyers, T. (1992). Course and correlates of postpartum depression during the transition to parenthood. *Development and Psychopathology, 4*, 29-47.

Chantilis, S. J., & Carr, B. R. (2000). Infertility. In E. J. Quilligan & F. P. Zuspan (Eds), *Current Therapy in Obstetrics and Gynecology* (5th ed., pp. 83-90). Philadelphia: W. B. Saunders.

Chaudron, L. H., & Pies, R. W. (2003). The relationship between postpartum psychosis and bipolar disorder: A review. *Journal of Clinical Psychiatry, 64*(11), 1284-1292.

Cohen, L. S., Friedman, J. M., Jefferson, J. W., Johnson, E. M., & Weiner, M. L. (1994). A re-evaluation of risk of in utero exposure to lithium. *Journal of the American Medical Association, 271*(2), 146-150.

Cohen, L. S., Nonacs, R., & Viguera, A. C. (2004). The pregnant patient. In T. A. Stern, G. L. Fricchione, N. H. Cassem, M. S. Jellinek, & J. F. Rosenbaum (Eds.), *Massachusetts General Hospital Handbook of General Hospital Psychiatry* (5th ed., pp. 593-611). Philadelphia: Mosby, an affiliate of Elsevier.

Crosignani, P. G., & Rubin, B. (1996). The ESHRE Capri Workshop. Guidelines to the prevalence, diagnosis, treatment, and management of infertility. *Human Reproduction, 11*, 1775-1807.

Dell, D. L. (2002). Gynecology. In S. G. Kornstein & A. H. Clayton (Eds.), *Women's Mental Health, A Comprehensive Textbook* (pp. 359-368). New York: Guilford.

DiRenzo, G. C., Luzietti, R., Gerli, S., & Clerici, G. (2001). The ten commandments in multiple pregnancies. *Twin Research, 4*(2), 159-164.

Domar, A. D. (2004). Impact of psychological factors on dropout rates in insured fertility patients. *Fertility and Sterility, 81*(2), 271-273.

Domar, A. D., Clapp, D., Slawsby, E. A., Dusek, J., Kessel, B., & Freizinger, M. (2000). Impact of group psychological interventions on pregnancy rates in infertile women. *Fertility and Sterility, 73*(4), 805-811.

Ellison, M. A., & Hall, J. E. (2003). Social stigma and compounded losses: Quality of life issues for multiple-birth families. *Fertility and Sterility, 80*(2), 405-414.

Forti, G., & Krausz, C. (1998). Clinical review 100. Evaluation and treatment of the infertile couple. *Journal of Clinical Endocrinology and Metabolism, 83*(12), 4177-4188.

Freeman, E. W., Rickels, K., Sondheimer, S. J., Polansky, M., & Xiao, S. (2004) Continuous or intermittent dosing with sertraline for patients with severe premenstrual syndrome or premenstrual dysphoric disorder. *American Journal of Psychiatry, 161*(2), 343-351.

Gregoire, A. J. P., Kumar, R., Everitt, B., Henderson, A. F., & Studd, J. W. (1996). Transdermal oestrogen for treatment of severe postnatal depression. *Lancet, 347*, 930-933.

Greil, A. L. (1997). Infertility and psychological distress: A critical review of the literature. *Social Science and Medicine, 45*(11), 1679-1704.

Hapgood, C. C., Elkind, G. S., & Wright, J. J. (1988). Maternity blues: Phenomena and relationship to later post-partum depression. *Australian and New Zealand Journal of Psychiatry, 22*, 299-306.

Harris, B., Lovett, L., Newcombe, R. G., Read, G. F., Walker, R., & Riah-Fahmy, D. (1994). Maternity blues and major endocrine changes. *British Medical Journal, 308*, 949-953.

Jennings, K. D., Ross, S., Popper, S., & Elmore, M. (1999). Thoughts of harming infants in depressed and non-depressed mothers. *Journal of Affective Disorders, 54*, 21-28.

Kendell, R. E., Chalmers, J. C., & Platz, C. (1987). Epidemiology of puerperal psychosis. *British Journal of Psychiatry, 150*, 662-673.

Kendell, R. E., Rennie, D., Clarke, J. A., & Dean, C. (1981). The social and obstetric correlates of psychiatric admission in the puerperium. *Psychological Medicine, 11*(2), 341-350.

Kendell, R. E., Wainwright, S., Hailey, A., & Shannon, B. (1976). The influence of childbirth on psychiatric morbidity. *Psychological Medicine, 6*(2), 297-302.

Kennerley, H., & Gath, D. (1989). Maternity blues: Associations with obstetric, psychological and psychiatric factors. *British Journal of Psychiatry, 155*, 367-373.

Khine, K., Luff, J. A., Rubinow, D. R., & Schmidt, P. J. (2003). The perimenopause and mood disorders. *Primary Psychiatry, 10*(12), 41, 44-47.

Knopps, G. G. (1993). Postpartum mood disorders: A startling contrast to the joy of birth. *Postgraduate Medicine, 93*, 103-116.

Kraeplin, E. (1921). *Manic-Depressive Insanity and Paranoia*. Edinburgh: E & S Livingstone.

Lam, R. W., Carter, D., Misri, S., Kuan, A. J., Yatham, L. N., & Zis, A. P. (1999). A controlled study of light therapy in women with late luteal phase dysphoric disorder. *Psychiatry Research, 86*, 185-192.

Lenzi, A., Lombardo, F., Salacone, P., Gandini, L., & Jannini, E. A. (2003). Stress, sexual dysfunctions, and male infertility. *Journal of Endocrinology Investigation, 26*(Suppl. to No. 3), 72-76.

Major, B., Cozzarelli, C., Cooper, M. L., Zubek, J., Richards, C., Wilhite, M., & Gramzow, R. H. (2000). Psychological responses of women after first trimester abortion. *Archives of General Psychiatry, 57*, 777-786.

McNaughton-Cassill, M. E., Bostwick, M., Vanscoy, S. E., Arthur, N. J., Hickman, T. N., Robinson, R. D., & Neal, G. S. (2000). Development of brief stress management support groups for couples undergoing in vitro fertilization treatment. *Fertility and Sterility, 74*(1), 87-93.

Miller, L. J. (1994). Use of electroconvulsive therapy during pregnancy. *Hospital and Community Psychiatry, 45*, 444-450.

Miller, L. J. (1998). Pharmacotherapy during the perinatal period. *Directions in Psychiatry, 18*, 49-63.

Miller, L. J. (2002). Post-partum depression. *Journal of the American Medical Association, 287*(6), 762-765.

Misri, S., & Kostaras, X. (2002). Postpartum depression: Is there an Andrea Yates in your practice? *Current Psychiatry, 1*(5), 23-29.

Monga, M., Alexandrescu, B., Katz, S. E., Stein, M., & Ganiats, T. (2004). Impact of infertility on quality of life, marital adjustment, and sexual function. *Urology, 63*(1), 126-130.

Neziroglu, F., Anemone, R., & Yaryura-Tobias, J. A. (1992). Onset of obsessive compulsive disorder in pregnancy. *American Journal of Psychiatry, 149*, 947-950.

Nonacs, R., & Cohen, L. S. (1998). Approach to the patient with infertility. In T. A. Stern, J. B. Herman, & P. L. Slavin (Eds.), *The MGH Guide to Psychiatry in Primary Care* (pp. 281-295). New York: McGraw-Hill.

Nonacs, R., & Cohen, L. S. (2002). Depression during pregnancy: Diagnosis and treatment options. *Journal of Clinical Psychiatry, 63*(Suppl. 7), 24-30.

Nonacs, R., Viguera, A. C., & Cohen, L. S. (2002). Psychiatric aspects of pregnancy. In S. G. Kornstein & A. H. Clayton (Eds.), *Women's Mental Health, A Comprehensive Textbook* (pp. 70-90). New York: Guilford.

O'Hara, M. W. (1991). Post-partum mental disorders. In N. Droegemueller & J. Sciarra (Eds.), *Gynecology and Obstetrics* (Vol. 6, pp. 1-13). Philadelphia: Lippincott.

O'Hara, M. W., Schlechte, J. A., Lewis, D. A., & Varner, M. W. (1991a). Controlled prospective study of post-partum mood disorders. *Journal of Abnormal Psychology, 100*, 63-73.

O'Hara, M. W., Schlechte, J. A., Lewis, D. A., & Wright, E. J. (1991b). Prospective study of postpartum blues: Biologic and psychosocial factors. *Archives of General Psychiatry, 48*, 801-806.

O'Hara, M. W., Stuart, S., Gorman, L. L., & Wenzel, A. (2000). Efficacy of interpersonal psychotherapy for post-partum depression. *Archives of General Psychiatry, 57*, 1039-1045.

Omtzigt, J. G., Los, F. J., Grobbee, D. E., Pijpers, L., Jahoda, M. J., Brandenburg, H., Stewart, P. A., Gaillard, H. L., Sachs, E. S., & Wladimiroff, J. W. (1992). The risk of spina bifida aperta after first trimester exposure to valproate in a prenatal cohort. *Neurology, 42*(Suppl. 5), 119-125.

Parry, B. L., Mahan, A. M., Mostofi, N., Klauber, M. R., Lew, G. S., & Gillin, J. C. (1993). Light therapy of late luteal phase dysphoric disorder: An extended study. *American Journal of Psychiatry, 150*, 1417-1419.

Peterson, B. D., Newton, C. R., & Rosen, K. H. (2003). Examining congruence between partners' perceived infertility-related stress and its relationships to marital adjustment and depression in infertile couples. *Family Process, 42*(1), 59-70.

Rapkin, A. J., Mikacich, J. A., & Moatakef-Imani, B. (2003). Reproductive mood disorders. *Primary Psychiatry, 10*(12), 31-40.

Resnick, P. J. (1969). Child murder by parents: A psychiatric review of filicide. *American Journal of Psychiatry, 126*(9), 325-334.

Robert, E., & Guibaud, P. (1982). Maternal valproic acid and congenital neural tube defects. *Lancet, ii*(8304), 937.

Rosa, F. W. (1991). Spina bifida in infants of women treated with carbamazepine during pregnancy. *New England Journal of Medicine, 324*, 674-677.

Schreiner-Engel, P., Walther, V. N., Mindes, J., Lynch, L., & Berkowitz, R. (1995). First trimester multifetal pregnancy reduction: Acute and persistent psychologic reactions. *American Journal of Obstetrics and Gynecology, 172,* 541-547.

Soares, C. N., Cohen, L. S., Otto, M. W., & Harlow, B. L. (2001). Characteristics of women with premenstrual dysphoric disorder (PMDD) who did or did not report history of depression: A preliminary report from the Harvard Study of Moods and Cycles. *Journal of Women's Health and Gender-Based Medicine, 10,* 873-878.

Spinelli, M. G. (1998). Psychiatric disorders during pregnancy and postpartum. *Journal of the American Medical Women's Association, 53*(4), 165-169, 186.

Steinberg, S., Annable, L., Young, S. N., & Liyanage, W. (1999). A placebo-controlled clinical trial of L-tryptophan in premenstrual dysphoria. *Biological Psychiatry, 45,* 313-320.

Steiner, M. (1990). Post-partum psychiatric disorders. *Canadian Journal of Psychiatry, 35,* 89-95.

Steiner, M., & Born, L. (2002) Psychiatric aspects of the menstrual cycle. In S. G. Kornstein & A. H. Clayton (Eds.), *Women's Mental Health, A Comprehensive Textbook* (pp. 48-69). New York: Guilford.

Steiner, M., & Tam, W. Y. K. (1999). Post-partum depression in relation to other psychiatric disorders. In L. J. Miller (Ed.), *Post-Partum Psychiatric Disorders* (pp. 47-63). Washington, DC: American Psychiatric Press.

Stewart, D. E. (1992). A prospective study of the effectiveness of brief professionally led infertility support groups. In K. Wijma & B. von Schoultz (Eds.), *Reproductive Life: Advances in Research in Psychosomatic Obstetrics and Gynecology* (pp. 151-165). Park Ridge, NJ: Parthenon Publishers.

Stotland, N. L. (1999). Obstetrics and gynecology. In J. R. Rundell & M. G. Wise (Eds.), *Essentials of Consultation — Liaison Psychiatry* (pp. 383-397). Washington, DC: American Psychiatric Press.

Thurtle, V. (1995). Post-natal depression: The relevance of sociological approaches. *Journal of Advanced Nursing, 22*(3), 416-424.

Troutman, B., & Cutrona, C. (1990). Non-psychotic post-partum depression among adolescent mothers. *Journal of Abnormal Psychology, 99,* 69.

Viguera, A. C., Nonacs, R., Cohen, L. S., Tondo, L., Murray, A., & Baldessarini, R. J. (2000). Risk of recurrence of bipolar disorder in pregnant and non-pregnant women after discontinuing lithium maintenance. *American Journal of Psychiatry, 157*(2), 179-184.

Weissman, M. M., Leaf, P. J., Tischler, G. L., Blazer, D. G., Karno, M., Livingston, B. M., & Florio, L. P. (1988). Affective disorders in five United States communities. *Psychological Medicine, 18,* 141-153.

Wisner, K. L., Parry, B. L., & Piontek, C. M. (2002). Clinical practice. Postpartum depression. *New England Journal of Medicine, 347*(3), 194-199.

Zuckerman, B., Amaro, H., Bauchner, H., & Cabral, H. (1989). Depressive symptoms during pregnancy: Relationship to poor health behaviors. *American Journal of Obstetrics and Gynecology, 160*(5, Pt. 1), 1107-1111.

Psychosocial Manifestations Of Organ Failure and Transplantation

Jerome J. Schulte, Jr.

The world's first heart transplant was performed on December 3, 1967, by Professor Christian Barnard on Louis Washkansky. Although the surgery was successful, Mr. Washkansky died 18 days later from an overwhelming infection due to a suppressed immune system secondary to the powerful medications necessary to stop his body's immune system from rejecting his new heart. Heart, liver, and renal transplantation would have stopped there if not for the development of medications, like cyclosporine in 1983 (Sangstat, 2004), which could stop rejection without causing the body to be as susceptible to overwhelming infection. Even with these advances in antirejection treatment, the specter of death from organ rejection or infection looms large and continuously in the minds of organ transplant recipients.

In spite of these hazards, the chance of organ transplantation gives hope. Hope not only of life, but of a fulfilling, normal, and productive life. Stories like that of Kelly Perkins, a 42 year old who suffered a viral syndrome that destroyed her heart, received a transplant, and scaled the 14,686-ft peak of the Matterhorn, is an inspiration to all and gives hope for an exceptional life to those awaiting transplantation (Associated Press, 2003).

The success of transplantation has created its own set of issues and concerns. The largest problem is a demand for transplantation that well outstrips the supply of transplantable donor organs. As of December 31, 2003, there were 82,884 patients, nationally, awaiting transplantation. Of the 25,455 transplants performed in 2003, 18,649 were from cadaveric donors and 6,806 from living donors. Over 6,000 patients died while waiting for transplantation in 2003 (Ustransplant.org, 2004b). Because demand is greater than supply, decisions must be made on prioritizing and rationing donor organs. Ethical and legislative decision making has had a large influence in determining who receives organs, and this decision-making process is constantly being refined.

Between the time of being diagnosed with organ failure and the time of relative safety from organ rejection (3 years after transplantation), patients experience the vicissitudes of the organ transplantation process. Each stage of the process—diagnosis, assessment for transplantation, acceptance for transplantation and being placed on a waiting list for an organ, transplantation, postoperative recovery, and postsurgical follow up—has its own trials and tribulations, and periods of hope and despair. This contribution will examine the psychosocial experience of patients undergoing organ failure and transplantation.

ORGAN FAILURE

As organs fail, besides feeling quite ill, the patient undergoes significant psychosocial changes. Common to all types of organ failure is decline in functional status and change in role functioning (Surman & Prager, 2004). A patient's occupation must often be abandoned because of insufficient energy to meet occupational demands and also because of the time requirement to maintain health. Family functioning may suffer not only because of time spent on health concerns instead of with the family, but because of changes in family roles. Not only does the patient have less time and energy to be a parent and spouse, but there is a shift from the family member being a support supplier to the one who needs support. Overshadowing the family is the real chance of death in the foreseeable future. These predisposing factors increase the risk for adjustment disorders, depression, and anxiety. These issues have specific implications for each of the prototypical types of organ failure: renal failure, heart failure, and liver failure.

CHARACTERISTICS OF SPECIFIC TYPES OF ORGAN FAILURE

Renal Failure

The most common causes of renal failure are hypertension, diabetes mellitus, or collagen vascular diseases (such as systemic lupus erythematosus). Renal failure stands out as different from other organ failures in that patients with renal failure may live for years by using dialysis to supply artificial kidney function. Dialysis is time-consuming, with patients spending 12 hours a week, spread over three sessions, being dialyzed. After dialysis, patients often experience nausea and dizziness. Also, dialysis patients must strictly follow a special renal diet. These all-consuming stressors, coupled with the loss of autonomy, can lead to depression. Depression in patients on dialysis is associated with an increase in mortality (Kimmel, Weihs, & Peterson, 1993). Uremia (a metabolic disturbance associated with renal failure with symptoms of nausea, vomiting, fatigue, anorexia, weight loss, muscle cramps, severe itching, and cognitive impairment) can be an organic cause of depression and also causes delirium. In the presence of uremia, dialysis should be performed.

Treatment of depression, anxiety, and cognitive impairment in renal failure necessitates careful dosing of psychiatric medications that are eliminated by the kidneys (Cohen et al., 2004). Supportive psychotherapy and cognitive therapy can be helpful in the treatment of depressive and anxiety symptoms. Needle phobia can be quite problematic for the renal failure patient, with the necessity of insertion of a large-bore needle three times a week to provide dialysis. Hypnosis and behavioral interventions can be quite helpful here (Fernandes, 2003; Surman & Tolkoff-Rubin, 1984).

Another area where psychiatric or psychological assessment may be needed is in the determination of dialysis treatment termination. Patients who are unable to receive a transplanted kidney may decide that the quality of their life is unacceptably poor and they wish to end dialysis. Assessment for depression and these patients' capacity for informed medical decision making must be performed prior to ending dialysis (Hirsch, 1989; Neu & Kjellstrand, 1986). Often a trial of antidepressant medication is performed before dialysis is terminated if the patient suffers from depression.

Heart Failure

Heart failure is the decreased ability of the heart to adequately pump blood to other organs in the body, thereby depriving them of needed oxygen. Unlike renal failure, where there is at least some independence, in end-stage heart failure, functioning is so impaired that patients often need to be hospitalized in an Intensive Care Unit (ICU) to stay alive while awaiting an available heart. ICU care allows for intravenous medication to stimulate the heart as well as electrical monitoring of the heart to prevent and treat lethal arrhythmias (abnormal heart electrical stimulation). Symptoms of severe heart failure result from a body organ not receiving enough oxygen. For example, chest pain occurs when the heart itself has insufficient oxygen to maintain its pumping action. Muscle pain occurs when skeletal muscles being used are deprived of oxygen. Cognition is impaired when the brain lacks sufficient oxygen. To compensate for the lack of oxygen, shortness of breath develops, triggering an increased respiratory rate in an attempt to increase oxygen flow. Generalized hypoxia causes chronic fatigue and weakness. Common causes of heart failure are myocardial infarction (heart attack with death of heart muscle) secondary to coronary artery disease (blockage in the arteries that supply blood to the heart) and cardiomyopathy (disease of the heart muscle).

Liver Failure

The liver is involved in storing and releasing sugar when we need it, detoxifying drugs and ammonia, making important proteins, making clotting factors to prevent bleeding, and aiding in the absorption of certain vitamins and storing iron. Initial symptoms of liver failure such as fatigue, loss of appetite, nausea, and diarrhea are common to many different medical complaints and therefore do not help much in early diagnosis. Symptoms of serious liver failure (when 80% of the liver has been affected) are jaundice, bleeding problems, a swollen abdomen, confusion, and sleepiness that may progress to coma.

Liver failure is the result of acute or chronic causes. The most common acute cause of liver failure is intentional acetaminophen (Tylenol) overdose. Other causes are hepatitis virus, medication-induced liver inflammation, and ingesting mushrooms that are toxic to the liver. Treatment of acute liver failure is aimed at preserving as much healthy liver as possible. If identified early, acetaminophen overdose can be treated easily, but if the patient delays coming for treatment there is no cure for the liver failure except transplantation. If caught early, viral hepatitis can be treated with supportive care as the virus runs its course. In these cases the liver may recover on its own. The most common causes of chronic liver failure in the United States are related to excessive alcohol consumption: alcoholic cirrhosis and alcoholic hepatitis. Other chronic causes of liver failure include hepatitis B and C, malnutrition, and hemochromatosis (an illness that causes the body to absorb too much iron, which is deposited in the liver).

Beyond an often slow and painful death, patients with liver failure secondary to acetaminophen overdose often think they are ingesting a benign substance only to find out they may really die. Because of the self-inflicted nature of their condition, the staff caring for these patients often experience significant countertransference feelings toward them, especially if they are moved to the top of a transplant list ahead of patients that have been waiting longer.

Depression is common in liver failure (Collis & Loyd, 1992). This may be directly due to liver failure, the unmasking of a mood disorder that had been masked by alcoholism, or due to medication side effects. For example, medications like alpha-interferon, which is used to treat viral hepatitis, have a high rate of causing depression (Lerner, Stoudemire, & Rosenstein, 1999).

THE PROCESS OF ORGAN TRANSPLANTATION AND THE PSYCHOSOCIAL MANIFESTATIONS OF TRANSPLANTATION

The Concept of Team Evaluation

Patients with end-stage organ failure are referred for transplant by their primary physician, usually a specialist in the failed organ. They are then evaluated by different members of the transplant team who eventually meet and discuss together whether to select the patient for transplant. The team involves specialists in transplant medicine: surgeons, medical specialists, nurse transplant coordinators, and mental health professionals. Each has his or her own job to do. The surgeon performs the actual transplantation surgery, and importantly is the leader of the transplantation team. The medical specialist is responsible for the medical management of the patient postoperatively and will assess the new organ's functioning, as well as monitor for infection and organ rejection. These specialists also serve as gatekeepers into the formal assessment process by performing a screening medical evaluation that determines when the full transplantation assessment will take place (Skotzko & Strouse, 2002).

Nursing coordinators then guide the patient through the formal selection process. They get to know patients quite well and are the patient's point of contact with the selection team members. Because of this, they often provide much supportive care to the patient and family during this very stressful process. They also provide much of the initial screening of the patient by obtaining basic medical and family information from the patient. The nurse coordinator also has an important educational role, teaching the patient and the family information about the transplant process and at the same time gathering information about the patient's and family's motivation for transplantation (Skotzko & Strouse, 2002).

Social workers, and less often psychiatrists and psychologists, provide the mental health assessment in the majority of programs (Levenson & Olbrisch, 1993). Assessments evaluate the following areas: psychiatric history, history of compliance with medical treatment, substance use history and current status, current mental status, social history and availability of support, family social and mental health history, perceived heath, coping style, and quality of life (Dew et al., 2000).

EVALUATION OF THE PATIENT

Evaluation/Selection of the Patient for Transplantation

Because more patients need organs than there are organs for transplantation, selection criteria are needed for patients needing transplantation. Over the past 15 years there has developed a fairly well-accepted prioritization of patients on transplant program wait lists. In general, the sickest patients and those with grave limitations in functional capacity, as well as those who have waited the longest, are highest on the list. There is much less consensus, however, regarding who should actually be placed on the list. Selection criteria for transplantation are usually exclusionary, thereby eliminating patients who medically cannot tolerate transplantation or because of psychosocial factors are unable to care for the organ after transplantation. Psychosocial factors associated with poor transplant outcome are poor social support, psychiatric disorders that could compromise postoperative compliance, alcohol and substance abuse, a past history of poor compliance with medical treatment, and maladaptive personality traits (Levenson & Olbrisch, 2000). Transplant programs each establish their own selection criteria, although criteria are also influenced by insurers and Medicare. In general, psychosocial selection criteria are based on an evaluation of how well patients will cope with surgery, an evaluation of premorbid psychiatric illness or substance dependence that would interfere with compliance, determination of whether the patient is capable of informed consent, and determination as to whether the patient can maintain a long-term relationship with the transplant team to help ensure compliance (Levenson & Olbrisch, 2000).

There is agreement among different transplant programs on certain psychosocial criteria. Because of the risk of noncompliance with antirejection medications, all programs, including those for heart, liver, and kidney transplantation, see current abuse of addictive drugs as disqualifying a patient for acceptance on the transplant list (Levenson & Olbrisch, 1993). Also, all programs agree that excessive caffeine use should have no bearing on whether a patient is accepted for transplantation. Beyond these, there is disagreement on criteria, with heart transplant programs being more restrictive and kidney transplant programs being less restrictive. Ninety percent of heart transplant programs see active schizophrenia as an absolute contraindication for transplantation as do 67% of liver and 72% of renal programs (Levenson & Olbrisch, 1993). Controlled schizophrenia is an absolute contraindication in a third of cardiac transplant programs, 15% of liver, and 6% of renal programs. A recent suicide attempt is an absolute contraindication in 51% of cardiac transplant programs, 17% of liver, and 28% of renal programs. The lower rate in liver programs is because Tylenol overdose commonly is the cause of liver failure and necessitates transplantation. There is even disagreement on how long an alcoholic needs to be abstinent prior to qualifying to be on the wait list for transplantation. Historically, 6 months of abstinence has been required, and for most programs this still is the standard. For the Ohio Solid Organ Transplantation Consortium, 3 months of abstinence is the standard (Ohio Solid Organ Transplantation Consortium, 2004). Other authors cite literature that shows conflicting results as to whether pretransplant abstinence predicts posttransplant abstinence (Bravata et al., 2001). Some advocate a case-by-case evaluation instead of a strict monthly abstinence-based criterion.

Evaluation of Living Donors

Living donors may wish to donate a kidney or part of their liver to someone in need of transplantation. Donors can live a normal life with just one kidney, and when part of a liver is donated, parts tend to regenerate in both recipient and donor. Because there is less chance of rejection from an organ donated by a relative, these are often the preferred organs for transplant. Harvesting organs from donors is not without risk. There is the usual pain and risk associated with any major surgery, and appropriate presurgical assessment should be performed. The evaluator should also consider the following factors in assessing potential organ donors: the potential for coercion, an implied obligation of the recipient to the donor, the potential belief by the donor that family or interpersonal problems will be "healed" by donating the organ, donor psychopathology that can be exacerbated by the stress of the donation, and ability of the donor to fully understand the consequences to themselves of organ donation (Skotzko & Strouse, 2002).

The Selection Committee

Most transplant programs meet regularly to decide who will be accepted for transplantation. Patients are presented with the indications for transplant, the medical and surgical risks, and the psychosocial assessment including the selection decision reached by the team (Skotzko & Strouse, 2002). At Massachusetts General Hospital a working committee developed selection criteria. This group found that the core requirement for selection is that the patient could be medically managed following transplantation (Surman & Prager, 2004). The mental health practitioner on the selection committee should understand the impact of personality style, decision-making power, countertransference, and group dynamics so that he or she can facilitate the group process when problems occur (Skotzko & Strouse, 2002).

The Selection Decision

After the long and involved selection assessment, the patient must await the decision of the selection committee. During this period of anxious anticipation, patients know that their death or survival depends upon being accepted for transplantation. The family, who has experienced this with the transplant candidate, often mirrors the feelings. If the patient is rejected by the selection committee, both must process the loss of hope for a new life and the anticipation of death and dying. If, on the contrary, the patient is accepted for transplantation, the patient and family all expect improvement in the transplant candidate's situation (Kuhn, Myers, & Davis, 1988a), but usually face the opposite because the patient often deteriorates while awaiting transplantation.

WAITING FOR TRANSPLANTATION

Patients may wait months for transplantation. As they wait, organ failure worsens, role functioning changes, and functioning declines, often requiring ICU admission for extended periods of time. Their quality of life worsens and medical costs increase dramatically. Beyond functional decline and role loss is the issue of separation from family by the necessary ICU stay. There is often anxiety due to fear that the transplant may not take place in time or that there will be organ rejection once the transplant does occur. A sense that time is running out often results in anger and frustration, while at the same time there is a morbid preoccupation that someone must die in order for the patient to live (Vlay et al., 1989). Supportive psychotherapy can be very helpful for these waiting patients, restoring a sense of hope as well as combating loneliness. Countertransference issues (J. Kay & R. Kay, 2003; Surman & Prager, 2004) can be quite intense during psychotherapy with the realization that the therapist is building a relationship with someone who may be dead tomorrow, as is illustrated in the following case:

> Dr. J was treating a 30-year-old depressed cardiac transplant patient in brief psychotherapy. The onset of the patient's depression coincided with clinical evidence that his new heart was being rejected. The patient's course deteriorated rapidly, and he was hospitalized. Dr. J continued to see the patient as he awaited the highly unlikely possibility of a new donor. After each of the sessions, Dr. J noted that he was exceptionally tired. On the way to his session with the patient that occurred on Christmas Eve, Dr. J stopped at the nursing station and prepared a plate of Christmas cookies for the patient, something he had never done for a patient regardless of the treatment setting. (J. Kay & R. Kay, 2003, p. 1702)

As cardiovascular status continues to decline, confusion and disorientation may develop secondary to decreased cerebral profusion or medication side effects. It is difficult to perform psychotherapy in this situation, and this syndrome is difficult to treat medically. It greatly disturbs therapists and family members as they sense the patient is slipping away. During the wait for transplant, one of every four patients dies. Surman and Prager (2004) identify preoperative psychotherapeutic issues for wait listed patients as: hope versus loss, preparation for living versus dying, the stress of "false starts," survivor guilt, and consideration of depression and anxiety due to the preceding problems. Patients hope for renewed life when selected for transplantation, but they experience loss as well, losing function and autonomy while trying to maintain hope in the face of ongoing deterioration. As patients wait, they prepare for conflicting outcomes: life with transplantation or death if the transplant does not occur in time. False starts are frequent. Patients often feel they need to remain at home near the phone or at least near the hospital so they can be there at a "moment's notice" if an organ becomes available. Many fear "missing the call" (Skotzko & Strouse, 2002) after waiting months for an organ. There is reality to this fear. Patients must be within hours of their transplant center in order to receive an organ when it is procured. The reason for this has to do with the concept of cold ischemia time. This is a time interval that begins when an organ is cooled with a cold perfusion solution after organ procurement surgery and ends when the organ is implanted (Ustransplant.org, 2004a). Times vary per organ: 90% of hearts are transplanted within 4½ hours, 90% of livers within 12 hours, and 90% of kidneys within 27 hours (Ustransplant.org, 2004a).

False starts are common; many times patients receive a call and rush to the hospital, only to find out that an organ did not become available or went to someone else. One case was noted where the patient actually went under anesthesia, only to find out upon awakening that the donor organ was inadequate for transplantation. That patient died before receiving transplantation (Surman & Prager, 2004). The progression of illness with its effect on other organ systems may make the patient, who has waited for months, now ineligible for transplantation. This "death sentence" has a devastating effect on the patient, the family, the treatment team, and other patients awaiting transplant (Skotzko & Strouse, 2002). Patients also experience guilt as they wait for a transplant when they consider that someone else must die in order for them to live. They often become preoccupied with the news, looking for tragic outcomes of others (Weems & Patterson, 1989). They also grieve the loss of other organ failure patients, whom they have gotten to know during their lengthy hospitalizations.

Frustration and demoralization associated with waiting can lead to depression, anxiety, and regression. As patients linger on the wait list hoping for an organ, they tend to become dysphoric with the continuing loss of function and mounting fear of approaching death. In particular, patients with cardiac disease are at increased risk of depression (Robinson & Levenson, 2004). When they get the phone call that an organ has been procured, they often react with anxiety (Surman & Prager, 2004). There are many causes for anxiety, including their prior experience with false starts and the realization that "This is it"; once their heart is taken, there is no turning back. Under this kind of stress, regression, especially in patients with premorbid personality issues, may result in problematic behavior (Kuhn, Davis, & Lippmann, 1988b; Phipps, 1991).

During this time of waiting, social support is very important for patients and their families to combat depression and anxiety and to prevent regression. This support can come from nonmental health professionals belonging to the treatment team and from support groups or from psychotherapeutic intervention from treatment team social workers, psychologists, or consult psychiatrists (Suszycki, 1986). Specific symptoms of anxiety or dysphoria may be treated with behavioral interventions and relaxation techniques (Skotzko & Strouse, 2002). Pharmacotherapy can also be extremely helpful. In general, medications must not worsen the already present end-organ failure. Short-acting benzodiazepines with inactive metabolites such as lorazepam or oxazepam are preferred for the treatment of anxiety (Robinson & Levenson, 2004). Selective serotonin reuptake inhibitors (SSRIs) are safe in patients with cardiac disease, as are tricyclic antidepressants (TCAs) (J. Kay et al., 1991), but they take weeks to work. Psychostimulants such as methylphenidate are safe and can relieve depression quickly (Robinson & Levenson, 2004).

THE TRANSPLANT SURGERY AND THE IMMEDIATE POSTOPERATIVE PERIOD

Transplant surgery is stressful for patients knowing, as they are being wheeled in for the surgery, that "This is it." Hope of this being the beginning of a new life is experienced at the same time as the fear of "dying on the table." The families of patients must wait for news of success or failure. The first milestone after surgery is extubation, which generally happens 1 to 2 days after surgery and allows the patient to communicate again with family and medical providers. Family expectations for a speedy recovery are often confronted by postoperative problems. Common postoperative problems are delirium (confusion and disorientation, with the patient appearing agitated or depressed), infection, bleeding, metabolic disturbances, reactions to medication, and new organ dysfunction. All of these may cause confusion in a patient already debilitated by months of organ failure. Once delirium clears, the patient and the family are often confronted by organ rejection and infection.

Fighting Postoperative
Rejection and Infection

Rejection, the patient's body recognizing that the new organ is different from the body and trying to kill it, is common posttransplant and has historically been, along with infection, the major cause of death in transplant patients. Up to nine different medications may be used to fight rejection. Side effects of these medications are dose dependent, so the goal of treatment is to use the lowest dose that will prevent rejection. Cyclosporine, the backbone of antirejection treatment, has the following dose dependent side effects: seizure, delirium, anxiety, tremor, dysarthria (speech and articulation problems), visual hallucinations, blindness, numbness and tingling sensations, unbalanced gait, coma, paralysis, and a sense of internal restlessness (Robinson & Levenson, 2004). Physicians carefully monitor laboratory tests and take biopsies of the new organ to monitor for rejection. When rejection does occur, larger doses of antirejection medications are used, and the number of medications used is increased. This increases the likelihood of side effects.

Rejection is a common occurrence in transplantation and is one of the most feared events by patients. Patients are vigorously educated on the signs and symptoms of rejection so they can report problems quickly to their doctors. Also, they have frequent routine follow-up, so rejection can be identified at the earliest possible stage. However, in the newly transplanted patient the news of rejection is often met by the patient and the family with fear and denial. "We have come so far, how can this happen now?" The patient fears rejection progressing to damaging or even killing the new organ. If rejection progresses to killing the new organ, there will be need for retransplantation. Fear of rejection may lead to panic level anxiety and depressed mood in the patient and the family. There is also knowledge that the result of fighting rejection by increasing the strength and numbers of antirejection drugs may lead to compromising the immune system too much, leading to infection. Patients understand that infection can kill them also. The realization that there is this delicate balance between rejection and infection can be difficult for patients to tolerate.

Other Medical Complications
During the Postoperative Period

Besides rejection and infection, many other complications may occur postoperatively. Graft failure and vascular occlusion may occur, which often necessitates retransplantation. Emergent retransplantation has poor results and usually is not performed (Skotzko & Strouse, 2002). The sadness, grief, and let-down for patients and family is profound in those circumstances where the new organ fails. Now patient and family must prepare for death. Sometimes the failure of the new organ may be slow enough to find a new organ and prepare the patient for retransplantation. Reexperiencing the vicissitudes of the past months in a compressed time period because of the renewed need for transplantation with the specter of death hanging over the patient and family can be traumatizing. In this setting the patient may decline retransplantation; this decision is usually supported unless a treatable depressive or anxiety syndrome is present (Skotzko & Strouse, 2002). Psychotherapeutic intervention is also often necessary and effective as seen in the following clinical case (J. Kay, 2001, p. 7):

Mr. C was a 28-year-old married father who had undergone liver transplantation. Eight months postoperatively he began to reject his new liver, was hospitalized, and became severely depressed. His depression was marked by crying spells, anhedonia, sleeplessness, suicidal ideation, and pervasive hopelessness. At the transplant surgeon's request, the psychiatrist visited the patient in the hospital and found him to be despondent, tearful, and hopeless. He was difficult to engage, spoke very softly, and avoided nearly all eye contact. His surgeon had informed him that he would undoubtedly require a second transplant, but the patient adamantly refused another operation. Given his difficulty in speaking to the psychiatrist, it was decided (with the patient's consent) first to initiate antidepressant therapy, then to explore the basis of his refusal of further surgery. Within 2 weeks Mr. C's depression began to lift; however, his surgeon was becoming increasingly irritated with him because of his continued refusal to undergo retransplantation.

In an attempt to obtain a better understanding of the patient's position, the psychiatrist saw the patient daily. Although the patient denied any fear of dying under surgery, he was able to recall a highly traumatic incident that occurred when he was 16, at which time he nearly drowned while swimming in a rock quarry. When the psychiatrist asked what was the most frightening aspect of the event, the patient described intense panic when he had swallowed large amounts of water and was unable to breathe. When questioned about the possible relationship between this event and his position on retransplantation, Mr. C shared that the most terrifying aspect of the first transplant operation had been his inability to breathe postoperatively because of the numerous tubes in his mouth and nose. Psychoanalytically oriented focal psychotherapy allowed the patient to understand his resistance and to agree to a second operation—providing that his surgeon was aware of and sensitive to his concern.

Transplant Team Stress

The transplant team develops an emotionally strong long-term relationship with patients and their families. They understand the patient's medical history and what the patient has been through in the course of the illness and the transplant process. The team also has an intimate knowledge of the patient's psychosocial make-up. As the transplant team becomes important to the patient and family for support through the organ transplant process, the reverse also occurs: The patient becomes important to the transplant team.

Because of the attachment of the treatment team, when a patient they know well dies, there is often bereavement. The team as a whole is often saddened, and the nursing staff who worked closest with the patient is most affected. When this happens repeatedly it can lead to staff burnout. It is helpful to facilitate mourning by using memorial services or use of the chaplain service (Skotzko & Strouse, 2002). Mental health providers to transplant patients are also at risk for dysphoria when a patient dies because they often have very close relationships to the patients they have seen for supportive therapy. The loss of hope that was expected from the transplantation may increase the sense of loss.

The circumstances of the patient's death, or even if a patient the staff knows well is doing poorly, can be profoundly stressful for the transplant staff. Transplant patient care, especially postoperative care, is complicated, potentially involving multiple organ systems at once, is very fast paced, and requires close monitoring for evidence of rejection, infection, or other postoperative problems. Over time, this may become overwhelming for nursing staff, especially if a mistake costs someone's life.

Nursing coordinators are particularly vulnerable to stress and burnout, because they have the closest relationship with the patients and their families. They are the providers who initially contact patients for evaluation, walk them through the process, and monitor their follow-up. They are the information source about the process and its complications for patients and families (Skotzko & Strouse, 2002). Throughout this process a strong and supportive relationship develops. Also, they may be the bearer of "bad" news to patients about laboratory tests or biopsies. As with other team members, but more so because of their close relationship with patients, nurse coordinators suffer grief and loss when patients die.

RESUMING LIFE

Predischarge

The task of the predischarge period is to educate patients on caring for their new organ. This involves understanding the new complex medication regimen they will have to take for the rest of their life. They need to understand the real risk of rejection, the need to take medications to prevent rejection, the side effects of the medications, and the necessity of keeping records of their medication use so that the treatment team can monitor their clinical status. Instruction and training must be given to the family for any intravenous forms of medication that will be given at home (Skotzko & Strouse, 2002). Education about rejection and infection may be experienced as intense and may trigger anxiety in patients that have already been through a significantly stressful emotional time with transplantation (Surman & Prager, 2004). Denial of the risk of rejection may appear.

Discharge and Resuming Life

Anxiety may also occur as discharge approaches; the adjustment to postdischarge life may be problematic (Freeman et al., 1988a, 1988b; Surman et al., 1987). The patient has been dependent on the transplant team for months, and adjustment to caring for oneself and the new organ may feel overwhelming. Adding to the stress is not only the thought of the risk of rejection or infection, but feeling overwhelmed by having to monitor and adhere to a complex medication regimen (Skotzko & Strouse, 2002). There is also the knowledge that patients must be regularly monitored for rejection, that many patients go through at least one rejection episode during their first postoperative year, and that this will require a change in their medication regimen to increase immunosuppressive therapy when it occurs (Sangstat, 2004).

There are data that it takes an extended period of time for posttransplant patients to readjust to normal life. The first anniversary of the transplant is a major milestone for full adjustment (Kuhn et al., 1988b). Major fears in the time after discharge are rejection and infection. Rejection is the most common fear for patients at 2- and 4-year follow-up (Sutton & Murphy, 1989). Many other issues confront patients after discharge; the expectation of the patient or family that life is now supposed to be normal may cause anxiety when it seems life may never be normal. Stressors include the loss of disability insurance after transplantation and not being able to qualify for health insurance should they return to work because of having a "prior condition" (Thomas, 1996). Antirejection medication is quite expensive: The cost to the patient of immunosuppressive therapy is estimated at $12,000 to $15,000 in the first year following transplant, and approximately $10,000 to $12,000 each year thereafter (Sangstat, 2004). Other stressors for patients are readjustment to family roles, tolerating the side effects of medications, and meeting the expectations of the medical staff (Craven, 1990). Anxiety seems to be better at discharge than 4 and 12 months after transplant (Jones et al., 1988; Skotzko & Strouse, 2002). But anxiety does seem to decrease after the first posttransplant year, indicating that adjustment does take place but the process is long and involved (Jones et al., 1992).

CONCLUSION

The gift of transplantation has been life saving for thousands of patients. New advances are continuously made to help those in organ failure live longer, allowing longer wait list survival and a greater chance for transplantation. With the fairly fixed supply of donor organs, there are many more in need of organs than the supply of organs. As reviewed here, waiting is stressful for patients and families, as is transplant surgery and the postsurgical recovery period. Readjustment to life posttransplant also has its vicissitudes. However, in the end, although it takes considerable time, many patients return to a full, satisfying, and lengthy life.

CONTRIBUTOR

Jerome J. Schulte, Jr., MD, is the Medical Director, Mental Health Inpatient Unit, Good Samaritan Hospital, Dayton, Ohio and Assistant Professor, Department of Psychiatry, and head of Consultation Psychiatry at Wright State University, Dayton, Ohio. Dr. Schulte supervises the indigent inpatient psychiatry service at Good Samaritan Hospital supervising psychiatric residents, internal medicine residents, and medical students. He has been the recipient of the Wright State University School of Medicine Teaching Excellence Award on multiple occasions, most recently in 2004. He is past recipient of the Arnold P. Gold Foundation Humanism in Medicine Award from the Healthcare Foundation of New Jersey in 2002. He is also a NASA mission operations consultant for astronaut selection for space shuttle and space station and Flight Medicine consultant for the U.S. Airforce in psychiatry through his reserve duty at the Aerospace Medicine Consultation Service, Brooks AFB, Texas. Dr. Schulte may be contacted at Good Samaritan Hospital, MHIPU, 2222 Philadelphia Drive, Dayton, OH 45406. E-mail: jschulte@shp-dayton.org

RESOURCES*

Associated Press. (2003, August 27). *New Heart, New Mountain to Climb.* Retrieved October 14, 2004, from the CBS News website: http://www.cbsnews.com/stories/2003/08/27/health/main570389.shtml

Bravata, D., Olkin, I., Barnato, A., Keeffe, E., & Owens, D. (2001). Employment and alcohol use after liver transplantation for alcoholic and nonalcoholic liver disease: A systematic review. *Liver Transplantation, 7,* 191-203.

Cohen, L., Tessier, E., Germain, M., & Levy, L. (2004). Update on psychotropic medication use in renal disease. *Psychosomatics, 45,* 34-48.

Collis, I., & Lloyd, G. (1992). Psychiatric aspects of liver disease. *British Journal of Psychiatry, 161,* 12-22.

Craven, J. (1990). Psychiatric aspects of lung transplant: The Toronto Lung Transplant Group. *Canadian Journal of Psychiatry, 35,* 759-764.

Dew, M., Switzer, G., DiMartini, A., Matukaitis, J., Fitzgerald, M., & Kormos, R. (2000). Psychosocial assessments and outcomes in organ transplantation. *Progress in Transplantation, 10,* 239-259.

Fernandes, P. (2003). Rapid desensitization for needle phobia. *Psychosomatics, 44,* 253-254.

Freeman, A., Folks, D., Sokol, R., & Fahs, J. (1988a). Cardiac transplantation: Clinical correlates of psychiatric outcome. *Psychosomatics, 29,* 47-54.

Freeman, A., Sokol, R., Folks, D., McVay, R., McGiffin, A., & Fahs, J. (1988b). Psychiatric characteristics of patients undergoing cardiac transplantation. *Psychiatric Medicine, 6,* 8-23.

Hirsch, D. (1989). Death from dialysis termination. *Nephrology Dialysis Transplantation, 4,* 41-44.

Jones, B., Chang, V., Esmore, D., Spratt, P., Shanahan, M., Farnsworth, A., Keogh, A., & Downs, K. (1988). Psychological adjustment after cardiac transplantation. *Medical Journal of Australia, 149,* 118-122.

Jones, B., Taylor, F., Downs, K., & Spratt, P. (1992). Longitudinal study of quality of life and psychological adjustment after cardiac transplantation. *Medical Journal of Australia, 157,* 24-26.

Kay, J. (2001). Integrated treatment, an overview. In J. Kay (Ed.), *Integrated Treatment for Psychiatric Disorders: Review of Psychiatry Series* (Vol. 20, pp. 1-29). Arlington, VA: American Psychiatric Press.

Kay, J., Bienenfeld, D., Slomowitz, M., Burk, J., Zimmer, L., Nadolny, G., Marvel, N., & Geier, P. (1991). Use of tricyclic antidepressants in recipients of heart transplants. *Psychosomatics, 32,* 165-170.

Kay, J., & Kay, R. (2003). Individual psychoanalytic psychotherapy. In A. Tasman, J. Kay, & J. Lieberman (Eds.), *Psychiatry* (2nd ed., pp. 1699-1772). London: John Wiley and Sons.

Kimmel, P., Weihs, K., & Peterson, R. (1993). Survival in hemodialysis patients: The role of depression. *Journal of the American Society of Nephrology, 4,* 12-27.

Kuhn, W., Davis, M., & Lippmann, S. (1988b). Emotional adjustment to cardiac transplantation. *General Hospital Psychiatry, 10,* 108-113.

Kuhn, W., Myers, B., & Davis, M. (1988a). Ambivalence in cardiac transplantation candidates. *International Journal of Psychiatry in Medicine, 18,* 305-314.

Lerner, D., Stoudemire, A., & Rosenstein, D. (1999). Neuropsychiatric toxicity associated with cytokine therapies. *Psychosomatics, 40,* 428-435.

Levenson, J., & Olbrisch, M. (1993). Psychosocial evaluation of organ transplant candidates: A comparative survey of process, criteria, and outcomes in heart, liver, and kidney transplantation. *Psychosomatics, 34,* 114-123.

---

* Although all websites cited in this contribution were correct at time of publication, they are subject to change at any time.

Levenson, J., & Olbrisch, M. (2000). Psychosocial screening and selection of candidates for organ transplantation. In P. Trzepacz & A. Dimartini (Eds.), *The Transplant Patient* (pp. 21-41). New York: Cambridge University Press.

Neu, S., & Kjellstrand, C. (1986). Stopping long-term dialysis. *New England Journal of Medicine, 314*, 14-20.

Ohio Solid Organ Transplantation Consortium. (2004). *Hepatic Patient Selection Criteria.* Retrieved October 15, 2004, from http://www.osotc.org/cr_hp.htm

Phipps, L. (1991). Psychiatric aspects of heart transplantation. *Canadian Journal of Psychiatry, 36*, 563-568.

Robinson, M., & Levenson, J. (2004). Psychopharmacology in transplantation. In J. Levenson (Ed.), *The American Psychiatric Press Textbook of Psychosomatic Medicine* (pp. 151-172). Arlington, VA: American Psychiatric Press.

Sangstat. (2004). *Solid Organ Transplantation: The History of Cyclosporine.* Retrieved October 15, 2004, from the Sangstat website: http://www.sangstat.com/resource/solid_history.asp

Skotzko, C., & Strouse, T. (2002). Solid organ transplantation. In M. Wise & J. Rundell (Eds.), *The American Psychiatric Press Textbook of Consultation-Liaison Psychiatry: Psychiatry in the Medically Ill* (2nd ed., pp. 623-655). Arlington, VA: American Psychiatric Press.

Surman O., Dienstag, J., Cosimi, A., Chauncey, S., & Russell, P. (1987). Liver transplantation: Psychiatric considerations. *Psychosomatics, 28*, 615-618.

Surman, O., & Prager, L. (2004). Organ failure and transplantation. In T. Stern, G. Fricchione, N. Cassem, M. Jellinek, & J. Rosenbaum (Eds.), *Massachusetts General Hospital Handbook of General Hospital Psychiatry* (pp. 641-669). St. Louis, MO: Mosby.

Surman, O., & Tolkoff-Rubin, N. (1984). Use of hypnosis in patients receiving hemodialysis for end-stage renal disease. *General Hospital Psychiatry, 6*, 31-35.

Suszycki, L. (1986). Social work groups on a heart transplant program. *Journal of Heart and Lung Transplantation, 5*, 166-170.

Sutton, T., & Murphy, S. (1989). Stressors and patterns of coping in renal transplant patients. *Nursing Research, 38*, 46-49.

Thomas, D. (1996). Returning to work after liver transplant: Experiencing the roadblocks. *Journal of Transplant Coordination, 6*, 134-138.

Ustransplant.org (2004a, October). *Center and OPO Specific Reports, July 2004.* Retrieved October 16, 2004, from http://www.ustransplant.org

Ustransplant.org (2004b, October). *Fast Facts About Transplants.* Retrieved October 15, 2004, from http://www.ustransplant.org

Vlay, S., Olson, L., Fricchione, G., & Friedman, R. (1989). Anxiety and anger in patients with ventricular tachyarrhythmias: Responses after automatic internal cardioverter defibrillator implantation. *Pacing and Clinical Electrophysiology, 12*, 366-373.

Weems, J., & Patterson, E. (1989). Coping with uncertainty and ambivalence while awaiting a cadaveric renal transplant. *American Nephrology Nurses Association (ANNA) Journal, 16*, 27-31.

Assessment and Treatment of Psychosocial Issues With Cardiac Patients

Mark A. Williams and M. Gillian Steele

Cardiovascular disease (CVD) is the leading cause of death for both men and women in the United States. It is a myth that heart disease is primarily a man's disease. In fact, since 1984, CVD has taken the lives of more females than males. Prior to menopause, the incidence of CVD is lower in women than men. However, after middle age the incidence rates begin to even out. After the age of 75, the prevalence of CVD among women is actually higher than among men (American Heart Association [AHA], 2003).

Data from the Framingham Heart Study (Hurst, 2002), a longitudinal, population-based study of heart disease in the United States, indicates that for men in the 35- to 44-year-old age group, the incidence of a first major cardiovascular event is 7 per 1,000. The incidence rate increases in the 85- to 94-year-old group to 68 per 1,000. With the aging of the population, we are facing an increased burden of disability due to heart disease and its associated conditions (e.g., diabetes, hypertension, cerebral vascular disease).

Current prevalence data from the American Heart Association (AHA, 2003) include the following statistics:

- 50,000,000 Americans have high blood pressure.
- 13,200,000 Americans have been diagnosed with coronary heart disease.
- 7,800,000 Americans have had a myocardial infarction.
- 6,800,000 Americans suffer from angina pectoris.
- 1 in 5 American adults has some form of CVD.
- On average, one American dies every 34 seconds from CVD.
- Blacks have a substantially higher death rate from CVD compared to whites.
- The estimated 2004 direct and indirect cost of CVD in the U.S. is $368.4 billion.
- In 1999, $26.3 billion in Medicare payments was made on behalf of patients discharged from hospitals with a primary diagnosis of CVD.

These statistics clearly show the large burden that heart disease has on individuals, as well as the economic costs to society. Fortunately, much has been learned about the cause of heart disease. Medical treatments have improved substantially in recent years, and there is a substantial role for prevention efforts as well as rehabilitation. Areas of primary, secondary, and tertiary prevention and rehabilitation will be best accomplished by the involvement of individuals from multiple professions. In this contribution we will be making the argument that persons who work in the areas of behavior change and behavioral health promotion have a substantial role to play in the prevention, treatment, and rehabilitation of persons with heart disease.

RISK FACTORS

Several medical and lifestyle factors have been shown to increase one's risk for heart disease (AHA, 2003). Recent research has shown that 80% or more of persons with coronary heart disease (CHD) have at least one of the traditional risk factors: hypertension, hyperlipidemia, smoking, or diabetes (Greenland et al., 2003).

Recent data (AHA, 2003) indicate that one's risk of CHD is increased by 30% due to exposure to environmental tobacco smoke. Smoking itself is estimated to cost the U.S. $157 billion in health-related expenses per year.

Cholesterol levels are the most common laboratory-evaluated risk factor for CHD. Treatment outcome studies have demonstrated that cholesterol-lowering drugs decrease the incidence of heart disease and future morbidity and mortality among patients with CHD. However, both medication access and compliance with taking cholesterol-lowering medications over substantial time periods has been problematic. For example, studies have shown that fewer than half of persons whose clinical profile would warrant a treatment including cholesterol-lowering drugs are actually prescribed these. Also, only about 50% of persons prescribed lipid-lowering drugs are still taking them after a 6-month time frame (AHA, 2003).

Diabetes mellitus is another common risk factor for CHD. Death rates among individuals with CHD are increased two to four times when diabetes is present. Also, 65% to 75% of individuals with diabetes mellitus will die from some kind of vessel disease. These statistics are more alarming when one considers that there has been a 50% increase in the prevalence of diabetes mellitus over the past decade (AHA, 2003).

The "metabolic syndrome" represents a constellation of medical findings that places one at risk for diabetes, CVD, and mortality. The syndrome is defined as including at least three of the following (AHA, 2003):

1. Waist circumference greater than 40 inches in men and greater than 35 inches in women.
2. Serum triglyceride level of 150 mg/dL or higher.
3. HDL cholesterol level less than 40 mg/dL in men and less than 50 mg/dL in women.
4. Blood pressure of 130/85 or higher.
5. Fasting glucose level of 110 mg/dL or higher.

Current estimates indicate that about 47 million Americans meet the definitional criteria for the metabolic syndrome (AHA, 2003).

Being overweight or obese is another risk factor for CVD. Commonly the definition of "overweight" is having a Body Mass Index (BMI) of 25 to 29.9. Persons with a BMI of 30.0 or higher are labeled "obese." Based on these criteria, 2001 data indicate that 64.5% of U.S. adults are either overweight or obese. Thirty percent of U.S. adults are obese. A typical 20-year-old male with a BMI of 45 has an average reduction of life span of 13 years. A female with the same BMI has an average reduction of life span of 8 years. Obesity-related medical disorders cost the U.S. about $100 billion per year (AHA, 2003).

Physical inactivity is a substantial public health problem and a risk factor for many diseases, including CVD. Studies suggest that physical inactivity increases the risk of CHD by a multiple of 1.5 to 2.4. This is comparable to the level of increased risk from high blood pressure, high cholesterol, or cigarette smoking (Pate et al., 1995). Data from 1997 to 1998 indicated that of Americans older than 18, 38% reported not engaging in physical activity. Fifty-five percent of Americans are not active enough to meet government established physical activity recommendations (AHA, 2003).

PSYCHOSOCIAL RISK FACTORS

In addition to the traditional risk factors for CVD noted above, there are several psychosocial factors that place persons at increased risk for developing CHD or increasing the morbidity and mortality of persons already diagnosed with CHD. These will be briefly discussed here and taken up again later in the contribution as targets for assessment and intervention.

Stress

Studies have shown a relationship between both chronic and acute stress and the development of CHD as well as increased morbidity and mortality among persons with already known heart disease (Muller, Tofler, & Stone, 1989; Rozanski, Blumenthal, & Kaplan, 1999).

Intense negative emotional experiences such as anger may cause heart attack or even sudden cardiac death among persons with preexisting CHD (Muller, 1999). Acute personal traumas (e.g., death of a spouse), natural disasters, and the stress of warfare have all been associated with an increased rate of heart attacks and sudden cardiac death (Cottington et al., 1980; Leor, Poole, & Kloner, 1996; Meisel et al., 1991).

Studies have shown that even the more typical stressors of daily life can trigger episodes of myocardial ischemia among cardiac patients. Stressful cognitive activities performed in a laboratory setting as well as procedures designed to provoke participants' anger have been shown to induce myocardial ischemia (Gabbay et al., 1996; Ironson et al., 1992). Studies examining the relationship between occupational stress and CVD have generally found that positions with lower control over job demands predict later development of heart disease. Additional exacerbating factors include high job demands, and for women, unsupportive bosses and high family demands (Haynes & Feinleib, 1980; Karasek & Theorell, 1990).

Stress is a difficult construct to measure because persons vary in their behavioral, emotional, and physiological reaction to events. Some researchers have suggested that greater cardiovascular reactivity and endocrine responses to stress may be an independent risk factor for development of CHD (Krantz & Manuck, 1984; Rozanski et al., 1999). For example, researchers examined the amount of blood pressure reactivity to a cold pressor task (holding one's hand in a container of ice-cold water) among a group of healthy young men. Follow-up data 23 years later revealed that the magnitude of diastolic blood pressure reactivity seen in response to the cold pressor task significantly predicted later development of cardiac disease (Keys et al., 1971). Other studies have shown that heightened reactivity to laboratory stressors is positively associated with increased myocardial ischemia during daily life activities and normal stressors. This increased reactivity is associated with a higher occurrence of heart attacks among patients with CHD (Blumenthal et al., 1995; Krantz et al., 1996).

The Type-A Behavior Pattern (TABP) and Hostility

The TABP is a familiar concept to laypersons and health care professionals alike. Thousands of studies on TABP, including those relating TABP to CHD, have been published (Matthews, 1988). Historically, the TABP has been defined as persistent behavioral characteristics that include incessant striving to accomplish more and more, chronically feeling a sense of time urgency in performing tasks, being prone toward feelings of hostility and outward expressions of anger, restlessness, impatience, competitiveness, a vague mistrust of others, and perfectionism (Sotile, 1996). Although some early cross-sectional studies that examined the relationship between TABP and CHD found positive correlations, more recent prospective studies have not found a significant link between the full TABP constellation of characteristics and development of CHD (Matthews, 1988). However, more recent prospective studies have found that persons with high levels of hostility do have an increased risk for developing CHD or hypertension (Matthews, 1988; Yan et al., 2003).

How is it that hostility is damaging to one's heart? There are several possible answers to this question. One possibility is that hostility has a direct negative impact on the body. The behavioral expression and subjective report of hostility has been associated with increased cortisol levels, increased lipid levels in the blood, increased physiological reactivity, and decreased immune functions (R. B. Williams, Barefoot, & Shekelle, 1985). A second explanation is that hostile individuals may live in more stressful and anger-producing environments, and they may have fewer supports or opportunities for respite from their stress leading to a chronic stress reaction. Persons with higher hostility appear to react with stronger physiological reactivity in response to interpersonal conflicts (Smith & Brown, 1991; Smith & Sanders, 1986). It has also been proposed that persons with high hostility are at greater risk for disease because they have poorer health habits (Leiker & Hailey, 1988). Some research has shown that these individuals consume more caffeine, use more nicotine, drink more alcohol, consume more calories, and have fewer health-promotive behaviors such as regular exercise and adequate sleep (Smith, 1992).

Inadequate Social Support

The term "social support" is multifactorial. Generally, the term can be divided into three categories. First, "social network" refers to the quantity of social contacts one reports having. Second, "social relationships" are concerned with the perceived nature of the social contacts one reports having. Finally, "specific social supports" reflect the actual resources one has available to draw from (e.g., emotional support, information, practical assistance) (House & Kahn, 1985). Studies examining the relationship between health and measures of social support have found that, generally, measures that evaluate one's perceptions of support as compared to more objective measures of support and health are more highly correlated (Antonucci & Israel, 1986).

Studies have shown that persons with more social isolation and less support have an increased likelihood of developing CHD (Shumaker & Cjakowski, 1994). Two pathways have been proposed as to how low social support may increase one's risk for CHD. First, the "direct effects model," which relies heavily upon animal research, argues that humans have an innate need for social attachments. When these needs are not met, physical dysfunction and emotional distress occur (Baumeister & Leary, 1995). The "buffer hypothesis" (Cohen & Wills, 1985) proposes that social support helps to shield an individual from the effects of stressful life events. Social support may buffer the impact of stress by helping one to appraise a situation as more manageable. Alternatively, the support may involve extending pragmatic assistance to an individual to help solve stress-producing situations. Support that specifically matches one's needs (e.g., emotional support for uncontrollable loss or practical support for controllable stressful life demands) are arguably of the most help. In other words, generic emotional support may not always be helpful if it does not match up with the needs of the individual.

Depression

Several studies have found depression to be a risk factor for cardiac events following coronary artery bypass grafting (CABG). Perhaps the best study to date included a sample of 817 patients who were evaluated for depression with the Center for Epidemiologic Studies Depression Scale (CES-D) prior to the CABG, reevaluated 6 months following surgery, and followed for up to 12 years. The mean follow-up was 5 years. Results found that 38% of patients met criteria for depression (CES-D >/= 16) prior to surgery. Persons with either mild, moderate, or severe depression at baseline that persisted to the 6-month follow-up had a higher death rate than those with no depression (adjusted hazard rate 2.2) (Blumenthal et al., 2003). Another recent study (Lesperance et al., 2002) found that improvement in symptoms of persons initially diagnosed with mild depression within the first year following a heart attack was associated with decreased long-term mortality (5-year survival data). However, patients with higher initial depression scores during admission for heart attack did not show a decreased mortality rate at the 5-year follow-up, regardless of whether depression symptom scores declined at the 1-year follow-up.

As with stress, depression may negatively impact heart functioning in a variety of ways. Depression may have a direct effect on the physiological mechanisms underlying heart disease (Merz et al., 2002). Medication compliance has been found to be lower among depressed patients with coronary artery disease (Carney et al., 1995). Depressed cardiac patients are likely to have less social support (Holahan et al., 1995). Individuals with dispositional optimism, a personality trait believed to reduce the odds of developing depression, have been found to show a faster physical recovery and faster return to normal life activities following CABG surgery (Scheier et al., 1989).

Neuropsychological Status

Individuals with CVD have an increased risk for acquired cognitive deficits (Putzke et al., 1997). These are presumed to be of diverse etiology including history of cerebral vascular disease, hypoxic/anoxic events, medication side effects, or other causes. Following CABG surgery it is common for patients to have clinically notable cognitive deficits. This oftentimes improves rather quickly, but a small percentage of CABG patients appear to have residual neuropsychological deficits that persist for months and at times are permanent (Keith et al., 2002). Regardless of the cause of cognitive deficits in heart disease patients, it is important to appreciate the nature and extent of a patient's cognitive functioning such that medical management can appropriately be adapted and increased practical support from family members or others can be arranged.

THE CASE FOR PSYCHOSOCIAL ASSESSMENT AND INTERVENTION

It seems logical that because many studies have shown that stress, depression, hostility, low social support, and unhealthy lifestyles increase the incidence of heart disease, interventions targeting these factors should decrease the incidence of heart disease and improve the morbidity and mortality of persons already diagnosed with heart disease. Numerous psychosocial interventions that have included stress management training, health education, and targeted risk factor reduction (e.g., decreased hostility, smoking cessation, weight management, emotional management, life skills training) have been studied with cardiac patients. A 1999 meta-analysis of 37 studies concluded that these programs reduced cardiac mortality by 34%, reduced recurrent myocardial infarction by 29%, and had a significant effect on lowering traditional risk factors such as blood pressure, cholesterol, body weight, smoking, physical inactivity, and poor eating habits (Dusseldorp et al., 1999). Studies to date have not used dismantling research designs. Therefore, it is unclear as to which components of these multicomponent treatment programs are responsible for the positive outcomes. At this point, a multicomponent stress management and health education program that includes components of relaxation training, cognitive therapy, and patient-specific targeted treatments (e.g., depression, anxiety, hostility, smoking cessation, weight management) is recommended.

Blumenthal et al. (2002) examined the effectiveness of a stress management program on 94 patients with coronary artery disease (CAD) who were established prior to the interventions to have stress-induced myocardial ischemia. The patients were assigned to one of three groups. The first group received a structured stress management program that lasted 1.5 hours per week for 16 weeks. The second group participated in an exercise program three times a week for 4 months. The third group received standard medical follow-up similar to the other groups, but did not participate in a formal exercise or stress management program. At the 5-year follow-up, those who participated in the stress management program were found to have significantly fewer clinical CAD events compared to the usual care group. Subsequent analysis of the estimated economic cost of the three groups found that the patients who participated in the stress management group had lower medical expenditures. The average cost per patient per year during the 5-year follow-up was $5,998 for the patients in the stress management group, $8,689 for those in the exercise group, and $10,338 for those who received usual medical care (American Psychological Association [APA] Practice Directorate, 2005).

At present the literature is promising in its support for the effectiveness of psychosocial and behavioral interventions for the treatment of cardiac disease. Recent economic analyses suggest a potential added benefit of decreasing overall health care cost while improving medical outcomes. The remainder of this contribution will focus on specific assessment and treatment tools that the behavioral health clinician may wish to draw from in working with cardiac patients.

ASSESSMENT OF THE CARDIAC PATIENT

Cognitive Assessment

The need for cognitive assessment and the extent of testing indicated will vary depending upon multiple factors. A review of the patient's medical history and daily functioning will aid in determining whether cognitive assessment is indicated. Examples of medical histories that increase the probability of cognitive disorder are history of coronary bypass grafting surgery, cardiopulmonary arrest, known cerebral vascular disease, history of other primary brain events (e.g., traumatic brain injury, epilepsy, tumor, infectious processes, brain irradiation, hypoxic-anoxic events, etc.), history of substance abuse, or use of multiple medications. Also, patients with congestive heart failure may develop temporary electrolyte imbalances leading to confusion or delirium. Educational and occupational history should be reviewed to rule out low cognitive capacities or learning disabilities that are developmentally based. Cognitive impairments may have a detrimental impact on medical compliance and ability to appreciate treatment options. Common benefits of cognitive assessment include being able to adjust the manner in which information is provided to the patient, obtain additional support from family members or others in a caretaking role, or assist with teaching certain compensatory strategies. Targets of compensatory strategies often include medication compliance, keeping a symptom log, or providing simplified information regarding dietary modifications. Under some circumstances, repeat cognitive testing may be indicated. For example, many patients show cognitive deficits during the acute recovery stage following a CABG, but most of them improve substantially within a few weeks to months.

Putzke et al. (1997) have published a large descriptive study of the performance of a large group of heart transplant candidates on a broad range of cognitive tests. These include tests of attention, concentration, mental processing speed, learning efficiency, fine motor functions, visual-constructional, language, problem-solving, and executive functions. As a group, the patients ranged from unimpaired to having severe cognitive deficits. Clinically, it can be helpful to consider how a patient is functioning compared to both a nonpatient normative reference group and a mixed cardiac patient group such as that provided by Putzke et al. One can generally obtain a fairly broad assessment of a patient's cognitive functioning adequate for screening purposes with an assortment of tests taking between 45 to 75 minutes to administer. Of course, additional time will be needed for the patient interview, chart review, scoring, report preparation, and feedback to the referral source and the patient.

Stress Assessment

Social Readjustment Rating Scale (SRRS)

The Holmes and Rahe (1967) Social Readjustment Rating Scale (SRRS) is perhaps the oldest of the commonly used stress assessment scales. The scale design reflects the stimulus view of stress: that certain life events have inherent challenging impact on the individual, without consideration of moderating factors such as coping abilities or external supports. It is a self-report questionnaire consisting of 43 items reflecting life change events. Some of these are generally perceived as negative life events (e.g., death of a spouse, divorce, loss of job), and some of the items reflect generally positively perceived life events (e.g., marriage, starting a new job, etc.). Its primary advantage is that it can give the clinician a general idea of the nature and number of potentially stressful life events the patient has faced over a specified time frame. Its major disadvantage is that it does not take into account the individual's own appraisal of the life events, coping resources, or external supports.

Life Experiences Survey (LES)

The LES (Sarason, Johnson, & Siegel, 1978) is a 57-item self-report scale that asks respondents to indicate which life events they have experienced during a specified time frame. Some of the items are negative events and some of the items are positive events. The scale differs from the SRRS in that the respondent is asked to indicate on a 7-point Likert-type scale the items' desirability and the perceived degree of impact.

Hassles Scale (HS)

The HS (Kanner et al., 1981) scale was developed in response to studies that suggested that minor day-to-day stressors may negatively impact health more than major life events. The HS is a 117-item self-report questionnaire that uses a 3-point Likert-type scale to rate the severity and frequency of minor stressors over the previous month.

Daily Stress Inventory (DSI)

The DSI (Brantley et al., 1987) measures minor daily stressors with a 58-item questionnaire. The respondent rates the frequency and perceived impact of stressors likely to occur on a daily basis.

Perceived Stress Scale (PSS)

The PSS (Cohen, Kamarck, & Mermelstein, 1983) is a global measure of a respondent's perceived stress that is not focused on specific events. The PSS is likely strongly correlated with other measures of emotional distress such as negative affectivity, anxiety, and depression. Although its construct validity may be low, its usefulness as a more individual measure of perceived stress independent of life events can be useful for clinical analysis and treatment outcome measurement.

Coping Assessment

Coping abilities moderate the impact of life events on the individual's experience of stress and subsequent negative outcomes in regard to emotional, behavioral, and physical functioning. Like stress, the concept of coping is broad. Generally, coping is considered to include both one's appraisal of situations (cognitive component) and one's ability to effectively manage stressful situations (behavioral component). Coping may reduce the impact of stress through a number of mechanisms, including engaging in strategies that prevent exposure to stressors (proactive coping), removing the stressful demand, modifying the appraisal of the situation such that it is perceived to be more manageable, or minimizing the stress response by using strategies such as relaxation, meditation, and seeking social and practical support. Gathering information about an individual's coping abilities provides important information for the clinician that will aid in treatment planning.

Ways of Coping Questionnaire (WCQ)

The WCQ (Folkman & Lazarus, 1988) is the most widely used measure of coping (R. Schwarzer & C. Schwarzer, 1996). The scale presents to the respondent a large list of items that reflect cognitive and behavioral coping responses. The respondents use a 4-point Likert-type scale and rate their use of these various coping resources during a stressful situation. The scoring of the scale results in eight dimensions that are generally conceptualized by two factors: problem-focused versus emotion-focused coping techniques. The major advantage of scales such as the WCQ is that it aids the clinician in determining the most typical coping responses of the individual. For example, individuals with relatively narrow ranges of coping responses may be helped by being taught additional coping strategies. Similarly, individuals who rely too heavily on either a problem-focused or emotion-focused set of coping strategies may find that they are well equipped to manage certain types of stressors but not others. There is no one type of coping strategy that is universally effective, and multiple factors interact to determine which coping strategies may be optimal at any given point in time. However, in general, research suggests that when persons are faced with controllable stress, they are more likely to show more favorable mental and physical health outcomes when they emphasize problem-focused coping strategies. Likewise, persons facing uncontrollable stressful situations appear to have better outcomes when they are able to emphasize emotion-focused coping strategies (Martin & Brantley, 2004).

Social Support Assessment

Social support assessment measures can differ substantially in their focus. Some are helpful for determining the depth of one's social network, others focus more on the nature of the relationships and the respondents' perception of support received, while still others are more targeted for specific types of support.

Social Network List (SNL)

The SNL (Stokes, 1983) is a social network measure. The respondents are asked to list as many as 20 people involved in their lives. They are then asked to indicate which of these individuals they feel they could confide in or turn to for help in a time of need. The SNL can be helpful in obtaining a specific understanding of who the patient relies upon. It can also be used informally as a tool for discussing levels of interpersonal closeness and the importance of learning to open up to others.

Inventory of Social Supportive Behaviors (ISSB)

The ISSB (Barrera, Sandler, & Ramsey, 1981) evaluates one's perceptions of actual support received during the past month. Using a 40-item questionnaire, respondents indicate the frequency with which they received specific behaviorally oriented assistance from others. Examples of specific items include receiving money or receiving physical affection. Measures such as these may help to identify persons who report having an adequate social network and who do not complain of low support on more general measures, but, when specifically asked to indicate the frequency of actual behavioral support received recently, may show evidence of relatively low support. These persons may perceive themselves to be independent and reserved, and may resist asking for help from others. Although these characteristics have many positive benefits in a competitive society, they also contribute to increased risk of isolation, loneliness, and depression during times of physical illness. Therefore, this behavioral style may need to be a focus of intervention.

Interpersonal Support Evaluation List (ISEL)

The ISEL (Cohen et al., 1985) is a 40-item questionnaire that measures one's perceived available support. This scale measures not only tangible support but also intangible support leading to a sense of belonging and increased self-esteem.

Anger/Hostility Assessment

The anger-hostility construct can be considered according to various components. Most studies that have examined the relationship between anger-hostility and CHD have used global measures. From a clinical perspective it may be helpful to consider the different dimensions of the anger-hostility construct to include the attitude component, the mode of expression (e.g, anger-in or anger-out), and measures of the frequency, intensity, and duration of anger reactions (Siegel, 1986).

Cook and Medley Hostility Scale (Ho)

The Ho scale (Cook & Medley, 1954) is composed of 50 items from the MMPI. The items reflect hostile affect, cynicism, and aggressive behavior. The scale has been included in many studies that have found a relationship between hostility and CHD.

Multidimensional Anger Inventory (MAI)

The MAI (Siegel, 1986) is a 38-item Likert-type self-report scale. However, the scale has also been rewritten in the third person for studies that have examined spousal ratings of anger. The MAI provides information about reported level of arousal experienced with anger (frequency, duration, and magnitude). Additional dimensions include Hostile Outlook, Anger-In, and Anger-Out. A major advantage of the MAI in clinical use is the ability to compare the patient's self-report with the spousal or observer's ratings. Studies have shown that self-reports on hostility scales (and other self-report scales) can be lowered by a defensive response set. In fact, Helmers et al. (1995) found that patients with high hostility scores combined with high defensiveness exhibited the most frequent ischemic episodes during ambulatory electrocardiographic monitoring.

General Psychological Screening

It is desirable to have all cardiac patients complete at least a brief measure of global psychological symptoms. The relationship between depression and increased morbidity and mortality among heart disease patients has been adequately established to recommend that a depression screen should be a standard part of patient follow-up with the primary care provider. However, there are multiple other emotional, behavioral, or situational factors that may interfere with optimal medical treatment. Therefore, our recommendation is to encourage the use of broad-based symptom and problem checklists in the primary care setting. Table 1 (p. 94) presents recommendations for both general and more specific screening instruments.

PSYCHOSOCIAL TREATMENT COMPONENTS

Empirically evaluated psychosocial treatments for patients with heart disease have included multiple components that have varied from study to study. It is difficult to determine which aspects of the effective studies are critical for reducing cardiac-related morbidity, mortality, or improved quality of life. However, components common to these treatment studies are various stress management techniques, health education, and interventions targeted toward discontinuing unhealthy habits such as smoking, physical inactivity, and poor eating habits. Appropriate identification and treatment of depression should also be a core component of a psychosocial treatment plan. Below we will describe common stress management techniques and point the reader to resources for further information on these techniques. Stress management techniques are generally appropriate for most cardiac patients. For patients with clinically significant mental health problems, more individualized treatments will be necessary.

TABLE 1: General Screening Instruments and Selected Specific Instruments

General Screening Tools
    Brief Symptom Inventory (Derogatis & Spencer, 1982)
    Kellner Symptom Questionnaire (Kellner, 1987)

Depression Screening Tools
    Beck Depression Inventory (Beck, 1978)
    Center for Epidemiologic Studies Depression Scale (Radloff, 1977)

Anxiety Screening Tool
    State Trait Anxiety Scale (Speilberger, Gorsuch, & Luschene, 1970)

Alcoholism Screening Tools
    Michigan Alcohol Screening Test (Selzer, 1971)
    The CAGE Questionnaire (Ewing, 1984)

Adjustment to Illness Tools
    Psychosocial Adjustment to Illness Scale (Derogatis & Lopez, 1983)
    Cardiac Health Concerns Questionnaire (Stanton et al., 1984)
    Medical Outcomes Study-Short Form SF-36 (Mahler et al., 1992)

Family Assessment Scales
    Family Assessment Measure (Skinner, Steinhauer, & Santa-Barbara, 1983)
    Family Adjustment to Medical Stressors Scale (Koch, 1983)
    Miller Social Intimacy Scale (Miller & Lefcourt, 1982)
    Marital Conflict Scale (Waltz & Badura, 1988)
    Spousal Coping Instrument (Nyamathi, Dracup, & Jacoby, 1988)

Prior to beginning stress-management training, specifically relaxation training, it is helpful to teach patients about the physical effects of stress. Many patients will have some familiarity with the term "fight or flight response," and we recommend using this explanatory concept. Handouts or a chart depicting the physical changes that occur when we are faced with stressful situations should be presented. Detailed information can be obtained from resources listed in Table 2 (see p. 95). The important point to make is that stress causes our bodies to react in a fashion that in the short run can be protective, but if allowed to persist too long can lead to physical, emotional, and cognitive dysfunction. The concept of the "relaxation response" (Benson, 2000) should then be presented. This is the concept that our bodies also have the ability to undo the effects of stress and return to a healthier state. While the "fight or flight" response causes our bodies to raise blood pressure, increase heart rate, increase rate of breathing, and so on, the "relaxation response" allows us to reverse the effects of stress by decreasing heart rate, blood pressure, breathing rate, and so forth. The concept is that too much stress is bad for us and that by learning to elicit the relaxation response more effectively, we can reduce the negative impact of stress on our bodies and minds.

Progressive Muscle Relaxation

Progressive muscle relaxation (PMR) is a commonly used technique for inducing a relaxed state. Usually individuals are able to achieve a notable relaxation response the first time they are led through a PMR exercise. For this reason, we prefer to teach PMR exercises as the first step in learning a series of techniques for achieving the relaxation response. The exercise typically requires 15 to 30 minutes.

PMR involves the systematic tensing and relaxing of muscle groups. Patients are instructed to focus their awareness on the difference between the feelings of tension and relaxation in

---

TABLE 2: Bibliography of Recommended Books and Websites

Recommended Books

Anger Kills (R. W. Williams & V. Williams, 1993)
Coping With Heart Illness (Sotile, 1995)
Dr. Dean Ornish's Program for Reversing Heart Disease (Ornish, 1990)
Full Catastrophe Living (Kabat-Zinn, 1990)
Heart Illness and Intimacy: How Caring Relationships Aid Recovery (Sotile, 1992)
Meditation for Dummies (Bodian, 1999)
Psychosocial Interventions for Cardiopulmonary Patients (Sotile, 1996)
The Relaxation Response (Benson, 2000)
Stress Management for Dummies (Elkin, 1999)
The Wellness Book (Benson & Stuart, 1992)
Wherever You Go There You Are (Kabat-Zinn, 1994)

Recommended Websites*

American Association of Cardiovascular and Pulmonary Rehabilitation (www.aacvpr.org)
American Dietetic Association (www.eatright.org)
American Heart Association (www.americanheart.org)
Center for Mindfulness (http://www.umassmed.edu/cfm/)
Centers for Disease Control and Prevention (www.cdc.gov)
Food and Nutrition Information Center (www.nal.usda.gov/fnic/)
Medline Plus (www.nlm.nih.gov/medlineplus/heartdiseases.html)
The Mended Hearts, Inc. (www.mendedhearts.org)
The National Coalition for Women With Heart Disease (www.womenheart.org)
National Heart, Lung, and Blood Institute (www.nhlbi.nih.gov)
National Institute for Fitness and Sport (http://www.nifs.org/medical/cardio_rehabilitation.asp)
Nutrition, Health and Heart Disease (www.health-heart.org)
The Psychology of "Stress" (http://www.guidetopsychology.com/stress.htm)
Stress Management from MindTools (http://www.mindtools.com/smpage.html)
Tufts University Nutrition Navigator (http://navigator.tufts.edu/)
University of California Irvine Heart Disease Prevention Program (www.heart.uci.edu)

---

* Although all websites cited in this contribution were correct at time of publication, they are subject to change at any time.

---

each of the muscle groups as the therapist systematically leads patients through the exercise. With practice, patients are able to become more aware of the presence of muscle tension in their daily life and will be able to practice strategies for reducing muscle tension and achieving a more relaxed state.

To begin PMR training it is necessary to find a private and quiet place. A reclining chair is desirable but not necessary. Patients are asked to sit or lie back in a comfortable position and close their eyes. During the initial training session the therapist should talk patients through the exercise. We have found that the timing of the exercise is best performed when the therapist participates in the PMR exercise while verbally leading patients through the exercise. Afterward, a tape-recorded PMR session can be given to the patient for practice at home. Variations of the PMR technique have been described, and modifications may be necessary for patients with certain joint conditions, jaw problems, or if wearing contact lenses (they will not want to squeeze the eyes tightly). We generally tell patients to tense specified muscles to about 75% of their maximum. They are instructed that the goal is to produce enough tension as to be able to focus on the difference between the sensations of tension and relaxation but not so much as to cause pain.

We generally like to begin the exercise by having patients make a fist with both hands and squeeze. They are instructed: *"Feel the tension, hold it, hold it, and now relax. Allow the tension to flow out of your hands, leaving your hands feeling very calm and relaxed. Become aware of the difference between the feelings of tension and relaxation in your hands."* As a flexible rule we have patients hold the tension for about 7 seconds, and the relaxation phase lasts for about 30 seconds. We generally like to lead patients through two sets of tension and relaxation phases for each of the muscle groups. We also like to remind patients at various times: *"We are in no hurry; just allow yourself to enjoy the sensation of relaxation, and if your mind wanders, just gently redirect your attention toward focusing on the sensations of relaxation and tension."*

Using narrative guidance in a fashion similar to that described above, the therapist leads patients through the other muscle groups:

- *"Now bend your arms, bring your fists up to your shoulders, and tighten your upper arms. . . ."*
- *"Now shrug your shoulders up toward your ears and tighten your upper back. . . ."*
- *"Now close your eyes tightly and tense your forehead. . . ."*
- *"Now tightly press your lips together, tensing the muscles in your lower face. . . ."*
- *"Now squeeze the muscles in your abdomen. . . ."*
- *"Now raise both legs, pointing your toes out, and tighten the muscles in your upper and lower legs. . . ."*

It is our experience that most patients will be able to obtain a satisfying experience from the first PMR exercise. However, a few patients require more practice sessions prior to being able to achieve a relaxation response. Also, a small number of individuals will be made anxious by the procedure. They typically report having a sensation of losing control. Allowing patients to keep their eyes open during the initial session may adequately suppress the anxiety.

Guided Imagery

The second relaxation technique that we like to teach patients is guided imagery. Generally, we will introduce guided imagery to patients after they have obtained a relaxed state using the PMR technique. They are instructed that they are going to be using the richness of their imagination to obtain a deeper and more peaceful state of relaxation.

The technique begins by making sure that patients are in a comfortable position and in a quiet environment. Prior to beginning, the therapist should ask the patients what kind of imaginary scene they would like to practice, remembering that the goal will be to obtain an increased sense of relaxation and a peaceful state of mind. Scenes involving nature are commonly used and may be suggested to the patient. Imagining sailing on a boat, lying under an umbrella on the beach, resting in a hammock at the lake, or relaxing in front of a fireplace in a secluded cabin are examples of scenes that many persons will find appealing.

During the initial part of the imagery training exercise, the therapist should describe for patients what the therapist wants patients to imagine. This models for patients an approach that incorporates all of the five senses into the imagined scene. It also paces patients to take their time and to develop the imagery in rich detail. As the session progresses the therapist can ask patients to continue the scene and to describe to the therapist in detail what they are experiencing. The therapist may ask questions such as, *"What are you seeing, hearing, feeling on your face, tasting, (etc.)?"* At least 15 to 20 minutes will be required to perform the exercise. As it feels appropriate, the therapist may make suggestions during the exercise such as, *"Allow yourself to fully enjoy the feeling of relaxation and peacefulness. There is plenty of time. If your mind wanders, just gently redirect yourself to this peaceful place (etc.)."*

Patients should be encouraged to use all of the relaxation techniques daily in one form or another. Having patients keep a daily log documenting their relaxation exercises is important. This can also be used for documenting specific events that can be discussed in the cognitive restructuring component of the stress-management training.

Diaphragmatic Breathing

Diaphragmatic breathing involves relaxing the belly and inhaling as the belly expands. As the belly moves outward, the diaphragm pushes on the abdomen from above. As the diaphragm expands further, the lungs gather more air, which in turn is expelled on exhalation. This breathing technique allows for deeper, fuller, and slower breaths and disrupts the muscle tension that often occurs in the diaphragm (Kabat-Zinn, 1990).

When learning diaphragmatic breathing, patients should begin by sitting straight in a chair or lying back comfortably in a recliner. Instruct patients to place one hand on their belly and the other on their chest. The therapist should also do this and model for patients the diaphragmatic breathing technique. Patients are instructed to notice that during the inhalation, the hand covering the belly rises, while the hand covering the chest does not move. Also, during the exhalation, the hand covering the belly will fall back toward the body while the hand covering the chest remains level (Elkin, 1999).

Diaphragmatic breathing elicits the relaxation response. After a few cycles of breathing in this fashion patients should be able to notice an increased sense of relaxation and reduced physical tension. Physical relaxation prepares the body for improved concentration and capacity for sustained focus. Diaphragmatic breathing, PMR, and guided imagery can all be combined to assist patients in learning to obtain a deeper relaxation response. These are also tools that can be used in most settings and require little time to elicit the relaxation response once one has gained a small amount of practice. Patients are encouraged to call upon relaxation techniques at points in their day when they sense increased tension, physiological arousal, anxiety, anger, impatience, or other experiences that lead to the stress response.

Mindfulness Meditation

In our busy society multitasking has become a way of life. Many find themselves in a position of having little time that can be set aside for meditation or relaxation. The concept of Mindfulness Meditation is quite simple. It involves attempting to fully concentrate on the present moment and focus attention only on one experience at a time (Hafen et al., 1996). Mindfulness Meditation can be practiced anywhere and at any time. It may be more accurately described as a way of being rather than as a technique that can be rigidly outlined. One may choose to focus intently on features of one's physical experience such as breathing, or the taste of food, or a specific emotion or thought. Similarly, one may focus on some specific features of the surrounding environment. With the practice of intense, sustained focus, one's awareness is increased and personal insights may be discovered. Kabat-Zinn (1990) notes that as we practice becoming more mindful of our experiences, we begin a process that allows us to cope with life on a continual basis with the "owning of each moment of our experience, good, bad or ugly" (p. 11).

Mindfulness is founded in Buddhist practice as a method for increasing our awareness of conscious and unconscious experience. However, its practice is independent of any specific dogma. Kabat-Zinn (1994) points out that meditation and relaxation are not the same thing. Mindfulness Meditation is about feeling the way you feel and being aware of yourself in that moment. It is possible to achieve a state of relaxation while becoming mindful of one's life and circumstances. However, the objective of mindfulness is not to have objectives as to how you will feel during or after meditation. The payoff, however, is increased self-discovery, self-acceptance, and subsequent behavior changes stemming from one's increased awareness. With the practice of being mindful we can become more aware of what is bothering us. This sets the stage for us to be able to identify and let go of certain self-defeating thoughts, to be more aware of how our actions impact others, and to take responsibility for our experience and reactions.

Anyone can learn to be more mindful. The practice should begin by taking a specified time, at least 15 minutes, and practice focusing on one thing throughout the exercise. Focusing intently on one's breathing is an example of a Mindfulness Meditation exercise. One attempts to become highly aware of the sensations that are produced with the inhalation and the exhalation. Attempts to control the breath are not important, only to be aware. As distracting thoughts enter the mind, they can be briefly noted, and one can then calmly return the focus to the breathing. One can focus on anything. With practice, it becomes easier to achieve an increased sense of focus or "being" as we go about living our lives and carrying out normal day-to-day activities. Beginning the practice of meditation can be aided by using commercially available audiotapes and CDs.

Cognitive Restructuring Interventions

It has been well established that the way in which we think contributes substantially to how we feel and behave. Heart patients with optimistic outlooks have been shown to recover quicker and to return sooner to previous activities. Persons with low self-efficacy are more likely to fail in attempts to modify habits such as quitting smoking, weight loss, and increasing physical activity. Cognitions have been established to be very important in mediating our emotional reactions. Furthermore, cognitive therapy techniques have been found to be effective for treating persons with an array of emotional and behavioral problems. Therefore, cognitive-based interventions should be a component of any broad-based psychosocial intervention for cardiac patients.

Numerous psychological issues that commonly arise in the heart patient can be addressed using cognitive therapy techniques. However, clinical judgment is required to determine when patients are ready to participate in this type of intervention. During a crisis period, such as in the early stages of recovery from a heart attack, it may be best to rely mostly on supportive interventions. During these times certain defenses such as denial may actually be of benefit to the patient, and the therapist may do best not to disrupt this coping strategy. However, with increased emotional stability and adjustment, the clinician will generally find that most patients become capable of benefiting from cognitive therapy.

Heart patients commonly face multiple issues that need to be evaluated and addressed. Emotionally, patients may present with chronic worry, fear of physical activity (including sexual activity), feelings of loss of self-worth, feelings of anger and self-blame, or feelings of loss and depression. Behaviorally, the clinician should be sensitive to behavioral characteristics that research has demonstrated to be risk factors for heart disease. These primarily include problems with anger, hostility, cynicism, and excessive physiological reactivity to stress. Associated behavioral characteristics such as time urgency, difficulties expressing feelings appropriately, impatience, perfectionism, dominance, denial, and rationalization are just a few examples of the many issues that may create problems for the patient. Patients often will not report emotional distress as a result of some of these problematic behavioral characteristics. Therefore, part of the task of the therapist is to help the patient understand that although some of the patient's behavior patterns may have been effective for certain aspects of his or her functioning, it is not good for his or her heart. Helping patients to identify the specific behavioral patterns that need to be modified and convincing them of its importance is one of the first challenges of the cognitive intervention. For example, one patient may show problems with excessive independence, trouble accepting and giving emotional support, having a cynical and defensive attitude, and suppressing negative feelings. Another patient may be too dependent on others and feel inadequate in his or her abilities for improving his or her situation. The important point is that each individual will present with a different package of needs, capabilities, defensiveness, and openness.

Although we do not have the space to go into detail on the multitude of cognitive techniques that may be of value, we have noted resources in Table 2 (see p. 95). As a component of a general cognitive restructuring intervention with heart patients, one may begin by introducing the importance of our thoughts, attitudes, and beliefs in determining how we feel and react (both behaviorally and physiologically) to events. The following 10 examples of common "cognitive distortions" (Burns, 1980; Sotile, 1996) may be reviewed with the patient.

1. <u>All-or-Nothing Thinking</u>. This is basically black-or-white thinking.

   a. Example: *"If I can't exercise the way I used to, I won't exercise at all."*
   b. Restructured: *"I may not be able to do everything that I used to do, but with consistent efforts, I may be able to do quite a lot."*

2. <u>Overgeneralization</u>. Involves thinking that an undesirable event will occur frequently when in fact it is likely to occur infrequently.

   a. Example: *"A neighbor of mine died from a heart attack while having sex. I'm not sure that I'll be able to take that risk."*
   b. Restructured: *"I have some concern about what level of physical exertion is safe and whether or not I can have sexual relations safely. I need to gather more information and talk with my doctor about this."*

3. <u>Selective Perception</u>. This involves filtering information in such a way that only the potentially negative aspects of the experience are focused on.

   a. Example: *"I feel like a failure; I missed 2 days of exercise last week."*
   b. Restructured: *"I wish I hadn't missed those 2 days of exercise; however, I've been making adequate progress. Maybe I can include additional forms of exercise to make the activity more appealing."*

4. <u>Mind Reading</u>. Involves drawing premature conclusions without checking out the facts with others.

   a. Example: *"I've not heard from my friend John in over 3 weeks. He must not care to socialize with me anymore."*
   b. Restructured: *"I need to call John and see if we can get together over the weekend. He'll probably be happy to hear from me."*

5. <u>Catastrophizing</u>. Involves thinking that the worst case scenario is likely to occur in the absence of reasonable factual information to support this.

   a. Example: *"I probably won't live to see my grandchildren."*
   b. Restructured: *"More than ever, it's clear to me what's important in life. I'm going to try to live a loving and happy life every day."*

6. <u>Discounting</u>. Involves diminishing the positive aspects of a situation and even turning them into a negative situation.

   a. Example: *"I've lost too little weight for all of the effort that I've put forth this past month."*
   b. Restructured: *"My endurance, strength, and exercise consistency have been good. I may want to talk with the dietician about ideas for losing more weight."*

7. <u>Magnification and Minimization</u>. Magnification usually occurs when one focuses too much on one's weaknesses, limitations, or fears. Symptoms or physical limitations can also be magnified and produce unnecessary disability. Minimization may involve not giving oneself enough credit for one's abilities and strengths.

    a.   Example: *"I'm of no use to my family anymore. I can't even mow the grass."*
    b.   Restructured: *"I wish that I could still do everything that I used to do. But I still have plenty to offer, and I'm thankful for the family and friends I have."*

8. <u>Emotional Reasoning</u>. Occurs when strong negative feelings cloud one's ability to think more rationally.

    a.   Example: *"I feel so irritable since I stopped smoking. Maybe I'd be better off just going ahead and smoking again. They can't guarantee me that I'll live any longer without the cigarettes."*
    b.   Restructured: *"My outlook is really being affected by these withdrawal symptoms. They tell me that this is a normal experience. Maybe I should go to those smoking cessation groups. It is important for my health and day-to-day functioning capacity to kick this habit."*

9. <u>Labeling and Mislabeling</u>. Involves the use of strong negative labeling of our failures, mistakes, or personal characteristics, or those of someone else.

    a.   Example: *"These doctors don't really care about me; they're greedy, self-absorbed, and don't have time for me."*
    b.   Restructured: *"I'm not really sure why Dr. Smith seems to be so rushed during our office visits. I am feeling better, and the cardiac rehabilitation program that he referred me to has been helpful. At this point I suppose my complaints are not substantial, and it would be unfair to label him as unconcerned."*

10. <u>Personalizing Blame</u>. Involves taking too much harsh responsibility for negative events. Although recognizing one's capacity for personal control in many situations is good, taking excessive blame may serve to keep patients overly focused on the past and interfere with moving forward.

    a.   Example: *"I'm such an idiot. I knew that I should have taken better care of myself. I have no self-control. What a slob I am."*
    b.   Restructured: *"Well I've certainly made some mistakes in the past, and it probably contributed to my current health problems. I can't change the past, but I can try to learn from my experiences and take better care of myself now."*

As a homework assignment, patients may be instructed to keep a diary of negative emotional or undesirable behavioral events they have witnessed in themselves. They should be asked to bring their diary into the clinic where it can be reviewed with the therapist and serve as a set of situations for applying the strategies of cognitive restructuring.

THE WHOLE ENCHILADA

The nature and extent of psychosocial interventions will need to be adapted according to a number of factors. Many times patients will be exposed to psychosocial treatments only as a brief psychoeducational intervention in a cardiac rehabilitation program. In these situations, common emotional adjustment issues should be discussed with patients, and group-administered stress management instruction can be given. It will be important to administer screening measures to identify those with possibly clinically significant depression, anxiety, or other psychiatric disorders in need of psychopharmacologic evaluation and referral for more intensive individual psychological treatment. Also, information on programs available for smoking cessation, substance abuse treatment, and weight management should be made available. Some patients may be able to gain access to more involved psychosocial treatment programs. In addition to the strategies already discussed, these programs may include specific interventions teaching assertiveness skills, communication skills, and problem-solving skills. These may be placed under the general category of life skills training. We also like to encourage heart patients and their families to participate in local associations designed in large part to provide ongoing encouragement, social support, and education related to living with heart disease. One such organization is The Mended Hearts, Inc. Their website is included in the list of resources in Table 2 (see p. 95).

Our goal in this contribution was to make a case for the value of psychosocial treatment programs and to provide a practical description of psychosocial assessment tools and interventions. In Table 2 we have included a list of resources that offer greater detail on the assessment and treatment of heart patients. Table 2 also includes a listing of websites and books from the popular press that clinicians and patients alike will find helpful in better understanding the importance of psychosocial issues in preventing and living with heart disease.

CONTRIBUTORS

Mark A. Williams, PhD, ABPP, is currently a practicing neuropsychologist with specific interests in the broader field of medical psychology. Dr. Williams was formerly an Assistant Professor in the departments of neurosurgery and psychology at the University of Alabama at Birmingham. For several years he served as a psychological consultant to the heart and lung transplantation program and the cardiopulmonary rehabilitation program at UAB. He has published numerous journal articles and book chapters in the areas of neuropsychology and medical psychology. Dr. Williams may be contacted at 131 Ionsborough, Mt. Pleasant, SC 29464. E-mail: mawphd@aol.com

M. Gillian Steele, BA, recently graduated from James Madison University with a major in Psychology and a minor in Spanish. She hopes to soon begin a doctoral training program in clinical psychology. Her areas of interest include use of stress management and behavior change techniques to improve physical and emotional health. She is also specifically interested in using her bilingual abilities to work with members of the Spanish-speaking community. Ms. Steele can be reached at 411 College Circle, Staunton, VA 24401. E-mail: G423chica@aol.com

RESOURCES

American Heart Association. (2003). *Heart Disease and Stroke Statistics–2004 Update*. Dallas, TX: American Heart Association.
American Psychological Association Practice Directorate. (2005). *Stress Management Significantly Reduces Long-Term Costs of Coronary Artery Disease* [Internet press release]. Retreived May 11, 2005, from http://www.apa.org/practice/stressmanagement.html
Antonucci, T. C., & Israel, B. A. (1986). Veridicality of social support: A comparison of principal and network member responses. *Journal of Consulting and Clinical Psychology, 54*, 432-437.

Barrera, M., Sandler, I. N., & Ramsey, T. B. (1981). Preliminary development of a scale of social support: Studies on college students. *American Journal of Community Psychology, 9*(4), 435-447.

Baumeister, R. F., & Leary, M. R. (1995). The need to belong: Desire for interpersonal attachments as a fundamental human motivation. *Psychological Bulletin, 117*(3), 497-529.

Beck, A. T. (1978). *Depression Inventory*. Philadelphia: Center for Cognitive Therapy.

Benson, H. (2000). *The Relaxation Response*. New York: Harpertorch.

Benson, H., & Stuart, E. M. (1992). *The Wellness Book*. New York: Birch Lane Press.

Blumenthal, J. A., Babyak, M., Wei, J., O'Connor, C., Waugh, R., Eisenstein, E., Mark, D., Sherwood, A., Woodley, P. S., Irwin, R. J., & Reed, G. (2002). Usefulness of psychosocial treatment of mental stress-induced myocardial ischemia in men. *The American Journal of Cardiology, 89*, 164-168.

Blumenthal, J. A., Jiang, W., Reese, J., Frid, D. J., Waugh, R., Morris, J. J., Coleman, E., Hansen, M., Babyak, M., Thyrum, E. T., Krantz, D. S., & O'Connor, C. (1995). Mental stress-induced ischemia in the laboratory and ambulatory ischemia during daily life: Association and hemodynamic features. *Circulation, 92*, 2102-2108.

Blumenthal, J. A., Lett, H. S., Babyak, M. A., White, W., Smith, P. K., Mark, D. B., Jones, R., Mathew, J. P., & Newman, M. F. (2003). Depression as a risk factor for mortality after coronary artery bypass surgery. *Lancet, 362*, 604-609.

Bodian, S. (1999). *Meditation for Dummies*. New York: Wiley.

Brantley, P. J., Waggoner, C. D., Jones, G. N., & Rappaport, N. (1987). A Daily Stress Inventory: Development, reliability, and validity. *Journal of Behavioral Medicine, 10*, 61-73.

Burns, D. (1980). *Feeling Good: The New Mood Therapy*. New York: New American Library.

Carney, R. M., Freedland, K. E., Eisen, S. A., Rich, M. W., & Jaffe, A. S. (1995). Major depression and medication adherence in elderly patients with coronary artery disease. *Health Psychology, 14*, 88-90.

Cohen, S., Kamarck, T., & Mermelstein, R. (1983). A global measure of perceived stress. *Journal of Health and Social Behavior, 24*, 385-396.

Cohen, S., Mermelstein, R., Karmack, T., & Hoberman, H. B. (1985). Measuring the functional components of social support. In I. G. Sarason & B. Sarason (Eds.), *Social Support: Theory, Research and Applications* (pp. 73-94). The Hague, Netherlands: Martinus Nijhoff.

Cohen, S., & Wills, T. A. (1985). Stress, social support and the buffering hypothesis. *Psychological Bulletin, 109*, 5-24.

Cook, W., & Medley, D. (1954). Proposed hostility and pharasaic-virtue scales for the MMPI. *Journal of Applied Psychology, 38*, 414-418.

Cottington, E. M., Matthews, K. A., Talbott, E., & Kuller, L. H. (1980). Environmental events preceding sudden death in women. *Psychosomatic Medicine, 42*, 567-574.

Derogatis, L. R., & Lopez, M. C. (1983). *Psychosocial Adjustment to Illness Scale*. Riderwood, MD: Clinical Psychometric Research.

Derogatis, L. R., & Spencer, P. M. (1982). *Brief Symptom Inventory*. Riderwood, MD: Clinical Psychometric Research.

Dusseldorp, E., van Elderen, T., Maes, S., Meulman, J., & Kraaij, V. (1999). A meta-analysis of psychoeducational programs for coronary heart disease patients. *Health Psychology, 18*, 506-519.

Elkin, A. (1999). *Stress Management for Dummies*. New York: Wiley.

Ewing, J. A. (1984). Detecting alcoholism: The CAGE Questionnaire. *Journal of the American Medical Association, 252*, 1905-1907.

Folkman, S., & Lazarus, R. S. (1988). *Manual for the Ways of Coping Questionnaire*. Palo Alto, CA: Consulting Psychologists Press.

Gabbay, F. H., Krantz, D. S., Kop, W. J., Hedges, S. M., Klein, J., Gottdiener, J. S., & Rozanski, A. (1996). Triggers of myocardial ischemia during daily life in patients with coronary artery disease: Physical and mental activities, anger, and smoking. *Journal of the American College of Cardiology, 27*, 585-592.

Greenland, P., Knoll, M. D., Stamler, J., Neaton, J. D., Dyer, A. R., Garside, D. B., & Wilson, P. W. (2003). Major risk factors as antecedents of fatal and nonfatal coronary heart disease events. *Journal of the American Medical Association, 290*(7), 891-897.

Hafen, B. Q., Karren, K. J., Frandsen K. J., & Smith, N. L. (1996). *Mind/Body Health*. Boston: Allyn and Bacon.

Haynes, S. B., & Feinleib, M. (1980). Women, work, and coronary disease: Prospective findings from the Framingham Heart Study. *American Journal of Public Health, 700*, 133-141.

Helmers, K. F., Krantz, D. S., Merz, C. N. B., Klein, J., Kop, W. J., Gottdiener, J. S., & Rozanski, A. (1995). Defensive hostility: Relationship to multiple markers of cardiac ischemia in patients with coronary disease. *Health Psychology, 14*(3), 202-209.

Holahan, C. J., Moos, R. H., Holahan, C. K., & Brennan, P. L. (1995). Social support, coping, and depressive symptoms in a late-middle-aged sample of patients reporting cardiac illness. *Health Psychology, 14*, 152-163.

Holmes, T. H., & Rahe, R. H. (1967). The Social Readjustment Rating Scale. *Journal of Psychosomatic Research, 11*, 213-218.

House, J. S., & Kahn, R. L. (1985). Measures and concepts of social support. In S. Cohen & S. L. Syme (Eds.), *Social Support and Health* (pp. 83-108). Orlando, FL: Academic Press.

Hurst, W. (2002). *The Heart, Arteries and Veins* (10th ed.). New York: McGraw-Hill.

Ironson, G., Taylor, C. B., Boltwood, M., Bartzokis, T., Dennis, C., Chesney, M., Spitzer, S., & Segall, G. M. (1992). Effects of anger on left ventricular ejection fraction in coronary artery disease. *American Journal of Cardiology, 70*, 281-285.

Kabat-Zinn, J. (1990). *Full Catastrophe Living*. New York: Dell.

Kabat-Zinn, J. (1994). *Wherever You Go There You Are*. New York: Hyperion.

Kanner, A. D., Coyne, J. C., Schaefer, C., & Lazarus, R. S. (1981). Comparison of two modes of measurement: Daily hassles and uplifts versus major life events. *Journal of Behavioral Medicine, 46*, 7-14.

Karasek, R. A., & Theorell, T. G. (1990). *Health, Work, Stress, Productivity, and the Reconstruction of Working Life.* New York: Basic Books.

Keith, J. R., Puente, A. E., Malcolmson, K. L., Tartt, S., Coleman, A. E., & Marks, H. F. (2002). Assessing postoperative cognitive change after cardiopulmonary bypass surgery. *Neuropsychology, 16,* 411-421.

Kellner, R. (1987). *Manual of the Symptom Questionnaire.* Albuquerque, NM: University of New Mexico.

Keys, A., Taylor, H. L., Blackburn, H., Brozeck, J., Anderson, J., & Simonson, E. (1971). Mortality and coronary heart disease among men studied for 23 years. *Archives of Internal Medicine, 128,* 201-214.

Koch, A. Y. (1983). Family adjustment to medical stressors. *Family Systems Medicine, 1*(4), 74-87.

Krantz, D. S., Kop, W. J., Santiago, H. T., & Gottdiener, J. S. (1996). Mental stress as a trigger of myocardial ischemia and infarction. *Cardiology Clinics, 14,* 271-287.

Krantz, D. S., & Manuck, S. B. (1984). Acute psychophysiologic reactivity and risk of cardiovascular disease: A review and methodological critique. *Psychological Bulletin, 96,* 435-464.

Leiker, M., & Hailey, B. J. (1988). A link between hostility and disease: Poor health habits? *Behavioral Medicine, 3,* 129-133.

Leor, J., Poole, W. K., & Kloner, R. A. (1996). Sudden cardiac death triggered by an earthquake. *New England Journal of Medicine, 334,* 413-419.

Lesperance, F., Frasure-Smith, N., Talajic, M., & Bourassa, M. G. (2002). Five year risk of cardiac mortality in relation to initial severity and one-year changes in depression symptoms after myocardial infarction. *Circulation, 105*(9), 1049-1053.

Mahler, D., Faryniarz, K., Tomlinson, E., Colice, G. L., Robins, A. G., Olmstead, E. M., & Conner, G. T. (1992). Impact of dyspnea and physiologic function on general health status in patients with chronic obstructive pulmonary disease. *Chest, 102,* 395-401.

Martin, P. D., & Brantley, P. J. (2004). Stress, coping, and social support in health and behavior. In J. M. Raczynski & L. C. Leviton (Eds.), *Handbook of Clinical Health Psychology* (Vol. 2, pp. 233-267). Washington, DC: American Psychological Association.

Matthews, K. A. (1988). Coronary heart disease and Type A behaviors: Update on and alternative to the Booth-Kewley and Friedman (1987) quantitative review. *Psychological Bulletin, 104,* 373-380.

Meisel, S. R., Kutz, I., Dayan, K. I., Pauzner, H., Chetboun, I., Arbel, Y., & David, D. (1991). Effect of Iraqi missile war on incidence of acute myocardial infarction and sudden death in Israeli civilians. *Lancet, 338,* 660-661.

Merz, C. N. B., Dwyer, J., Nordstrom, C. K., Walton, K. G., Salerno, J. W., & Scheider, R. H. (2002). Psychosocial stress and cardiovascular disease: Pathophysiological links. *Behavioral Medicine, 27,* 141-147.

Miller, R. S., & Lefcourt, H. M. (1982). The assessment of social intimacy. *Journal of Personality Assessment, 46,* 514-518.

Muller, J. E. (1999). Circadian variation and triggering of acute coronary events. *American Heart Journal, 137,* S1-S8.

Muller, J. E., Tofler, G. H., & Stone, P. H. (1989). Circadian variation and triggers of onset of acute cardiovascular disease. *Circulation, 79,* 733-743.

Nyamathi, A., Dracup, K., & Jacoby, A. (1988). Development of a Spousal Coping Instrument. *Progress in Cardiovascular Nursing, 3,* 1-6.

Ornish, D. (1990). *Dr. Dean Ornish's Program for Reversing Heart Disease.* New York: Ballantine Books.

Pate, R. R., Pratt, M., Blair, S. N., Haskell, W. L., Macera, C. A., Bouchard, C., Buchner, W., Ettinger, W., Heath, G. W., & King, A. C. (1995). Physical activity and public health: A recommendation from the Centers for Disease Control and Prevention and the American College of Sports Medicine. *Journal of the American Medical Association, 273*(5), 402-407.

Putzke, J. D., Williams, M. A., Millsaps, C. L., Azrin, R. L., LaMarche, J. A., Bourge, R. C., Kirklin, J. K., McGiffin, D. C., & Boll, T. J. (1997). Heart transplant candidates: Neuropsychological descriptive data base. *Journal of Clinical Psychology in Medical Settings, 4,* 343-355.

Radloff, L. S. (1977). The CES-D Scale: A self-report depression scale for research in the general population. *Applied Psychological Measure, 1,* 385-401.

Rozanski, A., Blumenthal, J. A., & Kaplan, J. R. (1999). Impact of psychological factors on the pathogenesis of cardiovascular disease and implications for therapy. *Circulation, 99,* 2192-2217.

Sarason, I. G., Johnson, J. H., & Siegel, J. M. (1978). Assessing the impact of life changes: Development of the Life Experiences Survey. *Journal of Consulting and Clinical Psychology, 46,* 348-349.

Scheier, M. F., Matthews, K. A., Owens, J. F., Magovern, G. J., Lefebvre, R. C., Abbott, R. A., & Carver, C. S. (1989). Dispositional optimism and recovery from coronary artery bypass surgery: The beneficial effects on physical and psychological well-being. *Journal of Personality and Social Psychology, 57,* 1024-1040.

Schwarzer, R., & Schwarzer, C. (1996). A critical survey of coping instruments. In M. Zeidner & N. S. Endler (Eds.), *Handbook of Coping: Theory, Research, and Applications* (pp. 107-132). New York: Wiley.

Selzer, M. L. (1971). The Michigan Alcoholism Screening Test: The quest for a new diagnostic instrument. *American Journal of Psychiatry, 127,* 1653-1658.

Shumaker, S. A., & Cjakowski, S. M. (1994). *Social Support and Cardiovascular Disease* (Plenum Series in Behavioral Psychophysiology and Medicine). New York: Plenum Press.

Siegel, J. M. (1986). The Multidimensional Anger Inventory. *Journal of Personality and Social Psychology, 51,* 191-200.

Skinner, H. A., Steinhauer, P. D., & Santa-Barbara, J. (1983). The Family Assessment Measure. *Canadian Journal of Community Mental Health, 2,* 91-105.

Smith, T. W. (1992). Hostility and health: Current status of a psychosomatic hypothesis. *Health Psychology, 11*(3), 139-150.

Smith, T. W., & Brown, P. (1991). Cynical hostility, attempts to exert social control, and cardiovascular reactivity in married couples. *Journal of Behavioral Medicine, 14*, 579-590.

Smith, T. W., & Sanders, J. D. (1986). Type A behavior, marriage, and the heart: Person-by-situation interactions and the risk of coronary disease. *Behavioral Medicine Abstracts, 7*, 59-62.

Sotile, W. M. (1992). *Heart Illness and Intimacy: How Caring Relationships Aid Recovery*. Baltimore: Johns Hopkins University Press.

Sotile, W. M. (1995). *Coping With Heart Illness*. Champaign, IL: Human Kinetics.

Sotile, W. M. (1996). *Psychosocial Interventions for Cardiopulmonary Patients*. Champaign, IL: Human Kinetics.

Speilberger, C. E., Gorsuch, R. L., & Luschene, R. E. (1970). *Manual for the State Trait Anxiety Inventory*. Palo Alto, CA: Consulting Psychologists Press.

Stanton, B., Jenkins, C. D., Savageau, J. A., Harken, D. E., & Aucoin, R. (1984). Perceived adequacy of patient education and fears and adjustments after cardiac surgery. *Heart and Lung, 13*, 525-531.

Stokes, J. P. (1983). Predicting satisfaction with social support from social network structure. *American Journal of Community Psychology, 11*, 141-152.

Waltz, M., & Badura, B. (1988). Subjective health, intimacy and perceived self-efficacy after a heart attack: Predicting life quality five years afterwards. *Social Industrial Research, 20*, 303-332.

Williams, R. B., Jr., Barefoot, J. C., & Shekelle, R. B. (1985). The health consequences of hostility. In M. A. Chesney & R. H. Rosenman (Eds.), *Anger and Hostility in Cardiovascular and Behavioral Disorders* (pp. 173-185). Washington, DC: Hemisphere.

Williams, R. W., & Williams, V. (1993). *Anger Kills*. New York: Harper Collins.

Yan, L. L., Liu, K., Matthews, K. A., Daviglus, M. L., Ferguson, T. F., & Kiefe, C. L. (2003). Psychosocial factors and risk of hypertension: The coronary artery risk development in young adults (CARDIA) study. *Journal of the American Medical Association, 290*(16), 2138-2148.

Assessment and Treatment Of Child and Adolescent Eating Disorders

Eve M. Wolf and Crystal S. Collier

Childhood feeding disorders and adolescent eating disorders pose significant risks for the youth of today. Although pica, rumination disorder, and feeding disorder of infancy or early childhood have been identified as significant clinical problems in the *Diagnostic and Statistical Manual of Mental Disorders* (*DSM-IV-TR*; American Psychiatric Association [APA], 2000), clinical data is scarce in guiding the clinician in the assessment and treatment of these disorders. Although it is commonly acknowledged that symptoms of eating disorders may emerge in late childhood or early adolescence, published reports on the assessment and treatment of child and adolescent eating disorders are rare. The purpose of this contribution is to summarize information on the assessment and treatment of feeding and eating disorders in child and adolescent populations. In order to accomplish this task, the contribution will be organized into four sections. Section one will provide clinical descriptions, diagnostic considerations, epidemiological information, and etiological factors for child and adolescent eating disorders. Section two will address the role of cultural and developmental factors in the conceptualization and treatment of child and adolescent eating disorders. Section three will focus on assessment procedures specifically tailored to children and adolescents. Finally, section four will summarize key approaches to the treatment of child and adolescent eating disorders.

CLINICAL DESCRIPTIONS, DIAGNOSIS, EPIDEMIOLOGY, AND ETIOLOGY

Feeding and Eating Disorders of Infancy or Early Childhood

DSM-IV-TR (APA, 2000) identifies three eating disorders that are seen during childhood: pica, rumination disorder, and feeding disorder of infancy or early childhood. The essential feature of pica is persistent eating of nonnutritive substances for at least 1 month. Pica often starts in infancy and lasts for several months. It is considered developmentally inappropriate when the behavior persists beyond the age of 12 to 18 months. The typical substances ingested by infants and young children tend to be paint, plaster, string, hair, or cloth. Pica occasionally continues into adolescence, or less frequently, into adulthood. Older children, adolescents, and adults with pica typically eat animal droppings, sand, insects, leaves, cigarette butts, pebbles, clay, or soil (APA, 2000). Pica often goes unreported, so it is difficult to establish reliable rates of pica among children. It often goes undiagnosed in children of low socioeconomic status due to limited access to health professionals. The prevalence rate of pica among boys and girls is approximately equal. Pica is frequently associated with mental retardation and/or autistic disorder. It has been estimated to occur in 9% to 25% of individuals with intellectual disability residing in institutional settings (Matson & Bamburg, 1999). Pica can also co-occur with severe psychopathology such as schizophrenia; therefore, it should be assessed routinely in individuals with diagnoses of retardation, autism, or schizophrenia. Currently, there is no agreed-upon cause for pica. It has been suggested that pica is both a cause and effect of iron deficiency. Stressors such as maternal deprivation, parental separation, parental neglect, child abuse, and too little parental interaction have also been implicated as causes of pica. Additionally, low socioeconomic status, hunger, modeling, reinforcement, and direct teaching can also result in pica (Kronenberger & Meyer, 2001).

The essential feature of rumination disorder is the voluntary and pleasurable repeated regurgitation and re-chewing of food that develops in an infant or child after a period of normal functioning and lasts for at least 1 month. The food is typically ejected from the mouth or, more frequently, re-chewed or re-swallowed. There are two types of rumination disorder: psychogenic and self-stimulating. Psychogenic rumination is rare and occurs primarily in young male infants between the ages of 3 and 14 months. The rumination behavior with resultant weight loss and failure to thrive is believed to result from a seriously disturbed parent-child relationship. Mortality rate is reported to be as high as 25%. Self-stimulatory rumination is not uncommon and is seen in mentally retarded individuals of any age. It occurs even when parents are very nurturing and attentive. For both types of rumination, the disorder is 3.5 times more common in males than females. Infants with rumination are often described as quiet, sad, and singularly wide-eyed, and some are irritable and hungry between episodes. Rumination disorder is most commonly observed in infants but may be seen in older individuals, particularly those who also have mental retardation. Young infants are often found lying in a small pool of regurgitated liquid. They are observed to actively gag themselves either by manipulation of the tongue or with their pacifier or fingers. Finger mouthing and chewing movements often precede or accompany the regurgitation. The amount of food regurgitated may appear small but can result in significant nutrient loss. Repetitive regurgitation and re-swallowing of ingested liquids and solids, gagging, mouthing, constant head movement, and failure to thrive are the hallmarks of this condition.

Several factors have been hypothesized to account for rumination disorder. First, dietary factors such as food and liquid intake variables seem to influence rumination directly. Therefore, an individual is most likely to ruminate immediately after meals. Second, learning and conditioning factors may influence rumination. The behavior is thought to be maintained as a result of reinforcement. Operant research has shown that self-injurious behavior, such as rumination, can be maintained by three general sources of reinforcement: social positive reinforcement, social negative reinforcement, and automatic reinforcement. Social positive reinforcement may occur when an individual receives increased attention or more preferred food. Social negative reinforcement may occur when rumination allows the individual to escape or avoid aversive social or instructional situations. Automatic reinforcement may occur when rumination produces pleasing stimulation independent of the social environment (APA, 2000; Comerci, 1999; S. W. Ekvall, V. Ekvall, & Mayes, 1993; Vollmer & Roane, 1998).

Feeding disorder of infancy or early childhood (FDI) is a syndrome characterized by the persistent failure to eat adequately prior to age 6, causing significant failure to gain weight or significant weight loss over at least 1 month. The problematic behaviors of the FDI child, which are most apparent during the parent-child interaction, involve pushing food or utensils away from the mouth, refusal to open the mouth, throwing or spitting out food, screaming, squirming, turning the head away from food, trying to get out of the chair, or failure to attend to the food. Infants with feeding disorders are often irritable and difficult to console during feeding. They may appear apathetic and withdrawn. FDI occurs in less than 4% of the general population and may account for 2% to 5% of pediatric admissions. It is equally diagnosed in males and females. The typical age of onset is between 3 to 24 months of age. Onset sometimes occurs after a discrete event such as an illness, surgery, or switching to a different type of food. Malnutrition and developmental delay can result from poor intake and low weight.

No one factor has been found to account for FDI, which suggests that FDI is probably caused by several factors that interact in a unique fashion. In many cases of FDI, there seem to be problems in the parent-child relationship or problematic contingencies related to feeding such as ignoring the child during feeding or problems with scheduling. In other cases, parental psychopathology, low intellectual functioning, or inability to change behavior leads to maladaptive parent behavior at feeding times. Such maladaptive behaviors include but are not limited to the inability to read the child's cues, forcing the child to eat, not feeding the child properly, or establishing an inconsistent feeding schedule. Problems with swallowing mechanics or eating may also account for FDI. In this case, infants may have difficulty with chewing or swallowing, or have an oversensitive oral area or gag reflex. In some instances, FDI occurs after an illness or surgery that disrupts the child's schedule. If a child has a negative experience that involves the nose, mouth, or throat, a posttraumatic feeding disorder can develop in which the child gags and refuses food (APA, 2000; Kronenberger & Meyer, 2001).

Adolescent Eating Disorders

DSM-IV-TR (APA, 2000) identifies four separate but related eating disorders that are relevant to adolescents: anorexia nervosa (AN), bulimia nervosa (BN), eating disorder not otherwise specified (EDNOS), and binge eating disorder (BED). The essential features of AN are a failure to maintain body weight at or above the minimal level for age and height, fear of weight gain or being overweight, disturbance of body image, and, in females, absence of at least three consecutive expected menstrual cycles (amenorrhea). Although the most apparent symptom of AN is low body weight, intense fear of gaining weight and distorted body image are also key features. Children and adolescents with AN often fear that they will lose control of their hunger and eat until they become fat. This fear is reinforced by a narrow range of acceptable body size, with the children or adolescents viewing themselves as fat despite normative weight. Adolescents with AN typically lose weight through limiting total food intake, eating low-calorie foods, and excessive exercising. These individuals commonly qualify for the restricting type. Adolescents may also engage in binge eating and/or use of laxatives, diuretics, and self-induced vomiting, in which case they will qualify for the binge eating/purging type. Although surveys of child and adolescent populations are limited, prevalence data suggest that AN occurs in 0.5% to 1% in females and .02% in males. Because of the low occurrence in boys, AN is often viewed as a female disorder. The mean age of onset for AN is 17 years, with data suggesting bimodal peaks at ages 14 and 18. Research has identified common attributes in girls with AN, including high achievement, perfectionism, anxiety and depressive symptoms, and low self-esteem (APA, 2000; Kronenberger & Meyer, 2001).

The essential features of BN are binge eating and the use of extreme weight control measures in order to prevent weight gain from the eating binges. *DSM-IV-TR* (APA, 2000) defines binge eating as eating within a discrete period of time a quantity of food that is clearly larger than what most people would eat during a similar time frame and similar circumstances. The eating binge is also characterized by a lack of control over the eating. Despite attempts to expand the description of an eating binge, the *DSM-IV-TR* definition continues to be quite subjective. Common extreme weight control measures include fasting, overly restrictive dieting, excessive exercise, self-induced vomiting, and use of laxatives and diuretics in order to rid the body of excess calories. *DSM-IV-TR* also incorporates a duration and frequency criterion in stating that the eating binges and inappropriate compensatory behaviors must occur, on average, at least twice a week for at least 3 months. Final criteria specified by *DSM-IV-TR* address the fact that the individual's self-evaluation must be excessively influenced by body weight and shape, and that the bulimic behavior must not occur solely during episodes of AN.

DSM-IV-TR also specifies two subtypes of BN: the purging type is used for individuals who regularly engage in self-induced vomiting or laxative abuse following binge episodes; the nonpurging type is used for individuals who use fasting or excessive exercise, but not self-induced vomiting or laxative/diuretic use following binge episodes. Although BN has been found to have a 1% to 3% prevalence rate in females, data on high school girls indicate that the prevalence may be more accurately estimated at 8%. Similar to AN, BN is much more common in females than males. The mean age of onset of binge eating is typically reported as age 17, with purging symptoms beginning approximately 1 year following the onset of binge eating. The full syndrome of BN has been identified in girls as young as age 11. BN is often a hidden disorder and may occur in a variety of weight ranges depending on the amount of food consumed during eating binges and the effectiveness of the compensatory measures. Adolescents with BN at normal body weight are of particular concern as their symptoms may go undetected for extended periods of time. Parents and clinicians must take care to consider the possibility of significant eating issues, even in individuals with normative body weight. In addition to eating disorder symptomatology, BN is associated with depressive problems as well as problems in social relationships. Shoplifting as well as stealing food are common associated symptoms (APA, 2000; Kronenberger & Meyer, 2001).

EDNOS is a residual category in *DSM-IV-TR* used for disorders of eating that do not meet the criteria for any specific eating disorder. This category is commonly used for cases of AN in which there has been significant weight loss but the individual's current weight continues to fall within the normal range, or cases of BN that do not meet the frequency/duration criteria. It is not clear to what extent individuals diagnosed with EDNOS should follow similar conceptual and treatment paths as those diagnosed with AN and BN.

BED is a proposed diagnosis in *DSM-IV-TR*. The essential features are recurrent episodes of binge eating for which there is marked distress, in the absence of regular inappropriate compensatory behaviors. The binge eating is expected to occur, on average, at least 2 days per week for 6 months. Support for the BED research criteria are drawn from weight-control programs in which a mean prevalence rate of 30% has been reported. There is less of a gender split in BED, with females outnumbering males only 1.5:1. The prevalence rate for BED in non-patient community samples has been reported at 0.7% to 4%. The onset of BED is reported in late adolescence. BED is associated with a long history of dieting attempts. Individuals with BED report that their eating or weight interferes with their relationships with other people, with their work or school, and with their self-esteem. They also report body dissatisfaction, symptoms of depression and anxiety, somatic concerns, and interpersonal problems (APA, 2000; Kronenberger & Meyer, 2001).

Although a complete review of etiological factors for AN and BN is beyond the scope of this contribution, it is important to review recent research pertaining to the development of these disorders. The factors reviewed will undoubtedly have some application in the cases of EDNOS and BED, but the lack of diagnostic clarity regarding these categories prevents firm conclusions. In borrowing from Polivy and Herman's (2002) work, the causal factors will be organized into three clusters: sociocultural contributors to eating disorders, familial influences on eating disorders, and individual risk factors. Sociocultural factors address the fact that eating disorders do not present in all cultures at all times. Rather, eating disorders appear to present in cultures of abundance which value a thin-ideal. The media is often identified as an important contributory factor in promoting an unrealistic thin-ideal. Peer influence is also commonly cited as a contributor to eating disorders, because adolescent girls learn about the importance of being thin as well as extreme weight control measures from their peers. A number of familial factors that contribute to eating disorders have been identified. Family members may perpetuate an eating disorder by reinforcing attempts to be slender and perfectionistic. Family dynamics have been implicated, with eating-disordered families being described as enmeshed, intrusive, hostile, and negating of the individual's emotional needs. Moreover, the families have been described as critical, with coercive parental control and greater parental intrusiveness. Mothers of eating-disordered patients have been found to exhibit more eating-disordered symptoms themselves and are more dissatisfied with the family's general functioning.

Although negative family influences clearly contribute to the development of eating disorders, additional individual vulnerability factors are needed to explain the emergence of an eating disorder. Many individual factors have been proposed as contributing to the development of an eating disorder. Those interpersonal experiences most frequently cited include abuse, trauma, and teasing. Although teasing may lead to low self-esteem, depressed mood, and anxiety, abuse (physical, sexual, and emotional) may produce intolerable emotions and undermine identity. An eating disorder can assist individuals in dealing with emotional and identity problems by refocusing their attention on weight, shape, and eating and reestablishing a sense of control. Additional individual factors that have been identified as contributing to eating disorders include affective influences, particularly negative emotional states, low self-esteem, body dissatisfaction; and cognitive factors such as obsessive thoughts, inaccurate judgments, and rigid thinking patterns. Finally, individual biological factors have been proposed, including a genetic vulnerability to eating disorders, neuroendocrine factors linked to appetite, and a lack of internal awareness in accurately identifying internal states of hunger and satiety as well as emotional states (Polivy & Herman, 2002).

THE ROLE OF CULTURAL AND DEVELOPMENTAL FACTORS IN CHILD AND ADOLESCENT EATING DISORDERS

Cultural Factors

Historically, eating disorders have been viewed as a problem impacting White women. Early accounts of anorexia nervosa focused on European girls and women and highlighted Western culture as an important context for the disorder. Cross-cultural studies reported significantly higher prevalence rates for eating disorders among females in Western as opposed to non-Western societies. More recently, epidemiological studies have indicated that increasing numbers of Black American, Hispanic American, and Native American girls and women as well as girls and women in non-Western societies experience eating disorders (Smolak, Levine, & Striegel-Moore, 1996).

A key challenge to efforts to better understand eating disorders among ethnic groups is the fact that eating disorder diagnoses are based primarily on the clinical presentation of White girls and women. Little research has been done to clarify how symptom presentation may vary across ethnic groups. For example, key features of eating disorders in White populations, such as fear of fatness, feelings of loss of control, and body image distortion, may not be applicable to ethnic minorities. Three aspects of ethnicity that may have importance in understanding eating disorders among ethnic girls and women include (a) cultural norms about female beauty, (b) experiences associated with minority status, and (c) ethnic identity.

Cultural Norms About Female Beauty

There is substantial literature that has highlighted Western culture's thin-ideal, a focus on physical beauty as a central feature of femininity, and chronic dieting behavior as key risk factors in the development of eating disorders. Research focused on ethnic differences regarding ideal female beauty has yielded mixed results, with some ethnic groups reporting larger ideal body sizes than White populations and others choosing body shapes as thin as those chosen by White women. Although studies of White populations have consistently shown that overweight girls and women experience considerable social pressure in the form of weight-related teasing, criticism, and discrimination, studies of Black girls and women have identified less social pressure to conform to the thin-ideal than among White women (Smolak et al., 1996).

Experiences Associated With Minority Status

Ethnic girls and women are more likely than their White counterparts to experience stressful life conditions such as poverty and discrimination. As stressful life events have been found to be significantly correlated with subsequent psychiatric impairment, it is important to consider how stressful experiences related to minority status may function as a risk factor in the development of eating disorders. The stress of racially related insults and discrimination may result in feelings of frustration and isolation which may lead to binge eating. Pressure to assimilate to White culture may lead ethnic girls to abandon their culture's beauty ideals and adopt the thin-ideal and associated chronic dieting behavior of White culture. Ethnic girls finding themselves in the role of the "token" or "model" ethnic minority may become more perfectionistic, contributing to a vulnerability for the development of an eating disorder (Smolak et al., 1996).

Ethnic Identity

Harris and Kuba (1997) have focused extensively on the relationship between ethnocultural identity and eating disorders in women of color. Although their work has focused primarily on an adult population, their model is developmental in nature and thus has application in understanding eating disorder issues in adolescent girls. Harris and Kuba provide a framework for understanding eating disorders from a cultural perspective. They propose that "eating disorders may be symptomatic of conflicting cultural demands for beauty and acceptance. The suppression of these conflicting demands through internalized oppression may result in specific disordered eating symptoms. Understanding these demands is important for accurate identification and clinical treatment of eating disorders" (Harris & Kuba, 1997, p. 341). Thus, Harris and Kuba suggest that a key to eating disorders is found in the interaction between ethnocultural identity confusion and conflicts in cultural concepts of beauty or attractiveness. The personal definition of beauty and resulting self-image is initially guided by a woman's culture of origin. It may become problematic when her cultural concept of beauty is in conflict with the definition put forward by another culture. An eating disorder may be a means of suppressing one's ethnocultural concept of beauty by replacing it with a Eurocentric one of thinness. To help young women become more aware of these unconscious oppressive responses and their impact on identity development, an assessment of their ethnic identity development should be conducted.

Developmental Issues Relating to the Diagnosis of AN, BN, and BED

It is important to recognize that there has been little focus on diagnostic issues relating to AN, BN, and BED in children. Thelen, Lawrence, and Powell (1992) note diagnostic issues that may occur when attempting to assess eating disorder symptomatology in children. One problem relates to the validity of information obtained from children, as children will likely be hesitant to disclose binge eating and purging behavior for fear of negative consequences from parents. Moreover, children may have difficulty understanding the meaning of key terms such as binging and restricting caloric intake when utilizing self-report measures. Eating disorder symptomatology in children may present differently than that in older adolescents and adults. For example, children may display behaviors such as slow eating, food rituals, hoarding, scavenging, and hiding of food, but not express a fear of fatness, distorted body image, or fear of loss of control over their eating that is key to an eating disorder diagnosis. Finally, there is concern that although AN is sometimes detected in prepubertal children as a result of the marked weight loss that becomes obvious to parents and/or professionals, BN is less likely to be detected due to the potential absence of visible symptoms. Thus, BN as well as BED may be occurring in younger populations. An alternate reason for the low diagnosis of BN in children relates to the secrecy of this disorder. Given the limited resources of young children, they may not have access to the food and monetary resources required to engage in binge eating behavior nor have sufficient secrecy to maintain their binging and purging.

The Importance of a Developmental Model: The Early Adolescent Transition

Early adolescence is a period marked by significant developmental changes in physical growth, cognitive functioning, social roles and demands, peer and familial relationships, and identity issues. A developmental model is important in understanding why eating disorder concerns often emerge in adolescence (Brooks-Gunn & Attie, 1996; Smolak et al., 1996). It is important to understand eating problems in the context of challenges that confront individuals during this phase of development, namely, adjustment to the physical changes of puberty within a cultural climate that values the prepubertal figure over the mature female body, the loosening of ties to parents and transition toward increasing psychological and physical autonomy, and the development of a stable personality structure for regulating mood, impulse-control, and self-esteem. Moreover, early adolescence offers a unique opportunity for examining the development of eating problems within the framework of a model emphasizing changes in weight, in intimate relationships, and in achievement status. During puberty, body shape becomes increasingly important to self-esteem. Although many girls have positive feelings about breast development and increases in height, they typically report negative feelings about the weight gain and increase in fat deposits associated with this developmental stage. Not surprisingly, body image is the one aspect of self-esteem found to consistently decline in early adolescence. Coinciding with the weight gain in puberty is the adolescent girl's increased concern with appearance and desire to be popular. As most adolescent girls begin dating between the ages of 13 and 14, this can be a very stressful time. Because of the link between slenderness and attractiveness, many adolescent girls begin dieting at this time. Threats to an adolescent's sense of achievement include academic problems as well as threats of failure in athletic or extracurricular activities. Achievement threats are likely to predict disordered eating when the threats occur simultaneously with puberty and first dating, and when the adolescent has unrealistically high standards in a variety of areas. In this event, the threats to her high standards can result in feelings of anxiety, depression, feeling out of control, and feeling fat. When confronted with these negative emotions, adolescent girls may turn to thinness and weight control as the most clear-cut solutions (Smolak et al., 1996).

ASSESSMENT OF CHILD AND ADOLESCENT EATING DISORDERS

The purpose of this section is to address key issues in the assessment of eating disorder symptoms in child and adolescent populations. As childhood feeding disorders are relatively rare, few instruments are available to assist the practitioner in identifying key symptoms. Although numerous measures have been developed for the assessment of symptoms of AN, BN, and BED, these instruments have typically been developed for adult populations. As a result, the appropriateness of utilizing many of these measures with child and adolescent clients is questionable. Despite the fact that the majority of instruments have been normed on adult populations, there have been some attempts to develop instruments that are more developmentally appropriate for children and adolescents. Unfortunately, there is no general directory that summarizes these measures, and many of them are difficult to access. In the following section, we will address current attempts to assess eating disorder symptomatology in children and adolescents in four major categories: (a) self-report questionnaires, (b) clinical interviews, (c) self-monitoring, and (d) eating disorder-specific measures. Please note that this will not be an exhaustive review of all existing assessment measures that fall into each category. Rather, our attempt is to highlight key examples of measures in each category that attempt to be developmentally sensitive to child and/or adolescent populations. Narrative information on child and adolescent eating disorder measures can be found in the following text, and an abbreviated listing of the measures can be found in Table 1 below.

Self-Report Questionnaires

Self-report questionnaires in general are significantly limited by the fact that, although many of the core features of eating disorders are complex, definitions on questionnaires are often vague and subject to a wide variety of interpretations. Therefore, the accuracy of self-report instruments for children and adolescents is questionable. Consequently, accurate assessment needs to take into account the context in which the behavior occurred. There are a number of self-report questionnaires available for the assessment of eating disorders in children and adolescents.

The Bulimia Test-Revised (BULIT-R; Thelen et al., 1991) was developed to measure the symptoms of bulimia nervosa in individuals age 16 and older. The BULIT-R has 28 items that are scored and 8 items pertaining to weight-control behavior that are unscored. Questions are answered using a multiple-choice format. Questions are answered by choosing one of the following response options: always, almost always, frequently, sometimes, seldom, or never. Advantages of the BULIT-R include that it is very easy to read, the instructions are clear, and it can be administered in about 10 minutes. If you are interested in diagnosing bulimia nervosa, measuring the severity of bulimic symptoms, or measuring treatment outcomes, the BULIT-R is found to be particularly useful (McCarthy et al., 2002; Williamson & Netemeyer, 2000).

The Bulimic Investigatory Test, Edinburgh (BITE; Henderson & Freeman, 1987) is a 33-item self-report measure composed of yes/no questions as well as 5-, 6-, and 7-point Likert-type rating scales, designed to identify subjects with symptoms of bulimia or binge eating. It can be used to identify binge eaters or as a screening instrument for use in a clinical setting. In addition, it serves as a useful measure of severity and response to treatment. The BITE consists of two subscales: the Symptom Scale, which measures the degree of symptoms present, and the Severity Scale, which provides an index of the severity of binging and purging behavior as defined by their frequency. When the BITE is used as a screening instrument or in survey work, the subjects should be asked to complete the questionnaire based on their feelings and behavior over the past 3 months. When the BITE is used as a measure of response to treatment, only the past month should be considered. The BITE would be appropriate when used with subjects 16 years or older. The average time for completion of the questionnaire is less than 10 minutes. In addition, the BITE is easy to administer and simple to score. A copy of the BITE can be found in Henderson and Freeman's (1987) article as well as in the *Handbook of Assessment Methods for Eating Behaviors and Weight-Related Problems: Measures, Theory and Research* (Allison, 1995).

TABLE 1: Assessment Measures for Child and Adolescent Eating Disorders

DOMAIN	MEASURE	PROPERTIES	SOURCE
Self-Report Questionnaires			
	Bulimia Test-Revised (BULIT-R)	36 items Multiple choice 16+ years	Thelen et al. (1991)
	Bulimic Investigatory Test (BITE)	33 items Format varied 16+ years	Henderson and Freeman (1987)

TABLE 1 *(Continued)*

DOMAIN	MEASURE	PROPERTIES	SOURCE
Self-Report Questionnaires *(Continued)*	Children's Body Image Scale (CBIS)	4 items 7 side profiles 7-12 years	Truby and Paxton (2002)
	Children's Eating Attitudes Test (ChEAT)	26 items 6-point rating 8-13 years	Maloney, McGuire, and Daniels (1988)
	Eating and Me (E & M)	19 items 6-point rating 10-12 years	Sands et al. (1997)
	Eating Attitudes Test (EAT-26)	26 items 6-point ratings 14+ years	Garner et al. (1982)
	Eating Behaviors and Body Image Test for Preadolescent Girls (EBBIT)	38 items 4-point rating Fourth grade & up	Candy and Fee (1998a, 1998b)
	Eating Disorder Inventory-3 (EDI-3)	91 items 5-point rating 12+ years	Garner (2005)
	Eating Disorder Examination-Questionnaire (EDE-Q)	38 items Format varied 15+ years	Fairburn and Beglin (1994)
	Kids' Eating Disorders Survey (KEDS)	14 items Format varied 8-18 years	Childress et al. (1993)
	Questionnaire of Eating and Weight Patterns, Adolescent Version (QEWP-A)	27 items Format varied 12-18 years	Johnson et al. (1999)
Clinical Interviews			
	Eating Disorders Examination, Child Version (ChEDE)	62 questions Semistructured 7-14 years old	Bryant-Waugh et al. (1996)
	Eating Disorders Examination (EDE)	62 questions Semistructured 15+ years 7-point rating	Fairburn and Cooper (1993)
Eating Disorder-Specific Measures			
	Behaviors of Eating and Activity for Children's Health Evaluation System (BEACHES)	Observations Coding system 4-8 years	McKenzie et al. (1991)
	Children's Eating Behavior Inventory (CEBI)	40 items Format varied 2-12 years 5-point rating	Archer et al. (1991)
	Screening Tool of Feeding Problems (STEP)	23 items 3-point rating 14+ years	Matson and Kuhn (2001)

The Children's Body Image Scale (CBIS; Truby & Paxton, 2002) was developed to measure body size perception and body size dissatisfaction in girls and boys age 7 or older. The CBIS consists of seven figures of known body mass index (BMI), ranging from the "thinnest" to the "fattest." Children are asked questions regarding their perceived body figure as well as their ideal body figure. Additional information can be obtained in the Truby and Paxton (2002) article. A copy is presented on pages 125 to 126.

The Children's Eating Attitudes Test (ChEAT; Maloney, McGuire, & Daniels, 1988) was designed to assess children's attitudes toward their eating and dieting behavior. The authors modified the Eating Attitudes Test (EAT; Garner & Garfinkel, 1979), which was developed and tested on adolescents and adults. The ChEAT is a 26-item questionnaire that contains a 6-point, Likert-type rating scale on which respondents are required to mark their response to questions about perceived body image, obsessions/preoccupations with food, and dieting practices. The standardization sample consisted of 318 elementary school-aged children ranging in age from 8 to 13 years. The children were predominantly White and from middle to upper socioeconomic backgrounds. The time for completion of the ChEAT, including providing directions, is about 30 minutes. The ChEAT is appended in the Maloney et al. (1988) article as well as in the *Handbook of Assessment Methods for Eating Behaviors and Weight-Related Problems: Measures, Theory, and Research* (Allison, 1995).

The Eating and Me scale (E & M; Sands et al., 1997) was adapted from the Eating Disorder Inventory (EDI; Garner, Olmstead, & Polivy, 1983) and the Eating Attitudes Test (EAT; Garner & Garfinkel, 1979). The E & M scale consists of items drawn from the three subdomains of body dissatisfaction, dieting, and bulimia. The normative sample for the E & M consisted of elementary school-age children ranging in age from 10 to 12 years. The original EDI and EAT instruments were thought to be inappropriate for this preadolescent school-age population because of their length and complicated language. The E & M consists of 19 statements using a 6-point scale ranging from "never" to "always." The E & M scale is a useful tool for measuring eating/dieting behaviors of children. The authors (Sands et al., 1997) should be contacted for more information on the E & M scale.

The Eating Attitudes Test (EAT-26; Garner et al., 1982) is a 26-item measure developed as a clinical screening tool for the assessment of behaviors and attitudes characteristic of people with anorexia nervosa and bulimia nervosa. The EAT-26 is commonly used with individuals age 14 and above. Each item is answered on a 6-point, Likert-type rating scale. Administration of the EAT-26 takes less than 10 minutes. Additional information on the EAT can be found in the Garner et al. (1982) article.

The Eating Behaviors and Body Image Test for Preadolescent Girls (EBBIT; Candy & Fee, 1998a, 1998b) is a 38-item self-report questionnaire that consists of two factors. Factor one measures restrictive eating behaviors and body image dissatisfaction (Body Image Dissatisfaction/Restrictive Eating; BIDRE). Factor two is a measure of binge eating (Binge Eating Behaviors: BEB). The degree to which the respondent engages in the behaviors is assessed using a 4-point, Likert-type scale. The EBBIT has been studied in girls as young as fourth grade. The EBBIT appears to be more appropriate for preadolescent children than the EAT-26 or the Eating Disorder Inventory-2 (Garner, 1991b), but it has received less research or clinical attention. Additional information on the EBBIT can be obtained from the Candy and Fee (1998a, 1998b) article. A copy of the items and instructions for the administration, scoring, and interpretation are included in this volume on pages 231 to 238.

The Eating Disorder Inventory-2 (EDI-2; Garner, 1991b) is a 91-item self-report measure designed to assess psychological characteristics and symptoms common to anorexia and bulimia nervosa. The EDI-2 is appropriate for ages 12 and up. It is composed of 11 subscales. Three of the subscales were designed to assess attitudes and behaviors toward weight, body shape, and eating (Drive for Thinness, Bulimia, and Body Dissatisfaction). Five of the subscales measure more general psychological characteristics of persons with an eating disorder (Ineffectiveness, Perfection, Interpersonal Distrust, Interoceptive Awareness, and Maturity Fears). The remaining three subscales are Asceticism, Impulse Regulation, and Social Insecurity. Items on the EDI-2 are presented in a 6-point, forced choice format. Respondents rate whether each item applies "always," "usually," "often," "sometimes," "rarely," or "never." The EDI-2 is a widely used questionnaire that is easy to administer and score. The administration time for the EDI-2 is 20 minutes. The EDI-2 can be used as a screening instrument to detect at-risk populations, and it can be used for diagnosis. It also appears to be useful for differentiating level of severity and/or subtypes of anorexia or bulimia nervosa, and it can be used as a treatment outcome measure.

The Eating Disorder Inventory, child version (EDI-C; Garner, 1991a) is a modification of the EDI-2 that is formulated for children and adolescents. It is an extensive self-report assessment of eating disordered attitudes and behaviors and personality traits that is appropriate for children as young as 8 years old. While the majority of the questions remain the same as in the EDI-2, the wording of about one-third of the items has been changed to better suit younger respondents (Garner, 1991a). The EDI-C also has 91 items and reportedly has the same component subscales as the EDI-2. Recent research on the psychometric properties of the EDI-C indicates that instead of the original 11-factor structure of the EDI-2, only 5 reliable factors are evident on the EDI-C including Drive for Thinness, Emotional Disturbance/Affective Instability, Self-Esteem, Overeating/Binge Eating, and Maturity Fears. Thus while preliminary research indicates that many of the original items on the EDI-2 may have limited relevance among children, the 5 aforementioned factors appear to provide valuable information on eating disorder symptomatology in children (Eklund, Paavonen, & Almquist, 2005).

The Eating Disorder Inventory-3 (EDI-3; Garner, 2005) is a recent revision of the EDI-2 which retains the item set from the original EDI and EDI-2 while providing scales and composites more consistent with current theories and research on eating disorders. The EDI-3 consists of 91 items organized into 12 scales including 3 eating-disorder specific scales and 9 general scales. The EDI-3 also yields 6 composites including one that is eating-disorder specific (Eating Disorder Risk) and 5 that are general psychological constructs (Ineffectiveness, Interpersonal Problems, Affective Problems, Overcontrol, and General Psychological Maladjustment). Innovative aspects of the EDI-3 include a referral form (EDI-3 RF), a symptom checklist (EDI-3 SC), and a computer-based scoring program (EDI-3 SP). The EDI-3 RF can be administered to determine if an individual should be referred for a professional evaluation. The EDI-3 SC can facilitate systematic data gathering in order to determine whether the individual meets the criteria for an eating disorder diagnosis. The EDI-3 SP generates an individualized scoring report and clinical profile for each client (Garner, 2005). The EDI-3 can be purchased from Psychological Assessment Resources (www.parinc.com).

The Kids' Eating Disorders Survey (KEDS; Childress et al., 1993) is a 14-item self-report measure that includes a set of eight child figure drawings for each gender to graphically assess weight and body dissatisfaction. The KEDS is an easily administered screening instrument appropriate for children and adolescents between the ages of 8 and 18. The KEDS does not purport to make a diagnosis of an eating disorder, but is able to identify serious symptoms that warrant further investigation. Two factors have been identified by the KEDS: a weight dissatisfaction component and a purging/restricting component. A copy of the KEDS is appended to the Childress et al. (1993) article.

The Questionnaire on Eating and Weight Patterns, Adolescent Version (QEWP-A; Johnson et al., 1999) is based on the Questionnaire on Eating and Weight Patterns-Revised (QEWP-R; Spitzer, Yanovski, & Marcus, 1993) and differs from the original version in that simpler synonyms are substituted for a few difficult words. In addition, two items from the original QEWP (Questions 9 and 12) were combined to form a single, two-part question. The QEWP-A has 27 items that assess binge eating and purging. The measure is designed to identify individuals meeting criteria for binge eating disorder. The strength of the QEWP-A is that it is a criterion-based instrument that assesses the essential diagnostic criteria for purging and nonpurging bulimia as well as binge eating disorder. Additional information on the QEWP-A can be obtained from the Johnson et al. (1999) article.

Clinical Interviews

The clinical interview is the most common method of assessing eating-disordered behavior in children and adolescents and can vary from less structured formats, in which the clinician generates a series of questions in order to clarify the nature of the eating problems, to more structured interview formats such as the Eating Disorders Examination (EDE; Fairburn & Cooper, 1993) and the child version of the EDE (ChEDE; Bryant-Waugh et al., 1996). Regardless of the type of interview, it is essential that *DSM-IV-TR* diagnostic criteria are carefully reviewed. Specific questions must be asked about the nature, frequency, and course of the eating behavior. For example, when interviewing adolescents with BN, it is important to ascertain exactly what constitutes an eating binge as well as their pattern of use of extreme weight control measures. Although parents are typically interviewed regarding the feeding and eating disorders of infancy or early childhood, adolescents provide much of the specific information regarding AN, BN, and BED. The importance of establishing rapport and communicating a nonjudgmental attitude cannot be overemphasized, as adolescents will be understandably hesitant and resistant to provide specific information about their eating behavior. It is helpful for clinicians to communicate their experience and understanding of eating disorders and the fact that they are not shocked or surprised by the patient's particular behaviors. It is also important to communicate an understanding of the ambivalence adolescents may feel regarding changing their eating behavior. As adolescents with eating disorders are often unreliable informants, it may be helpful to verify information with collateral sources such as parents, other family members, or peers. Crowther and Sherwood (1997) provide an excellent discussion of process and content issues in eating disorder interviews that are relevant in working with children and adolescents. Specific questions must address weight and body image, such as the adolescent's current height and weight, highest and lowest weights, ideal weight, history of teasing or negative comments received regarding body shape or weight, and perceptions of one's weight. Crowther and Sherwood (1997) note that body image must be explored as a disturbance in perception (i.e., body image distortion), a disturbance in thoughts and feelings (i.e., body image dissatisfaction), and a disturbance in behavior (i.e., body image avoidance).

The Eating Disorders Examination (EDE; Fairburn & Cooper, 1993) is a semistructured interview for the assessment of eating disorders in individuals age 15 and above. The EDE contains 62 questions that are scored on a 7-point rating scale. For each item, there is at least one mandatory probe question and several optional questions. The EDE can be used both to assess the present state of symptoms over the previous 4 weeks and to generate operationally defined diagnoses for all of the eating disorders based upon assessment of a 3-month period. The EDE identifies three types of eating episodes: objective bulimic episodes, subjective bulimic episodes, and objective overeating. The EDE also provides a detailed assessment of dietary restriction. Items probe such areas as the avoidance of particular foods, self-imposed dietary rules and reactions to their violation, skipping meals, and preoccupation with food. The child version of the EDE is known as the ChEDE (Bryant-Waugh et al., 1996). It was adapted for children between the ages of 7 and 14 by slightly modifying the language to improve understanding by young children, assessing critical overevaluation of shape and weight through the use of a sort task, and taking special care to provide examples to help explain difficult concepts. Both the EDE and ChEDE are easily administered by a trained clinician and take from 30 minutes to 1 hour to complete. Additional information on the EDE and ChEDE can be found in the Fairburn and Cooper (1993) and Bryant-Waugh et al. (1996) articles. There is also a questionnaire form of the EDE known as the Eating Disorders Examination-Questionnaire

(EDE-Q; Fairburn & Beglin, 1994). It is a 38-item questionnaire used with adolescents 15 and above. Some of the items on the EDE-Q are rated in terms of number of days, and some individuals find this format to be difficult to use. In addition, determination of frequency of different types of eating episodes is more reliable with the EDE. Therefore, the EDE-Q may not be as valid as the interview measure. However, the EDE-Q may be useful to track change over time once clients have been instructed about the nature and size of binges.

Self-Monitoring

Self-monitoring of food intake and use of extreme weight control measures is an important part of the initial assessment as well as cognitive-behavioral interventions with children and adolescents diagnosed with AN, BN, and BED. Self-monitoring can provide information about the regularity of meals and snacks as well as eating binges and use of extreme weight control measures. In addition, information can be obtained regarding the amount and kind of food eaten, the time of day that the eating occurred, and thoughts and feelings associated with the eating episode (Crowther & Sherwood, 1997). Although clinicians use homemade self-monitoring forms or food diaries as well as ones that have been published, few forms have been created with a child and adolescent population in mind. An adaptation of a self-monitoring form originally created by Crowther, Lingswiler, and Stephens (1984) can be found on page 127. Although the basic structure of the form is unchanged, the language and format have been modified to make the self-monitoring form more engaging for individuals between the approximate ages of 10 and 18. (You may contact Dr. Wolf for a full-color electronic copy of the modified self-monitoring form.) When using the sample food diary, each form is to be completed for each eating occurrence in the course of a day by filling in the day and date as well as circling the time, location, mood, and individuals present during the eating episode and specifying the amount and type of food eaten. The sample form also includes questions regarding whether the food eaten was part of a meal and whether the individual binged or purged. It is important that clinicians not assume that clients will self-monitor accurately from the start. Rather, training in self-monitoring will have to occur and include such things as explanation of terms such as binge/purge, the importance of completing forms immediately after eating, the need of completing forms on all days rather than only when eating has been "good," and the tendency to feel ashamed of what one has eaten. Reinforcement for compliance with self-monitoring is recommended in the form of verbal praise, small prizes, or tokens. Although the length of self-monitoring varies among clinicians, the most common baseline period is 2 weeks.

Eating Disorder-Specific Measures

A variety of measures have been developed to assess particular aspects of eating disorders in children and adolescents as reported by their parents, guardians, or other informants such as health care professionals. The Behaviors of Eating and Activity for Children's Health Evaluation System (BEACHES; McKenzie et al., 1991) is a coding system that was developed to quantify direct observations of children's eating behavior and physical activity. Data are coded simultaneously on 10 different dimensions, including aspects of the physical environment, the child's level of activity and eating behavior, and the verbal and physical prompts and consequences that influence the child's consumption of food or activity level. BEACHES is appropriate for children 4 to 8 years of age. Observations are to be made once a week at the child's home or school over an 8-week period. Extensive training is necessary before observers' ratings are considered reliable, which can make BEACHES very expensive to use. A copy of BEACHES can be found in the *Handbook of Assessment Methods for Eating Behaviors and Weight-Related Problems: Measures, Theory, and Research* (Allison, 1995). Additionally, a brief description of the coding dimensions is presented in the McKenzie et al. (1991) article, or the complete coding definitions can be obtained from them.

The Children's Eating Behavior Inventory (CEBI; Archer, Rosenbaum, & Streiner, 1991) was designed to assess eating and mealtime behavior. The 40-item questionnaire contains yes/no questions and a 5-point, Likert-type rating scale and is divided into two domains: child and parent. In the child domain, 28 items are used to gather information about the child's food preferences and dislikes, self-feeding skills, and compliance during mealtimes. In the parent domain, the parents' interactions with family members are surveyed, along with their perceived stresses about mealtime events. The normative sample for the CEBI consisted of children ranging in age from 2 to 12 years of age. The CEBI has items that are easy to read with clear instructions for completing the questionnaire in about 15 minutes. The CEBI can be reproduced from the Archer et al. (1991) article. In addition, a revised, briefer version of the CEBI is reproduced in the *Handbook of Assessment Methods for Eating Behaviors and Weight-Related Problems: Measures, Theory, and Research* (Allison, 1995).

The Screening Tool of Feeding Problems (STEP; Matson & Kuhn, 2001) was designed for the purpose of quickly and efficiently identifying feeding and mealtime behavior problems in individuals with intellectual disabilities. The STEP consists of 23 items, each targeting a specific feeding problem. Staff familiar with the client being assessed are questioned about discrete behaviors they may have observed the client engage in during the last month they worked with him or her. The informants are instructed to respond to the items along two dimensions, frequency and severity. Each dimension is rated on a 3-point, Likert-type scale. The general categories of feeding problems include aspiration risk, selectivity, feeding skills, food refusal-related behavior problems, and nutrition-related behavior problems. The STEP can be administered to individuals as young as 14 years of age and takes approximately 4 minutes to complete. Additional information on the STEP can be found in the Matson and Kuhn (2001) article or by contacting Matson and Kuhn directly.

TREATMENT OF CHILD AND ADOLESCENT EATING DISORDERS

Treatment of Feeding and Eating Disorders of Infancy or Early Childhood

Pica

Although a number of treatments for pica have been described that use a variety of medical, nutritional, or behavioral interventions, it is clear that there is no single treatment of choice, and it is unlikely that any one single treatment strategy will effectively address the entire spectrum of pica behaviors. Because there are no clear guidelines, the selection of an appropriate treatment for a particular form of pica is a complex process. The nutritional and dietary approaches that have been used have demonstrated success in a limited number of cases, but in general, behavioral methods have been used most often and have resulted in the greatest reductions of pica.

Several behavioral techniques have been used in the treatment of pica. Antecedent strategies, such as environmental stimulation, discrimination training, and alternate sensory activities, involve the manipulation of conditions or stimuli that occur just before a behavior and are assumed to set the stage for the occurrence of that particular behavior. Modifying antecedent conditions is a socially acceptable form of treatment because it is nonintrusive, nonaversive, safe, and generally effective. For these reasons, antecedent strategies are often used as the initial form of treatment. Environmental stimulation has a positive impact on the occurrence of pica by making changes in the environmental conditions. Discrimination training attempts to directly modify the occurrence of the behavior by changing the individual's response to the antecedent stimulus. This procedure is based on the assumption that pica is less likely if the individual is able to discriminate between those items that are edible and those that are not. Discrimination training has been shown to be effective alone or in combination with other behavioral techniques. Alternate sensory activities are based on the idea that socially appropriate alternate activities can be used to set the occasion for less harmful sensory activities than pica through the use of sensory reinforcement. When using sensory reinforcement, it is important to remember that, once pica has been reduced to a satisfactory level, other procedures will be required to allow the individual to safely use age-appropriate materials. Response-contingent strategies, such as differential reinforcement procedures, screening procedures, aversive tastes, aversive odor and water mist, brief physical restraint, and overcorrection, involves the use of consequences that follow the occurrence of the undesirable behavior, or pica. Differential reinforcement techniques used in the management of pica range from general to very specific (Ellis, Singh, et al., 1997).

Rumination Disorder

Treatments for rumination disorder reflect the major features of the disorder. Considering that virtually all children with rumination disorder are cognitively limited by age or intellectual deficit, individual psychotherapy is rarely an option. Because medical causes for the behavior are ruled out in the process of formulating the diagnosis, medication alone is usually not effective in eliminating symptoms. Therefore, treatments for rumination disorder must rely on the child's environment and behavior to produce change. Specifically, this change can be achieved through the use of family and behavioral interventions (Kronenberger & Meyer, 2001).

Two family interventions used to treat rumination disorder are parent-child relationship therapy and family-marital therapy. Parent-child relationship therapy emphasizes the need for the infant to have a warm, stimulating environment and a supportive relationship with the parent. Staff provide parents with support and guidance and encourage parents to modify their behavior to meet the infant's emotional and bonding needs. The goal of this therapy is regular, nonthreatening, supportive interactions which occur initially under supervision, then later at home. This intervention may be combined with parent skills training which focuses on education about child development and parenting techniques as well as attending to any of the parents' adjustment problems.

Traditional family or marital therapy for parents of children with rumination disorder seeks to address familial problems that drive maladaptive and nonnurturing interactions between parents and children. The type of therapy specifically assesses the role of the child and the rumination disorder in the family system in order to provide the family with suggestions on how to modify the system to make it incompatible with the rumination behavior. In addition, there is a focus on keeping marital conflicts within the spousal subsystem, which insulates the infant from parental conflicts that may result in stress and less nurturing behavior. Both parent-child and family-marital therapy for rumination disorder have been criticized due to slow progress and high demands on staff. As a result, family-based interventions are often combined with other interventions (Kronenberger & Meyer, 2001).

A review of behavioral literature reveals several effective interventions based on the principles of dietary control, reinforcement, or punishment. Special feeding techniques used to treat rumination require the infant's active participation in the feeding process. Oral movements are required to express liquid from a nipple or to remove food from a spoon. Various means can be used to encourage oral activity including increasing the length of time the nipple or spoon is in the mouth and moving the nipple or spoon around in the mouth to increase taste and tactile sensation. These techniques are successful in reducing the frequency of rumination and are easily implemented by the usual caretakers of the infant in their natural setting and with minimal training. Food satiation is another technique used in the treatment of rumination. Because eating food is a pleasurable experience for many individuals with rumination, the repeated ingestion of regurgitated food serves as a positive reinforcer for the continued occurrence of the behavior. Food satiation interventions involve manipulation of the quantity of food an individual eats and are based on the assumption that the consumption of excessive amounts of food will cause the food to be less appealing. The decrease in the reinforcement value of the food subsequently results in a decrease in the occurrence of rumination. An advantage of the food satiation intervention is that it can be incorporated into an individual's mealtime routine because no special techniques or changes in the type of food served are required. Because the increased consumption of certain foods may result in excessive weight gain, consideration should be given to overall dietary management (Ellis, Parr, et al., 1997).

Several reinforcement procedures have also been implemented to decrease rumination. Overcorrection for rumination involves responses in which the child restores the environment to its previous state and practices desired responses. Specifically, the child must clean up the vomit, change clothes, brush teeth several times, and gargle with an oral antiseptic. Overcorrection for self-stimulating rumination has been shown to be effective and is often combined with other techniques. Extinction involves withholding the reinforcement that is maintaining the rumination behavior. Identification of the reinforcement is critical and usually requires careful behavioral assessment. Differential Reinforcement of Other Behavior (DRO) and Differential Reinforcement of Incompatible Behavior (DRI) are useful in providing the child with substitute responses for rumination (Kronenberger & Meyer, 2001).

Punishment strategies used to reduce the frequency of rumination can take several forms, including the presentation of an aversive stimulus, the removal of a positive stimulus, or the requirement that the individual engage in an effort-based activity following the occurrence of rumination or one of its precursors. Due to numerous legal and ethical issues, punishment is rarely used as a first-line treatment; however, it often leads to a more rapid reduction in rumination than other procedures, specifically when other treatments have proven ineffective or the rumination has become life-threatening. The most widely used and ethically acceptable aversive stimuli are strong negative-tasting liquids such as Tabasco sauce or highly concentrated lemon juice (Ellis, Parr, et al., 1997).

Feeding Disorder of Infancy or Early Childhood

Treatments for feeding disorder of infancy or early childhood (FDI) include medical evaluation/hospitalization, behavioral interventions, family interventions, and home monitoring and protective removal. The medical needs of the child with FDI must be the focus of initial treatment. As many of these children are undernourished or neglected, immediate medical evaluation and treatment are required. This treatment typically involves measures to monitor and increase nourishment and body weight, ranging from a specific diet and feeding plan to placement of a gastrostomy tube. If the case is severe, it may be necessary for the child to have supervised feeding during inpatient hospitalization. If the infant failed to gain weight at home but thrives in the hospital environment, it is essential to intervene with parents prior to hospital discharge in order to prevent a recurrence of weight loss and feeding problems. Behavioral treatments integrated with nutritional and medical recommendations to form a multidisciplinary plan are a universal part of treatment for FDI. Children with FDI should be encouraged to handle and play with food as a means to desensitize them to food and feeding cues. It is recommended that all interventions for FDI include support for and education of the parents. It is important that the parents are allowed to vent and receive support related to the difficulties of feeding a child with FDI. Educational techniques should provide parents with information about nutrition; child development, particularly feeding and temperament; behavioral parenting skills; and behavioral interventions for FDI. Specifically, parents should be educated on how to adjust their parenting behavior to fit the child's temperament. If the case of FDI is severe, more extreme interventions such as temporary separation of parent from child, required home visits by a social worker, or even removal of the infant from the parents' care, may be warranted. There are four factors that should be investigated when deciding the severity of a case of FDI: the severity of abuse/neglect, medical status of the child, willingness of the parent to change through psychological intervention, and psychological stability of the parent. A "parental holiday" may be suggested if the child refuses to eat during a hospitalization in an effort to break the cycle of negative parent-child interaction at mealtimes (Kronenberger & Meyer, 2001).

Treatment of Adolescent Eating Disorders

As a comprehensive review of treatment approaches for adolescent eating disorders is beyond the scope of this contribution, four commonly used treatment approaches will be addressed: cognitive-behavioral therapy (CBT), family therapy, interpersonal therapy (IPT), and pharmacological treatment. BN is the most researched eating disorder with respect to treatment efficacy (Williamson & Netemeyer, 2000; R. Wilson & Pike, 2001). Although numerous outcome studies have demonstrated the effectiveness of cognitive-behavioral strategies, the evidence for the effectiveness of CBT has been derived almost exclusively from studies involving adult populations (Ponton, 1996). As CBT has proven effective in the treatment of a wide array of child and adolescent problems such as depression, anxiety, attention-deficit/hyperactivity disorder, and behavioral problems, it is often the first choice of treatment for adolescent BN. Clinicians must use their knowledge of age-specific developmental stages and tasks to modify traditional CBT techniques so that they are appropriate to the emotional, interpersonal, and cognitive level of the adolescent clients. In addition, CBT may be combined with other modalities such as family therapy, interpersonal therapy, and pharmacological treatment.

CBT for BN, AN, and BED

As CBT is often the treatment of choice for BN, AN, and BED, Fairburn, Marcus, and T. Wilson's (1993) manualized approach will be described in some detail. The use of the CBT model will be delineated specifically for the treatment of BN, followed by remarks regarding modifications in the treatment of AN and/or BED. The CBT model focuses on the key role of cognitive and behavioral factors in maintaining the eating disorder. Major emphasis is placed on the value that adolescents place on achieving an idealized body weight and shape, as this is what leads individuals to rigidly restrict their food intake and makes them vulnerable to episodes of binge eating. Treatment typically encompasses 20 weekly individual sessions that focus on decreasing binge eating and purging; developing more healthy, regular eating patterns; and decreasing dysfunctional thoughts and feelings regarding the importance of body weight and shape.

CBT involves three stages of treatment. Stage one encompasses the first eight stages of treatment and focuses on establishing the therapeutic relationship, educating the client about the cognitive model and important factors in body weight regulation, beginning self-monitoring, setting a pattern of regular weekly weighing, establishing a pattern of regular eating, and developing self-control strategies that are incompatible with binge eating. Stage two encompasses the next eight stages and has an increasingly cognitive focus. Treatment focuses on eliminating dieting, as rigid dieting is a precipitant for binge eating. Clients are taught a variety of cognitive and behavioral procedures for reducing dietary restraint and resisting binge eating. Problem solving and cognitive restructuring skills are addressed as well as behavioral strategies that promote increased exposure to one's body as well as a variety of foods. Phase three incorporates the final phase of treatment in which the focus of treatment shifts to the use of relapse prevention techniques to ensure the maintenance of change following the end of treatment. G. Wilson, Fairburn, and Agras (1997) provide an excellent chapter which summarizes outcome data on CBT for BN as well as a summary description of the CBT treatment manual.

As both AN and BN have several common features, CBT has been found to be effective with clients diagnosed with AN. Cognitive restructuring has been recommended for both disorders in order to address unrealistic attitudes about body weight and shape. Psychoeducation, which addresses the importance of regular eating patterns, key principles in healthy body weight regulation, and the negative consequences of severe food restriction and purging behaviors, is also utilized for both BN and AN. Key differences in treatment between AN and BN occur in terms of motivation for change, targeting weight gain as a symptom, and in the pace and content of CBT. For example, patients with AN are extremely reluctant to commit to treatment because of their fear of the main goal of treatment, namely weight gain. Thus, although patients with BN and BED are reassured that treatment typically has little effect on body weight, patients with AN cannot be reassured in this way. In the treatment of BN, weekly weighing is often left up to the patient so that it does not dominate the session. In the treatment of AN, weight must be regularly checked by the therapist from another source than the patient, such as a physician or family member. Other modifications in the treatment of AN include a more gradual introduction of self-monitoring as motivation increases, a change in presenting the cognitive model of binging and purging for AN patients who do not binge, an incorporation of interpersonal themes in treatment, and integration of family therapy. There is a greater need for therapists treating AN to be aware of potential medical risks and the criteria for full or partial hospitalization. Although therapy is divided into three phases similar to those for BN, treatment for AN is typically longer, lasting from 1 to 2 years. Garner, Vitousek, and Pike (1997) provide an excellent summary of CBT for AN.

Family Therapy

Although outcome studies are limited in empirically validating family therapy as an effective treatment modality for AN and BN, it is often utilized with patients who are 18 or younger and living at home. Family therapy is an umbrella term, as specific family interventions vary widely and range from family therapy only, in which all treatment occurs in the family context, to periodic family sessions as an adjunct to individual therapy. Minuchin (Minuchin, Rosman, & Baker, 1978) was one of the first to advocate family therapy for eating disorders by stating that an eating disorder may reflect dysfunctional interaction patterns within a family and may function as a maladaptive solution to an adolescent's struggle to achieve autonomy. More recently, systematic studies of family treatment for AN have supported the efficacy of the Maudsley approach to family-based treatment (Dare & Eisler, 1997). This approach begins with the assumption that the cause of AN is unknown and that it is important to not view families as inherently flawed or pathological, as their guilt will then impede the family's ability to help the anorexic child. The Maudsley approach encompasses three clearly defined phases. In phase one, the clinician focuses on the dangers of severe malnutrition and attempts to create sufficient anxiety within the parental system to motivate parents to take action regarding the child's food refusal. Weight gain and separation of the child from her or his illness are the primary foci of phase one, which lasts approximately 4 to 6 months. When the patient is eating regularly and has gained sufficient weight, phase two of treatment begins. Sessions focus on the family's assessment of readiness to return control of eating to the adolescent and include various strategies for increasing the adolescent's control. Phase two usually lasts approximately 3 to 4 months and ends when the parents are satisfied that the adolescent can manage her or his eating independently. During phase three, treatment becomes less focused on food and weight gain and more focused on developmental issues of adolescence, such as puberty, social relationships, separation from parents, increased personal autonomy, and sexuality. Phase three typically lasts 2 to 3 months.

Family-based cognitive-behavioral therapy has been utilized for adolescents with BN. Building on the effectiveness of individual CBT in the treatment of adult BN, Lock (2002) has identified theoretical and practical reasons to include the family in CBT. Parents or guardians are legally responsible for minor patients and can provide powerful influence in support of (or opposition to) therapeutic goals. Parents have the ability to alter the behavioral milieu in terms of meal planning and foods readily available. They can assist in normalizing eating patterns, encourage self-monitoring, and encourage alternatives to binge eating and purging episodes. Family therapy can also be useful to family members who are often overwhelmed by issues presented by the eating-disordered patient and need assistance in learning how to most optimally interact at home. Lock (2002) has developed a modified version of Fairburn et al.'s (1993) manualized treatment for BN, which incorporates the family throughout treatment.

Interpersonal Therapy

IPT is a short-term, focal psychotherapy which aims to help patients identify and modify present interpersonal problems. It was developed in the mid-1960s for the treatment of adult clinical depression on the premise that interpersonal difficulties contribute to the development and maintenance of depressions, and that social support is associated with enhanced treatment gains. More recently, IPT has been utilized with other clinical problems including eating disorders. IPT has been successfully utilized in the treatment of BN and BED and has been incorporated as a key component in the treatment of AN. Clinical trials, which compare the effectiveness of CBT and IPT for adults with BN, have indicated that CBT produces more rapid remission and reduction of symptoms (Fairburn et al., 1995), with IPT showing equal effectiveness in the longer term at 8- and 12-month follow-up. Although research is needed to establish the effectiveness of IPT for adolescent eating disorders, the effectiveness of IPT in the treatment of adolescent depression suggests that this approach holds promise. In the treatment of eating disorders, IPT focuses on significant interpersonal relationships in the individual's life that appear to have caused and/or maintained the eating disorder. Little or no emphasis is placed on eating disorder symptoms or on the patient's preoccupation with dieting, weight, or shape (Fairburn, 1997).

IPT typically encompasses 15 to 20 sessions, each lasting 50 minutes, and extending for 4 to 5 months. Treatment consists of three stages. Stage one consists of three to four sessions, which address the rationale and nature of IPT, identify current interpersonal problems, and determine which interpersonal problems should become the focus of treatment. In the second stage of IPT, the adolescent is informed that treatment will change to being primarily patient-led. The therapist is active but not directive, encouraging the client to explore key problem areas and consider ways of changing. Formal problem solving is not used, though the therapist encourages the client to consider various options that are available. The general need to change is stressed throughout stage two, which incorporates 8 to 10 sessions. The third stage of IPT includes the last three to four sessions, which are often scheduled at 2-week intervals. Stage three focuses on two goals, namely to maintain treatment gains and to minimize relapse. Fairburn (1997) has written an excellent overview of interpersonal therapy for bulimia nervosa.

Psychopharmacological Treatment

Although the use of psychotropic medication is not considered a first-choice treatment in adolescent eating disorders, it may have a place in a comprehensive treatment package. Several types of medication have been used in the treatment of AN including neuroleptics, antidepressants, and appetite stimulants. Clinical trials demonstrating the efficacy of any of these medications for adolescents are very limited. Given the increased risk of medication-related side effects in severely malnourished patients, the regular use of drugs does not appear justified in the treatment of AN, and should be reserved for cases that are complicated as a result of comorbid diagnoses. For example, antidepressant medication such as amitriptyline, nortriptyline, and fluoxetine have been used in cases of AN with comorbid depression (Gowers & Bryant-Waugh, 2004; Kronenberger & Meyer, 2001).

More clinical trials have been conducted regarding the efficacy of medication in the management of BN, though most research has been conducted with adult populations. Antidepressants, particularly tricyclics and selective serotonin reuptake inhibitors, have been utilized as medications for BN and found to be effective in reducing bulimic symptoms. Specifically, fluoxetine, when administered at three times the dose recommended for depressive disorders, has been demonstrated to be effective in reducing bulimic behaviors in the short run and to be of potential value in relapse prevention. A recent study has highlighted the benefit of fluoxetine in the treatment of adolescent BN, with decreases in eating-disordered behavior and increases in general psychological functioning after 8 weeks of medication combined with supportive treatment (Kotler et al., 2003). Given the limited research, medication is not typically used as the sole or primary treatment for BN in children and adolescents. Medication is sometimes recommended for older adolescents with comorbid depression, though it should be avoided in cases with severe purging episodes, comorbid substance abuse, or low potassium levels (Robin, Gilroy, & Dennis, 1998). Further research is needed to clarify the impact of antidepressants on binge eating and mood in younger age clients (Gowers & Bryant-Waugh, 2004; Mitchell, 2001).

Children's Body Image Scale*

Instructions for the CBIS: Each child is asked to identify the body figure most like their own (perceived figure). They are then asked to nominate the body figure they would most like to have (ideal figure). The difference between the category numbers of their perceived and ideal figures is used as a measure of body size dissatisfaction (i.e., perceived-ideal discrepancy). This will provide a directional score such that a child wanting to be thinner will obtain a positive score, and a child wanting to be larger will obtain a negative score. Additionally, an absolute discrepancy score can be obtained (i.e., perceived-minus ideal) to provide a nondirectional indicator of body dissatisfaction.

The children can be asked two additional questions:

1) Do you think your body is (a) much too thin, (b) too thin, (c) just right, (d) a little too fat, or (e) much too fat?
2) Would you like your body to be (a) much thinner, (b) a little thinner, (c) stay the same, (d) a bit fatter, or (e) much fatter?

<u>Female Version</u>

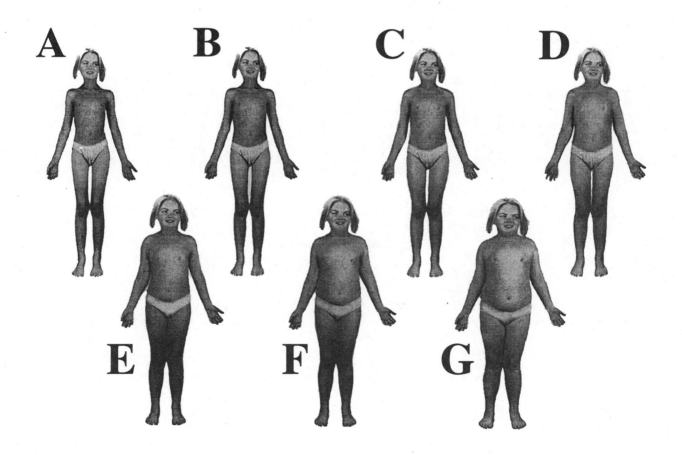

* Reproduced with permission from Dr. Helen Truby.

Male Version

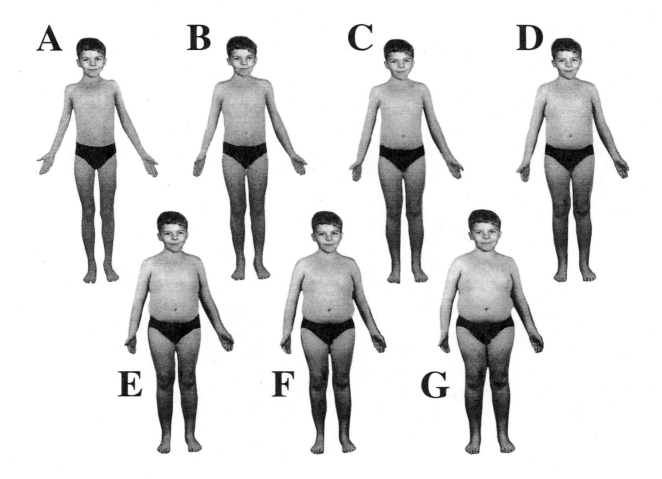

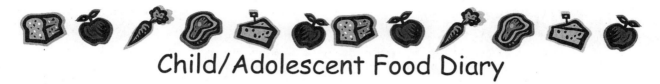

Child/Adolescent Food Diary

DATE:_____

TIME:

before 6 a.m.
6-7 a.m.
7-8 a.m.
8-9 a.m.
9-10 a.m.
10-11 a.m.
11-12 p.m.
12-1 p.m.
1-2 p.m.
2-3 p.m.
3-4 p.m.
4-5 p.m.
5-6 p.m.
6-7 p.m.
7-8 p.m.
8-9 p.m.
after 9 p.m.

PLACE:

HOME:
Kitchen
Dining Room
Living Room
Bedroom
Family Room
Yard/Porch

AWAY FROM HOME:
Cafeteria
Car/Bus/Train
Restaurant
Friend's Home

Other: _____

WHO WERE YOU WITH?

Parents
Friends
Alone
Other Family Members
Other: _____

FEELINGS:

Happy   Mad

Sad   Excited

Nervous   Tired

Bored

Amount:	Type of Food Eaten:

Was this food part of a meal?   Yes _____   No _____
Did you binge?   Yes _____   No _____
Did you purge?   Yes _____   No _____

CONTRIBUTORS

Eve M. Wolf, PhD, is an Associate Professor at the Wright State University School of Professional Psychology in Dayton, Ohio. For the past 20 years, she has been involved in clinical work and scholarship in the area of eating disorders. Currently, she supervises doctoral students in their clinical work at the University counseling center where eating problems and body image issues are common concerns. Dr. Wolf may be contacted at 220 Frederick A. White Health Center, 3640 Colonel Glenn Highway, Dayton, OH 45435. E-mail: eve.wolf@wright.edu

Crystal S. Collier, BA, is currently a fourth-year doctoral student at the Wright State University School of Professional Psychology where she is pursuing a PsyD degree. She received her bachelor's degree from the University of Kansas in 1996. Crystal is currently preparing to enter her internship year during the 2005-2006 academic year. Her interests include work with children, adolescents, and families. Crystal will complete her degree program in July 2006. She may be contacted by E-mail at collier.3@wright.edu

RESOURCES

Cited Resources

Allison, D. B. (1995). *Handbook of Assessment Methods for Eating Behaviors and Weight-Related Problems: Measures, Theory, and Research*. Thousand Oaks, CA: Sage Publications.

American Psychiatric Association. (2000). *Diagnostic and Statistical Manual of Mental Disorders* (4th ed. text rev.). Washington, DC: Author.

Archer, L. A., Rosenbaum, P. L., & Streiner, D. L. (1991). The Children's Eating Behavior Inventory: Reliability and validity results. *Journal of Pediatric Psychology, 16*, 629-642.

Brooks-Gunn, J., & Attie, I. (1996). Developmental psychopathology in the context of adolescence. In M. Lenzenweger & J. Haugaard (Eds.), *Frontiers of Developmental Psychopathology* (pp. 148-189). London: Oxford University Press.

Bryant-Waugh, R. J., Cooper, P. J., Taylor, C. L., & Lask, B. D. (1996). The use of the eating disorder examination with children: A pilot study. *International Journal of Eating Disorders, 19*, 391-397.

Candy, C. M., & Fee, V. E. (1998a). Reliability and concurrent validity of the Kids' Eating Disorders Survey (KEDS): Body Image Silhouettes with preadolescent girls. *Eating Disorders, 6*, 297-308.

Candy, C. M., & Fee, V. E. (1998b). Underlying dimensions and psychometric properties of the eating behaviors and body image test for preadolescent girls. *Journal of Clinical Child Psychology, 27*(1), 117-122.

Childress, A. C., Brewerton, T. D., Hodges, E. L., & Jarrell, M. P. (1993). The Kids' Eating Disorders Survey (KEDS): A study of middle school students. *Journal of the American Academy of Child and Adolescent Psychiatry, 32*, 843-850.

Comerci, G. D. (1999). Disordered eating behaviors: Anorexia nervosa, bulimia nervosa, cyclic vomiting syndrome, and rumination disorder. In M. Levine, W. Carey, & A. Crocker (Eds.), *Developmental-Behavioral Pediatrics* (pp. 380-391). Philadelphia: Saunders.

Crowther, J., Lingswiler, V., & Stephens, M. (1984). The topography of binge eating. *Addictive Behaviors, 9*, 299-303.

Crowther, J., & Sherwood, N. (1997). Assessment. In D. Garner & P. Garfinkel (Eds.), *Handbook of Treatment for Eating Disorders* (pp. 34-49). New York: Guilford.

Dare, C., & Eisler, I. (1997). Family therapy for anorexia nervosa. In D. Garner & P. Garfinkel (Eds.), *Handbook of Treatment for Eating Disorders* (pp. 307-324). New York: Guilford.

Eklund, K., Paavonen, E., & Almquist, F. (2005). Factor structure of the EDI-C. *International Journal of Eating Disorders, 37*(4), 330-341.

Ekvall, S. W., Ekvall, V., & Mayes, S. D. (1993). Rumination. In S. Ekvall (Ed.), *Pediatric Nutrition in Chronic Diseases and Developmental Disorders: Prevention, Assessment, and Treatment* (pp. 380-391). New York: Oxford University Press.

Ellis, C. R., Parr, T. S., Singh, N. N., & Wechsler, H. A. (1997). Rumination. In N. N. Singh (Ed.), *Prevention and Treatment of Severe Behavior Problems: Models and Methods in Developmental Disabilities* (pp. 237-252). Pacific Grove, CA: Brooks/Cole Publishing.

Ellis, C. R., Singh, N. N., Crews, W. D., Bonaventura, S. H., Gehin, J. M., & Ricketts, R. W. (1997). Pica. In N. N. Singh (Ed.), *Prevention and Treatment of Severe Behavior Problems: Models and Methods in Developmental Disabilities* (pp. 253-270). Pacific Grove, CA: Brooks/Cole Publishing.

Fairburn, C. G. (1997). Interpersonal psychotherapy for bulimia nervosa. In D. Garner & P. Garfinkel (Eds.), *Handbook of Treatment for Eating Disorders* (pp. 278-294). New York: Guilford.

Fairburn, C. G., & Beglin, S. J. (1994). Assessment of eating disorders: Interview or self-report questionnaire? *International Journal of Eating Disorders, 16*, 363-370.

Fairburn, C. G., & Cooper, Z. (1993). The Eating Disorders Examination (12th ed.). In C. G. Fairburn & G. T. Wilson (Eds.), *Binge Eating: Nature, Assessment, and Treatment* (pp. 317-360). New York: Guilford.

Fairburn, C., Marcus, M., & Wilson, T. (1993). Cognitive-behavioral therapy for binge eating and bulimia nervosa: A comprehensive treatment manual. In C. G. Fairburn & G. T. Wilson (Eds.), *Binge Eating: Nature, Assessment, and Treatment* (pp. 361-404). New York: Guilford.

Fairburn, C., Norman, P., Welch, S., & O'Connor, M. (1995). A prospective study of outcome in bulimia nervosa and the long-term effects of three psychological treatments. *Archives of General Psychiatry, 52*, 304-312.

Garner, D. M. (1991a). *Eating Disorder Inventory-C.* Odessa, FL: Psychological Assessment Resources.

Garner, D. M. (1991b). *Eating Disorder Inventory-2 Manual.* Odessa, FL: Psychological Assessment Resources.

Garner, D. M. (2005). *Eating Disorder Inventory-3.* Odessa, FL: Psychological Assessment Resources.

Garner, D. M., & Garfinkel, P. E. (1979). The Eating Attitudes Test: An index of the symptoms of anorexia nervosa. *Psychological Medicine, 9*, 273-279.

Garner, D. M., Olmsted, M. P., Bohr, Y., & Garfinkel, P. E. (1982). The Eating Attitudes Test: Psychometric features and clinical correlates. *Psychological Medicine, 12*, 871-878.

Garner, D. M., Olmsted, M. P., & Polivy, J. (1983). Development and validation of a multidimensional Eating Disorder Inventory for anorexia nervosa and bulimia. *International Journal of Eating Disorders, 2*, 15-24.

Garner, D. M., Vitousek, K. M., & Pike, K. M. (1997). Cognitive-behavioral treatment for anorexia nervosa. In D. Garner & P. Garfinkel (Eds.), *Handbook of Treatment for Eating Disorders* (pp. 94-144). New York: Guilford.

Gowers, S., & Bryant-Waugh, R. (2004). Management of child and adolescent eating disorders: The current evidence base and future directions. *Journal of Child Psychology and Psychiatry, 45*, 63-83.

Harris, D., & Kuba, S. (1997). Ethno cultural identity and eating disorders in women of color. *Professional Psychology: Research and Practice, 28*(4), 341-347.

Henderson, M., & Freeman, P. L. (1987). A self-rating scale for bulimia: The 'BITE.' *British Journal of Psychiatry, 150*, 18-24.

Johnson, W. G., Grieve, F. G., Adams, C. D., & Sandy, J. (1999). Measuring binge eating in adolescents: Adolescent and parent version of the questionnaire of eating and weight patterns. *International Journal of Eating Disorders, 26*, 310-314.

Kotler, L., Devlin, M., Davies, M., & Walsh, T. (2003). An open trial of fluoxetine for adolescents with bulimia nervosa. *Journal of Child and Adolescent Psychopharmacology, 13*, 329-335.

Kronenberger, W., & Meyer, R. (2001). *The Child Clinician's Handbook.* Needham Heights, MA: Allyn & Bacon.

Lock, J. (2002). Treating adolescents with eating disorders in the family context: Empirical and theoretical considerations. *Child and Adolescent Psychiatric Clinics of North America, 11*, 331-342.

Maloney, M. J., McGuire, J. B., & Daniels, S. R. (1988). Reliability testing of a children's version of the Eating Attitudes Test. *Journal of the American Academy of Child and Adolescent Psychiatry, 5*, 541-543.

Matson, J. L., & Bamburg, J. W. (1999). A descriptive study of pica behavior in persons with mental retardation. *Journal of Developmental and Physical Disabilities, 11*, 353-361.

Matson, J. L., & Kuhn, D. E. (2001). Identifying feeding problems in mentally retarded persons: Development and reliability of the Screening Tool of Feeding Problems (STEP). *Research in Developmental Disabilities, 22*, 165-172.

McCarthy, D., Simmons, J., Smith, G., Tomlinson, K., & Hill, K. (2002). Reliability, stability, and factor structure of the Bulimia Test-Revised and Eating Disorder Inventory-2 scales in adolescence. *Assessment, 9*, 382-389.

McKenzie, T. L., Sallis, J. F., Nader, P. R., Patterson, T. L., Elder, J. P., Berry, C. C., Rupp, J. W., Atkins, C. J., Buono, M. J., & Nelson, J. A. (1991). BEACHES: An observational system for assessing children's eating and physical activity behaviors and associated events. *Journal of Applied Behavior Analysis, 24*, 141-151.

Minuchin, S., Rosman, B., & Baker, L. (1978). *Psychosomatic Families: Anorexia Nervosa in Context.* Oxford: Harvard University Press.

Mitchell, J. (2001). Psychopharmacology of eating disorders: Current knowledge and future directions. In R. Striegel-Moore & L. Smolak (Eds.), *Eating Disorders: Innovative Directions for Research and Practice* (pp. 197-214). Washington, DC: American Psychological Association.

Polivy, J., & Herman, P. (2002). Causes of eating disorders. *Annual Review of Psychology, 53*, 187-213.

Ponton, L. (1996). Disordered eating. In R. DiClemente, W. Hansen, & L. Ponton (Eds.), *Handbook of Adolescent Health Risk Behavior* (pp. 83-113). New York: Plenum.

Robin, A., Gilroy, M., & Dennis, A. (1998). Treatment of eating disorders in children and adolescents. *Clinical Psychology Review, 4*, 421-446.

Sands, R., Tricker, J., Sherman, C., Armatas, C., & Maschette, W. (1997). Disordered eating patterns, body image, self-esteem, and physical activity in preadolescent school children. *International Journal of Eating Disorders, 21*(2), 158-166.

Smolak, L., Levine, M., & Striegel-Moore, R. (1996). *The Developmental Psychopathology of Eating Disorders: Implications for Research, Prevention, and Treatment.* Hillsdale, NJ: Lawrence Erlbaum Associates.

Spitzer, R. L., Yanovski, S. Z., & Marcus, M. D. (1993). *The Questionnaire on Eating and Weight Patterns-Revised (QEWP-R).* New York: New York State Psychiatric Institute.

Thelen, M. H., Farmer, J., Wonderlich, S., & Smith, M. (1991). A revision of the Bulimia Test: The BULIT-R. *Psychological Assessment, 3*, 119-124.

Thelen, M. H., Lawrence, C. M., & Powell, A. L. (1992). Body image, weight control, and eating disorders among children. In J. Crowther, D. Tennenbaum, S. Hobfoll, & M. Stephens (Eds.), *The Etiology of Bulimia Nervosa: The Individual and Familial Context* (pp. 81-101). Washington, DC: Hemisphere Publishing Corporation.

Truby, H., & Paxton, S. J. (2002). Development of the Children's Body Image Scale. *British Journal of Clinical Psychology, 41*, 185-203.

Vollmer, T. R., & Roane, H. S. (1998). Rumination. In L. Phelps (Ed.), *Health-Related Disorders in Children and Adolescents: A Guidebook for Understanding and Educating* (pp. 564-570). Washington, DC: American Psychiatric Association.

Williamson, D., & Netemeyer, S. (2000). Cognitive behavioral therapy. In K. Miller & S. Mizes (Eds.), *Comparative Treatments for Eating Disorders* (pp. 61-81). New York: Springer.

Wilson, G., Fairburn, C., & Agras, W. (1997). Cognitive-behavioral therapy for bulimia nervosa. In D. Garner & P. Garfinkel (Eds.), *Handbook of Treatment for Eating Disorders* (pp. 67-93). New York: Guilford.

Wilson, R., & Pike, K. (2001). Eating disorders. In D. Barlow (Ed.), *Clinical Handbook of Psychological Disorders: A Step-by-Step Treatment Manual* (pp. 332-375). New York: Guilford.

Additional Resources

Corcoran, K., & Fischer, J. (2000). *Measures for Clinical Practice, Volume 1* (3rd ed., pp. 531-533). New York: Free Press.

Kuhn, D. E., & Matson, J. L. (2002). A validity study of the Screening Tool of Feeding Problems (STEP). *Journal of Intellectual and Developmental Disability, 27*(3), 161-167.

Thelen, M. H., Mintz, L. B., & Vander Wal, J. S. (1996). The Bulimia Test-Revised: Validation with DSM-IV criteria for bulimia nervosa. *Psychological Assessment, 8*(2), 219-221.

WEBSITES*

Eating Disorder Websites

http://www.4woman.gov/bodyimage/bodyimage.cfm?page=125
http://www.aboutourkids.org/aboutour/articles/about_eating.html
http://www.anad.org/site/anadweb/
http://www.anred.com/
http://www.edreferral.com
http://www.hedc.org
http://www.keepkidshealthy.com/adolescent/adolescentproblems/eatingdisorders.html
http://www.mentalhealth.org/publications/allpubs/ken98-0047/default.asp
http://www.nationaleatingdisorders.org/p.asp?WebPage_ID=337
http://www.nimh.nih.gov/HealthInformation/ResourceList.cfm?Flowstate=4&DisOrdID=9
http://www.nimh.nih.gov/publicat/eatingdisorders.cfm
http://www.nlm.nih.gov/medlineplus/eatingdisorders.html
http://www.noah-health.org/english/illness/mentalhealth/eatingdisorders.html
http://www.noah-health.org/en/mental/disorders/eating/index.html
https://www.sjmcmd.org/eatingdisorders/

Websites Specifically for Parents

http://www.anred.com/prev.html
http://www.hedc.org/undrstnd/helpc.htm
http://www.kidshealth.org/parent/emotions/feelings/eating_disorders.html
http://www.nationaleatingdisorders.org/p.asp?WebPage_ID=289
http://www.pediatrics.about.com/cs/nutrition/l/blqz_eatdisorde.htm
http://www.psparents.net/eatingdisorders.htm

Websites Specifically for Children and Adolescents

http://www.hedc.org/undrstnd/helpself.htm
http://www.kidshealth.org/kid/health_problems/learning_problem/eatdisorder.html
http://www.nationaleatingdisorders.org/p.asp?WebPage_ID=292
http://www.noah-health.org/english/illness/mentalhealth/eatingdisorders.html#TEEN
http://www.noah-health.org/en/mental/disorders/eating/teen/index.html

---

* Although all websites cited in this contribution were correct at the time of publication, they are subject to change at any time.

Assessment and Treatment Of Children With Disabilities Who Have Been Abused

Leo M. Orange and Martin G. Brodwin

Every child is vulnerable to sexual abuse, but it is generally believed that children with disabilities are abused more frequently than children in the general population. Currently, studies are underway to determine more precisely the association between sexual abuse and disability. Research indicates that as many as one in four children who have disabilities will experience some form of sexual assault or abuse (Berliner & Elliott, 2001; Sobsey & Doe, 1991). When children and teenagers with disabilities are abused, the perpetrator is often someone they know and trust, such as a relative, family friend, or caregiver.

This contribution begins by discussing definitions of sexual abuse and the scope of this problem for children who have disabilities. Next, we review the various signs and symptoms to look for when assessing a child who may have been sexually abused. The emotional impact of abuse and factors related specifically to disability are described. Important areas discussed next include how to prevent abuse from occurring and how to protect children who have disabilities from abusive relationships. Prevention is described at the societal level, within the family, and with the child as a focus. Reactions to abuse and treatment modalities are explored. A wellness approach to the topic of sexual abuse is presented. Lastly, we provide several current websites for readers who seek additional information.

DEFINITION AND SCOPE OF SEXUAL ABUSE

Definition of Sexual Abuse

Sexual abuse is defined as being forced, threatened, or deceived into sexual activities ranging from looking or touching to intercourse or rape. Physical abuse is any form of violence against one's body, such as being hit, kicked, restrained, or deprived of food or water. Emotional abuse involves being threatened, terrorized, severely rejected, isolated, ignored, or verbally attacked. Maltreatment includes sexual abuse, physical abuse, neglect, and emotional maltreatment. Sexual abuse may also occur without touch, such as when someone exposes his or her genitals or forces or tricks an individual into exposing his or her own genitals. Another type of sexual abuse without touch involves a conversation or obscene telephone call, such as when a person calls and talks about sex (e.g., ways they would like to touch a person's body or be touched). Individuals with disabilities of all ages are at greater risk for all types of abuse and maltreatment than are those who do not have disabilities.

Sexual abuse of children involves someone too young to give informed consent but who has been involved in a sexual act. Exploitation of an individual who lacks adequate information to recognize such a situation or who is unable to understand or communicate (i.e., the child with a mental or physical disability) is also labeled sexual abuse. This kind of abuse is a violation of the whole person and is not restricted to a sexual act. It results in indignation and an overwhelming sense of violation and personal invasion that can affect the victim in physical, psychological, and social ways. Frequently, the aftermath of an assault or abuse is more severe than the actual event. This is particularly true of children with disabilities who cannot (or do not) access support systems and services that may otherwise be available.

The effects of these crimes may be short term, but in many cases the abuse causes irreparable emotional harm to the victim. The nature of some forms of sexual abuse also makes it difficult to observe and therefore more threatening to report. Fortunately, many professionals who work with children with disabilities recognize signs and symptoms of sexual abuse. Symptoms include behaviors, attitudes, psychosocial aspects, and physical manifestations. Some of these symptoms may be seen in all children who have been abused, but they can be more pronounced in children who have disabilities. These children already have issues and concerns related to their disabilities; abuse often leads to problems that are interrelated with disability. With sexual abuse, the normal adaptation to disability becomes more challenging, and the child may stop progressing toward adjusting to his or her disability.

Scope of the Problem

Until recently, the problem of abuse among people with disabilities received little attention. The few early publications typically studied adults, not children, and contained many methodological weaknesses. Essential constructs and variables important to statistical analysis were rarely defined. There was a particular lack of distinction among emotional, physical, and sexual abuse. According to Nosek, Howland, and Young (1998), researchers frequently used nonstandardized measurements and techniques. Global references were made to the type of abuse, for example, emotional versus sexual; yet there was little attempt to document or categorize specific incidents by perpetrators. Samples in these studies were generally quite heterogeneous in terms of disability type, age, and gender. Some researchers also used convenience sampling, such as using clients of intervention programs or those individuals listed in police reports, as opposed to representative or random sampling.

Researchers who study sexual violence against people with disabilities use a wide variety of definitions for sexual abuse, sexual assault, and rape (Berliner & Elliott, 2001; Sullivan & Knutson, 2003). Studies of sexual abuse in the general population usually distinguish between abuse during childhood and assault and rape during adulthood. Many acts of violence against people with disabilities are labeled abuse regardless of the victim's age or the specific offenses committed.

Comparing the percentage of sexual abuse victims who have disabilities with the percentage who do not have disabilities is difficult because of differences in terminology and methods used to determine these rates. However, data clearly indicate that people with disabilities are at higher risk for sexual violence than those without disabilities (Rogow & Hass, 1999). The risk and incidence for children who have disabilities is even greater (Mitchell & Buchele-Ash, 2000; Orange, 2002; Rogow & Hass, 1999).

SIGNS AND SYMPTOMS OF SEXUAL ABUSE

Every child is vulnerable to sexual abuse. As previously indicated, research has found that children with disabilities are more vulnerable to sexual abuse than children without disabilities (Ammerman, 1997; Crosse, Kaye, & Ratnofsky, 2001; Sullivan & Knutson, 2003). Parents must face the possibility that someone may hurt or take advantage of their child. As many as one out of every four children is a victim of sexual abuse (Steinberg & Hylton, 1998). Almost all of these children are abused by someone they know.

Sexual abuse involves forcing, tricking, bribing, threatening, or pressuring a person into heightened sexual awareness or activity (Mitchell & Buchele-Ash, 2000). Abuse may occur when an older or more knowledgeable child or adult uses a child for sex. The abuse often begins gradually and increases over time. Use of physical force is rarely necessary to engage a child in sexual activity because children, especially those with disabilities, are both trusting and dependent. Disability often results in greater dependence on and trust in those in authority (Crosse et al., 2001). These children want to please others and gain love and approval. Children are taught not to question authority, and they believe that adults are always right. Perpetrators of child sexual abuse are aware of this and take advantage of these vulnerabilities. Sexual abuse is an abuse of power over a child and a violation of a child's right to normal, healthy, trusting relationships (Sullivan & Knutson, 2003).

Because most children cannot or do not tell about being sexually abused, it is up to concerned adults to recognize signs of abuse. This is especially true for children with disabilities who may have difficulty communicating and having their needs understood. Physical evidence of abuse is rare. Therefore, one must look for behavioral signs. Unfortunately, there is no one behavior or behavioral pattern that can determine if a child has been sexually abused. The following are general behavioral changes that often are seen in children who have been sexually abused. Information that follows was obtained both from the Internet sources listed in the section titled "Websites" and from publications, such as Berliner and Elliott (2001), Rogow and Hass (1999), Sobsey (1994), Steinberg and Hylton (1998), and Sullivan and Knutson (2003).

Behavioral changes include fear or dislike of certain people or places, sleep disturbance, headaches, school problems, withdrawal from family and friends, disinterest in usual activities, excessive bathing or poor hygiene, depression, anxiety, and discipline problems (Rogow & Hass, 1999; Sobsey & Doe, 1991). Additional behaviors involve running away from home, physical complaints, eating disorders, passive or overly pleasing behaviors, delinquent acts, and excessive school absences. Perhaps most crucially, abused youth may show low self-esteem, self-destructive behavior, hostility, aggression, drug and alcohol problems, sexual activity or pregnancy at an early age, and suicidal ideation or actual attempts to end one's life (Ammerman, 1997; Crosse et al., 2001). In applying the above to children with disabilities, one needs heightened sensitivity to these signs and symptoms as children with disabilities may exhibit some of these as normally related to their disabilities and functional limitations.

Children who have been sexually abused frequently have more specific symptoms. Examples of these include copying adult sexual behavior; persistent sexual play with other children, themselves, toys, or pets; displaying sexual knowledge through language or behavior that is beyond what is normal for their age; unexplained pain, swelling, bleeding, or irritation of the mouth, genitals, or anal area; urinary infections; sexually transmitted diseases; and hints, indirect comments, and statements about the abuse (Ammerman, 1997; Rogow & Hass, 1999). Professionals need greater sensitivity to see these symptoms in children with disabilities, as physical limitations may mask some of these signs, while emotional and cognitive impairments often make communication more difficult.

Often children do not tell anyone about sexual abuse because they are too young to put what has happened into words, or they were threatened or bribed by the abuser to keep the abuse a secret, feel confused by the attention and feelings that accompany the abuse, or are afraid that no one will believe them (Sobsey & Doe, 1991). Children with disabilities who are dependent on caregivers may be abused by a care provider, and the child may not report the abuse because of dependency on and fear of the provider. Additionally, these children often blame themselves or believe the abuse is punishment for being "bad," feel too ashamed or embarrassed to tell, and show dependence on the abuser (a parent, guardian, or care provider) (Burrell, Thompson, & Sexton, 1994; Kragthorpe et al., 1997).

FEELINGS RESULTING FROM ABUSE

Children who have been sexually abused express many different, at times overwhelming, emotions. They already have heightened emotions because of their disabilities; the abuse further compounds these emotions. These include:

- **Fear** (of the abuser, of being perceived as causing trouble, of losing the support of adults important to them, of being taken away from home, and of being considered different or odd)
- **Anger** (at the abuser, at other adults around them who they feel did not protect them, and at themselves [feeling as if they were at fault])
- **Isolation** (assuming something is wrong with them, feeling alone in their experience, and having trouble talking about the abuse)
- **Sadness** (about having something taken from them, losing a part of themselves, feeling that they are growing up too quickly, and being betrayed by someone they trusted)
- **Guilt** (for not being able to stop the abuse, for believing they consented to the abuse, for reporting the abuse if they reported the abuse to someone, and for keeping the secret if they did not report the abuse)
- **Shame** (about being involved in the experience and about their bodies' response to the abuse)
- **Confusion** (they may still have positive feelings for the abuser, and their feelings change all the time) (Ammerman, 1997; Tobin, 1992).

Although these feelings are seen in children who have been abused, all children who demonstrate these symptoms have not necessarily been abused. These symptoms alone should not be used as proof of abuse. Most children demonstrate some of these symptoms from time to time, usually on a temporary basis. The extent and length of time these emotions are expressed needs careful and cautious assessment, as do other causative factors.

EMOTIONAL IMPACT OF ABUSE

It is well recognized that the factors of shame and guilt (either or both) are the primary psychological consequences of abuse. Both of these devastating emotions are the result of internalization of the offense. Victimized individuals frequently view themselves as the cause of the event and perhaps ultimately being a "bad" person (Young et al., 1997).

Shame is also commonly experienced and involves feelings of defeat and weakness in these highly traumatic and emotionally degrading situations (Santrock, 2004). There is a strong sense of loss of self-control with accompanying damage to self-esteem and a diminished concept of self. Victims may have been pressured, forced, or tricked but still believe they are partially to blame for the abuse, even though they did not consent or fully understand. Abusers dominate and manipulate their intended victims in overwhelming ways. The resulting shame and feelings of guilt can become incorporated into the victimized children's personalities (Tomison, 1996).

FACTORS RELATED TO DISABILITY

Many researchers believe that societal attitudes and beliefs play a significant role in placing children with disabilities at risk for maltreatment (Orange, 2002). Steinberg and Hylton (1998) contended that some societal beliefs, practices, and policies "devalue" children with disabilities. This is manifested in ways that indicate that children with disabilities are not as worthy of social, educational, and professional opportunities as children without disabilities. They may internalize societal attitudes and feel shame or believe themselves less worthy of being treated with respect (National Resource Center on Child Sexual Abuse, 1994). Segregating children with disabilities in school tends to increase the perception of differences and suggests that group membership and social distance influence attitudes about the acceptability of violence. "Attitudes about individuals or groups that tend to depersonalize, dehumanize, or distance them appear to make violence against them more acceptable" (Sobsey, 1994, p. 307).

Additionally, myths associated with children with disabilities increase risk. Sobsey (1994) discussed the misperception held by many that children with disabilities are not as vulnerable to being abused. Belief in this myth may result in a lack of awareness and attention to the problem. Steinberg and Hylton (1998) and Baladerian (1994) discussed three of these myths: (a) Children with disabilities are asexual and therefore do not need sex education (denying information that helps prevent abuse); (b) some children with disabilities are unable to manage their own behavior (resulting in care providers exerting unnecessary control); and (c) all care providers are special and good (resulting in a lack of awareness and attention to signs of abuse).

Because the care required for some children with disabilities is crucial to their survival, many have been taught to obey those in authority and comply with their care providers' requests and demands (Steinberg & Hylton, 1998). In fact, some children with disabilities may feel that their bodies do not belong to them. If a care provider behaves inappropriately, the child may not complain or resist because of the belief that care providers know what is best.

Many researchers have found that some children with disabilities lack the knowledge or understanding to realize when behavior is wrong or inappropriate (Ammerman, 1992; Steinberg & Hylton, 1998; Wolcott, 1997). Even if they do recognize behaviors as wrong, some children with disabilities may not attempt to stop the abuse or neglect because they fear losing the relationship. They are emotionally and/or physically dependent on their care providers (Tobin, 1992). In some cases, their disabilities may prevent them from being able to defend themselves or escape from the situation. Children who have difficulty communicating are at higher risk for maltreatment because potential perpetrators may believe they can "get away with it," thinking that the child will not be able to report the behavior (Ammerman & Patz, 1996; Wolcott, 1997). Children with disabilities may be perceived as being relatively "safe victims."

PREVENTION OF ABUSE

Protecting Children

Child sexual abuse can take place within the family, by a parent, stepparent, sibling, or other relative. It can occur outside the home by a neighbor, child care provider, teacher, or stranger. Often, a person who provides personal care for the child with a disability is most suspect. This occurs because the caregiver may have intimate contact when providing personal care and also spends a lot of time with the child (Struck, 1999). However, one must be careful not to simply blame the care provider.

No child, especially a child with a disability, is emotionally prepared to cope with sexual abuse. Sexual abusers can make the child extremely fearful of reporting the abuse, and only when a special effort by a parent or treating clinician has been made to make the child feel safe, can the child talk freely. If he or she admits to being molested, parents need to remain calm and provide reassurance that what happened was not the child's fault. If a child trusts someone enough to tell about the incident of sexual abuse, that person is in a position to help with the recovery process.

The following suggestions can help an individual provide positive support: keeping calm and not directing anger toward the child, believing what the child says, giving positive messages such as "I know you could not help it" or "I am proud of you for telling me," and explaining to the child that he or she is not to blame for what happened (Tobin, 1992). Additionally, recommendations for providing support include respecting the child's privacy and not discussing the abuse in front of others, being responsible and reporting the abuse to the proper law enforcement authorities, arranging a medical examination to assure there has been no permanent physical damage, and getting help from a professional therapist (Beach Center on Families and Disability, 1997).

Hewitt (1999) reported that low-risk children are those who are clear about their own boundaries and capable of stating them, have sufficient ability to verbalize, are capable of recognizing problems and talking about them, are assertive and confident in voicing their own particular views and concerns despite some adult opposition, and are usually older than preschool age. High-risk children tend to be passive, dependent, withdrawn, anxious, fearful, feel powerless, be unable to articulate concerns, and are not able to recognize problem behavior, much less report it.

As Ammerman and Baladerian (1993) stated, "The physical, emotional, and financial costs of abuse and neglect are so great as to make prevention the number one priority in the effort to eliminate maltreatment of children" (p. 9). If abuse or neglect does occur, one needs to report, investigate, and treat the problem. Society has an obligation to address efforts to prevent abuse and neglect. Prevention may be aimed at the general public (known as primary prevention) or targeted specifically to families considered at risk of child maltreatment (known as secondary prevention). A third form of prevention, known as tertiary prevention, is designed to prevent maltreatment on a societal level.

Because different, interrelated factors can contribute to sexual abuse, different, coordinated prevention strategies are needed (Rogow & Hass, 1999). A multifaceted approach is the most appropriate and effective. Approaches may be parallel, in which separate programs are implemented for children with disabilities, or integrated, in which the needs of children with disabilities are accommodated in generic programs serving all children.

Prevention at the Societal Level

One of the first steps in prevention is raising people's awareness of the problem. Heightened awareness can lead to additional funding for research and prevention programs and for implementation to combat the problem. The National Symposium on Abuse and Neglect of Children With Disabilities (1995) recommended that 10% of federal funds for child abuse awareness be devoted to disability issues.

Most experts in the field of abuse recommend coordination among the relevant parties to ensure that prevention efforts are comprehensive. Governmental agencies, service providers, and local communities can work together to support families that have children with disabilities, with collaboration among professionals from many fields (Rogow & Hass, 1999). Educators and health care professionals, who are often in contact with children with disabilities, can be trained to understand the problem and their role in prevention (Wolcott, 1997). One study found that 92% of special educators would attend specialized training on abuse prevention if it were made available (Orelove, Hollahan, & Myles, 2000).

At the societal level, prevention efforts often focus on changing societal attitudes about children with disabilities. The National Symposium on Abuse and Neglect of Children With Disabilities (1995) and Sobsey (1994) recommended promoting inclusion of children with disabilities into everyday life. Steinberg and Hylton (1998) added recommendations that included encouraging valuing children with disabilities, seeing them as individuals, and sharing responsibility for their well-being. Sobsey added recommendations including educating others specifically about people with disabilities, challenging negative attitudes and behaviors, and personalizing interactions.

Mitchell and Buchele-Ash (2000) advocated enacting legislation that supports prevention and protection of children with disabilities. For example, the Child Abuse Prevention, Adoption, and Family Services Act of 1998 was enacted to (a) increase awareness of crimes committed against children with disabilities, (b) collect data, and (c) develop strategies to address the special needs of this population.

Family-Focused Prevention Efforts

Families who have children with disabilities experience added stressors including (a) feeling unprepared to handle the care of a child who has a disability, (b) accepting that the child is "different," (c) having financial or time limitations stretched as additional medical and educational activities are needed, and (d) lacking the necessary social support or networks to work through the many challenges that arise in providing care for this child and the rest of the family. Because much of the maltreatment of children with disabilities occurs within families, prevention efforts have been focused on services to families. Goals of family-focused prevention efforts include increasing knowledge and understanding about child development; strengthening parenting skills; improving awareness of, and access to, resources; reducing isolation; and developing positive coping skills (Kragthorpe et al., 1997; Rycus & Hughes, 1998; Steinberg & Hylton, 1998). Services can be offered either to all families that have children with disabilities or to families considered to be at greater risk of maltreating their children.

One service offered to all families that have children with disabilities is the Individualized Family Service Plan (IFSP). The IFSP is required by the Individuals With Disabilities Education Act (IDEA; 1990) for families and their young children with disabilities from birth to age 5. The IFSP includes multidisciplinary assessment, goal setting and planning, linkage to community services, and coordination and monitoring of services provided (Jones et al., 1995). Parent involvement is crucial to ensure that the plan addresses all the family's identified needs.

The case management part of the IFSP is a major component. Case managers can advocate for and help coordinate a myriad of resources needed by families (Rycus & Hughes, 1998). These services include educational, medical, and recreational programs for children; financial assistance for families; respite care; counseling; and parenting programs (Ammerman, 1997). Parenting programs provide information about the child's disability and realistic expectations for growth and development, and teach positive parenting skills.

One kind of family-focused prevention program available to at-risk families with children who have disabilities involves home visits by trained professionals and para-professionals (Jones et al., 1995). Home visitation programs are available for many types of at-risk families. They often start before or soon after the birth of a child to help build family strengths from the beginning and may continue until the child is 5 years of age. Home-based services set the stage for services and support that are flexible, culturally competent, and responsive to family needs (Sandall, 1997).

Another type of family-focused programming is called Parent-to-Parent support. Parents of children with disabilities can exchange information on resources and problem-solve together when agency personnel are unavailable (i.e., after working hours). Parents who are at risk of maltreating their children with disabilities can benefit by talking with other parents in similar situations (Jones et al., 1995). They may express vulnerabilities and explore painful options with other parents in ways they would not feel comfortable when dealing with a professional. A survey conducted in 1996 found that "Parent-to-Parent support increases parents' sense of being able to cope [and] . . . increases parents' acceptance of their situation" (Santelli et al., 1997, p. 78).

When targeting prevention programs to at-risk families, Sobsey (1994) stated that it is important to identify the risk factors in families so programs can set priorities and tailor services to individual families. Many professionals have discussed the need to focus on reducing the effects of stress on families that have children with disabilities (Crosse et al., 2001). For example, Rycus and Hughes (1998) stated that services must address three factors in the stress equation: (a) reduce situational and psychological stress, (b) strengthen the family's ability to cope and to access supportive resources, and (c) help the family achieve a realistic perception of the situation.

A family-focused prevention service is an important component in the overall effort to prevent abuse and neglect of children with disabilities. Tomison (1996) stated that services should be available as long as a family needs them and whenever need occurs. Public funding and medical insurance coverage are key factors in the availability, accessibility, and longevity of services delivered to families of children with disabilities.

Child-Focused Prevention Efforts

Child maltreatment prevention programs are rarely made available or accessible to children with disabilities, often due to a lack of funding or a mistaken belief that this population does not need prevention information (Baladerian, 1994). In reality, "withholding knowledge from individuals with disabilities concerning self-protection increases their vulnerability to abuse and neglect" (Mitchell & Buchele-Ash, 2000, p. 235).

Child-focused prevention programs for children with disabilities should include sharing information about abuse (how to identify it, how to respond to it, how to tell others) and talking about feelings that occur when abuse is attempted. Parent involvement throughout the program is crucial to ensure that all family members are aware of and support the program's teachings.

A number of researchers have discussed the need for more appropriate and accessible programming for children with disabilities (Ammerman, 1997; Baladerian, 1994; Kragthorpe et al., 1997). Programs need to be inclusive and sensitive to ability levels, culture, age, and gender. Steinberg and Hylton (1998) recommended the use of developmentally appropriate concepts, concrete activities, and audiovisual aids. Prevention programs for children with disabilities need to be ongoing rather than a one-time effort; children with certain disabilities, such as cognitive, may need lessons repeated frequently.

Many programs provide specific information about abuse — what it is, how to recognize it, and what rights children have (Tobin, 1992). In addition to education, teaching assertiveness skills is often mentioned as a component of prevention efforts. Yet, Baladerian (1994) cautioned that simply telling children with disabilities to say "no" to an adult is often not beneficial, because they are taught to respect and comply with adults in authority. Abuse prevention programs also teach safety and self-defense skills (Wolcott, 1997). However, Sobsey (1994) stated, "It is important to recognize that many abused people with disabilities, as with other victims of abuse, face extreme power inequities that no amount of individual training can overcome" (p. 178).

REACTIONS TO SEXUAL ABUSE

An important part of treatment of victims of sexual abuse is to help them understand the meaning of abuse. This includes learning what is appropriate and inappropriate touching; what is wrong about sexual activity between adults and children, if they do not already know; why adults or a particular adult was sexual with them; and, in some cases, why they were chosen as targets and what that means to them. How these issues are addressed will vary with the disability and the child's developmental stage (Santrock, 2004). These issues may be more adequately dealt with in group treatment than individual therapy, and sometimes having the offender take full responsibility for the abuse in dyadic therapy with the victim is beneficial. Moreover, an adequate explanation for a child at a young age may not be sufficient as he or she grows older. Thus, this particular issue will need to be addressed at a more sophisticated level as the child matures, depending on the particular disability and cognitive limitations. This can be done by a parent but, in some cases, can best be done by a therapist.

Treatment of victimized children needs to include strategies for future protection. Teaching children to say no and learning how to inform someone about what happened may be useful, especially if the material is presented in a group setting and there are opportunities to role play how to resist and immediately report sexual advances. Specific protective strategies involving family members and helping professionals need to be developed in interfamilial sexual abuse situations. Additionally, the therapist must appreciate that placing even partial responsibility for self-protection on the person who has been victimized is potentially an overwhelming burden (Santelli et al., 1997).

TREATMENT OF SEXUAL ABUSE

Children with disabilities who have been sexually abused need help understanding the meaning of sexual abuse. Therapists have used a variety of methods and treatment programs for helping children with disabilities deal with the effects of sexual abuse. To be effective, therapists need an understanding of the child's particular disability. The most common treatment of sexual abuse involves dealing with feelings associated with the abuse. Resolving problems with acting out is the second most common treatment goal. Other treatment goals include dealing with fears, enhancing self-esteem, improving body image, resolving sexual acting out, and decreasing inappropriate sexual play (Mowbray, 1995).

Treatment structures also appear to be highly related. Therapists advocate that therapy focus on teaching the child with a disability acceptable ways to be sexual and setting appropriate limits on sexual behavior. It also may be useful to encourage regressive behavior in therapy, allowing the child to accomplish tasks and experiences in a healthy way which had been missed in earlier developmental stages (Berliner & Elliott, 2001).

WELLNESS APPROACH TO SEXUAL ABUSE

Parents can help prevent or lessen the chances of sexual abuse of their children who have disabilities by teaching them about sexual abuse to increase their awareness and coping skills. Without frightening their children, parents can provide them with appropriate safety information in a matter-of-fact way, along with other routine safety discussions about fire, water, health, and factors that may be specific to a particular disability. Although even the best educated child cannot always avoid sexual abuse, children with disabilities who are well prepared are more likely to avoid possible abusive situations or be able to inform a parent if abuse has occurred.

To protect children with disabilities from abuse, they need to be taught to feel good about themselves and know that they are loved, valued, and deserve to be safe. They need an understanding of the difference between safe and unsafe touching, of the proper names of all the body parts so they will be able to communicate clearly, and that safety rules apply to all adults. Children should know that their bodies belong to them and no one has a right to touch them inappropriately or hurt them. In addition, children can be taught that they must say "no" to suggestive behaviors of others if they feel uncomfortable, even to relatives and family friends; to report if any adult tells them to keep a secret; that they can rely on their parents to believe and protect them if they are abused; that they are not bad or at fault if sexual abuse occurs; and to inform a trusted adult about abuse even if they fear possible consequences (Beach Center on Families and Disability, 1997; Kragthorpe et al., 1997; Mitchell & Buchele-Ash, 2000).

Children with disabilities may be especially vulnerable because of physical, emotional, or cognitive limitations, depending on the particular disability, its severity, and the limitations it causes. It is imperative that family members, therapists, and those involved in the well-being of the child work together to let the child know that he or she is loved and did nothing wrong. Unconditional love and understanding is a key factor in developing self-worth and self-esteem (Corey, 2005). A child with a disability may be dealing with additional issues related to a particular disability (S. K. Brodwin, Orange, & M. G. Brodwin, 1994). By understanding their intrinsic value involving courageous self-discovery, and the love and respect of significant others in their lives, they are able to advance along a personal path of wellness knowing that they will be connected to people who love them.

CONCLUSION

Sexual abuse of children who have disabilities is a problem that is only beginning to attract the attention of researchers, service providers, and funding agencies. Researchers have not been able to gather precise information to determine the extent of sexual abuse among children who have disabilities. However, recent research has found that children with disabilities are sexually abused or maltreated 1.7 times the rate of other children (Berliner & Elliott, 2001; Crosse et al., 2001; Orelove et al., 2000). Other researchers suggest that children with disabilities may have increased vulnerability to sexual abuse because of society's responses to disability, rather than the disability itself (Hewitt, 1999; Mitchell & Buchele-Ash, 2000; Sullivan & Knutson, 2003).

For different disability types, varying dynamics of abuse come into play. For example, children with physical disabilities and limitations in physically escaping situations are in sharp contrast to children with hearing impairments, who may be able to escape but face communication barriers. Therapists need to pay particular attention to vulnerability factors that are disability related as opposed to those factors experienced by all children.

Children with disabilities are more at risk of abuse and neglect than children without disabilities. The factors that place these children at higher risk include those that place all children at risk of sexual abuse and maltreatment, in addition to other risk factors that are more directly related to disabilities. These include negative societal attitudes about disabilities; people's reactions to, and interactions with, children with disabilities (including family members and nonfamily caregivers); factors that relate to the particular disability itself; and program policies and procedures governing the care of children by others (Ammerman & Baladerian, 1993; Jones et al., 1995).

Primary prevention efforts will improve conditions for all families that have children with disabilities, and secondary prevention programs can target children and families who are at high risk of sexual abuse and maltreatment. Prevention strategies are aimed at improving the following: societal attitudes, federal policies, family dynamics, children's knowledge and safety skills, and program policies and procedures (Orelove et al., 2000; Struck, 1999).

To justify additional funding for prevention programs, including services for children and families and training for professionals, further research is needed to understand the scope and nature of this problem. Improved documentation of disabilities in the Child Protective Services system would assist in this process. Current prevention programming should be evaluated to determine its effectiveness. Finally, as Sobsey (1994) stated, "Before this problem can be successfully managed, society must adopt attitudes that allow all of its members to see the problem, recognize that it must be addressed, and believe that meaningful change is possible" (p. 304).

CONTRIBUTORS

Leo M. Orange, MS, is Coordinator of Disabled Students Programs & Services (DSP&S), at Oxnard College in Oxnard, California, and a part-time Assistant Professor at California State University, Los Angeles, in the Rehabilitation Counselor Education Program. Mr. Orange has published in counseling and rehabilitation journals on the subjects of reasonable accommodation, multicultural counseling, sexuality, abuse and maltreatment, and psychosocial aspects of disability. Additionally, he has presented professional papers and workshops at local, state, regional, and national conferences and conventions on various topics related to disability. Mr. Orange may be contacted at Oxnard College, Educational Assistance Center, 4000 Rose Avenue, Oxnard, CA 93033. E-mail: lorange.vcccd.net

Martin G. Brodwin, PhD, is Professor and Coordinator of the Rehabilitation Counselor Education Program at California State University, Los Angeles (CSULA). He frequently testifies as a Vocational Expert on disability determination for the Social Security Administration. Dr. Brodwin has coauthored 4 books and over 60 referred articles and book chapters on the subjects of rehabilitation counseling, abuse and neglect, reasonable accommodation, and cultural issues in relation to people who have disabilities. Between 1996 and 2005, he was the recipient of five prestigious awards for teaching and professional accomplishments. Dr. Brodwin can be reached at CSULA, 5151 State University Drive, Los Angeles, CA 90032. E-mail: mbrodwi@calstatela.edu

RESOURCES

Ammerman, R. T. (1992). Sexually abused children with multiple disabilities: Each is unique, as are their needs. *National Resource Center on Child Sexual Abuse (NRCCSA) News, 1*(4), 13-14.

Ammerman, R. T. (1997). Physical abuse and childhood disability: Risk and treatment factors. In R. Geffner, S. B. Sorenson, & P. K. Lundberg-Love (Eds.), *Violence and Sexual Abuse at Home: Current Issues in Spousal Battering and Child Maltreatment* (pp. 207-224). New York: Haworth Maltreatment and Trauma Press.

Ammerman, R. T., & Baladerian, N. J. (1993). *Maltreatment of Children With Disabilities*. Washington, DC: National Committee to Prevent Child Abuse.

Ammerman, R. T., & Patz, R. J. (1996). Determinants of child abuse potential: Contribution of parent and child factors. *Journal of Clinical Child Psychology, 25*(3), 300-307.

Baladerian, N. J. (1994). *Abuse and Neglect of Children With Disabilities*. Washington, DC: ARCH National Resource Center for Respite and Crisis Care Services.

Beach Center on Families and Disability. (1997). *How to Reduce Abuse and Neglect of Children With Disabilities*. Lawrence: University of Kansas.

Berliner, L., & Elliott, D. (2001). Sexual abuse of children. In J. Meyers, L. Berliner, J. Briere, C. T. Hendrix, C. Jenny, & T. Reid (Eds.), *APSAC Handbook on Child Maltreatment* (pp. 55-78). Thousand Oaks, CA: Sage Publications.

Brodwin, S. K., Orange, L. M., & Brodwin, M. G. (1994). Disabled clients: What every therapist needs to know. In L. VandeCreek, S. Knapp, & T. L. Jackson (Eds.), *Innovations in Clinical Practice: A Source Book* (Vol. 13, pp. 419-430). Sarasota, FL: Professional Resource Press.

Burrell, B., Thompson, B., & Sexton, D. (1994). Predicting child abuse potential across family types. *Child Abuse and Neglect, 18*(12), 1039-1049.

Child Abuse Prevention, Adoption, and Family Services Act of 1998, 42 U.S.C. § 5101 *et seq.*

Corey, G. (2005). *Theory and Practice of Counseling and Psychotherapy* (7th ed.). Belmont, CA: Thomson-Brooks/Cole.

Crosse, S. B., Kaye, E., & Ratnofsky, A. C. (2001). *A Report on the Maltreatment of Children With Disabilities*. Washington, DC: National Center on Child Abuse and Neglect.

Hewitt, S. K. (1999). *Assessing Allegations of Sexual Abuse in Preschool Children: Understanding Small Voices*. Thousand Oaks, CA: Sage Publications.

Individuals With Disabilities Education Act of 1990, 20 U.S.C. § 1400 *et seq.*

Jones, D., Peterson, D. M., Goldberg, P. F., Goldberg, M., & Smith, J. (1995). *Risky Situations: Vulnerable Children*. Minneapolis, MN: PACER Center.

Kragthorpe, C., Schmalzer, S., Xiong, D., Villasenor, J., Smith, J., Goldberg, P. F., & Goldberg, M. (1997). *Let's Prevent Abuse: A Prevention Handbook for People Working With Young Families*. Minneapolis, MN: PACER Center.

Mitchell, L. M., & Buchele-Ash, A. (2000). Abuse and neglect of individuals with disabilities: Building protective supports through public policy. *Journal of Disability Policy Studies, 10*(2), 225-243.

Mowbray, C. T. (1995). Treatment of children sexually abused in a daycare setting. *Journal of Child Sexual Abuse, 4*(3), 1-11.

National Resource Center on Child Sexual Abuse. (1994). *Responding to Sexual Abuse of Children With Disabilities: Prevention, Investigation, and Treatment*. Lawrence: Beach Center on Families and Disability, University of Kansas.

National Symposium on Abuse and Neglect of Children With Disabilities. (1995). *Abuse and Neglect of Children With Disabilities: Report and Recommendations*. Lawrence: Beach Center on Families and Disability, University of Kansas.

Nosek, M. A., Howland, C. A., & Young, M. E. (1998). Abuse of women with disabilities: Policy implications. *Journal of Disability Policy Studies, 11*(3), 158-175.

Orange, L. M. (2002). Sexuality and disability. In M. G. Brodwin, F. A. Tellez, & S. K. Brodwin (Eds.), *Medical, Psychosocial, and Vocational Aspects of Disability* (2nd ed., pp. 53-61). Athens, GA: Elliott & Fitzpatrick.

Orelove, F. P., Hollahan, D. J., & Myles, K. T. (2000). Maltreatment of children with disabilities: Training needs for a collaborative response. *Child Abuse and Neglect, 24*(2), 185-194.

Rogow, S., & Hass, J. (1999). *The Person Within: Preventing Abuse of Children and Young People With Disabilities.* Vancouver, BC, Canada: British Columbia Institute Against Family Violence.

Rycus, J. S., & Hughes, R. C. (1998). *Field Guide to Child Welfare, Volume III: Child Development and Child Welfare.* Washington, DC: Child Welfare League of America.

Sandall, S. R. (1997). Home-based services and supports. In A. H. Widerstrom, B. A. Mowder, & S. R. Sandall (Eds.), *Infant Development and Risk* (pp. 315-334). Baltimore: Paul H. Brookes.

Santelli, B., Turnbull, A., Marquis, J., & Lerner, E. (1997). Parent-to-parent programs: A resource for parents and professionals. *Journal of Early Intervention, 21*(1), 73-83.

Santrock, J. W. (2004). *Life-Span Development* (9th ed.). New York: McGraw-Hill.

Sobsey, D. (1994). *Violence and Abuse in the Lives of People With Disabilities: The End of Silent Acceptance?* Baltimore: Paul H. Brookes.

Sobsey, D., & Doe, T. (1991). Patterns of sexual abuse and assault. *Sexuality and Disability, 9*(3), 243-259.

Steinberg, M. A., & Hylton, J. R. (1998). *Responding to Maltreatment of Children With Disabilities: A Trainer's Guide.* Portland: Oregon Institute on Disability and Development, Child Development & Rehabilitation Center, Oregon Health Sciences University.

Struck, L. M. (1999). *Assistance for Special Educators, Law Enforcement, and Child Protective Services in Recognizing and Managing Abuse and Neglect of Children With Disabilities.* Virginia Beach: Virginia Department of Social Services, Child Protective Services.

Sullivan, P. M., & Knutson, J. F. (2003). Maltreatment and disabilities: A population-based epidemiological study. *Journal of Early Intervention, 27*(4), 21-33.

Tobin, P. (1992). Addressing special vulnerabilities in prevention. *National Resource Center on Child Sexual Abuse (NRCCSA) News, 1*(4), 5-12.

Tomison, A. M. (1996). Child maltreatment and disability. *Issues in Child Abuse Prevention, 7,* 1-11.

Wolcott, D. (1997). *Children With Disabilities: Risk Factors for Maltreatment.* Unpublished doctoral dissertation, University of Denver, Colorado.

Young, M. E., Nosek, M. A., Howland, C. A., Chanpong, G., & Rintala, D. H. (1997). Prevalence of abuse of women with physical disabilities. *Archives of Physical Medicine and Rehabilitation [Special issue], 78*(12, Suppl. 5), S34-S38.

WEBSITES*

Child Abuse Website
http://smhp.psych.ucla.edu/qf/sexassault.html

Child Sexual Abuse Help
www.medic8.com/healthguide/articles/childsexhelpabuse.html

Child Sexual Abuse/National Center for Post-Traumatic Stress Disorder (PTSD)
www.ncptsd.va.gov/facts/specific/fs_child_sexual_abuse.html

Crime and Misconduct Commission
www.cmc.qld.gov.au/SAPI.html

MedlinePlus: Child Sexual Abuse
www.nlm.nih.gov/medlineplus/childsexualabuse.html

Safe Network's Library of Child Sexual Abuse
www.safenetwork.org/Library1.html

Social Work Online
www.socialworker.com/websites.htm

Support Groups
www.healthcyclopedia.com/general-support-groups/sexual-abuse.html

---

* Although all websites cited in this contribution were correct at the time of publication, they are subject to change at any time.

Introduction to Section II: Practice Management and Professional Development

This section of *Innovations* includes contributions that assist practitioners in building and managing their practices in effective ways.

The first contribution, by Tawanda Greer, addresses the problems of health disparities among racial and ethnic minorities. Failure to improve culturally sensitive practices is a disservice to persons of color. The chapter discusses the disparities in health, and associated consequences, among racial and ethnic minorities, and it provides practical interventions to address these issues. A companion assessment tool, the "Index of Race-Related Stress–Brief Version (IRRS-B)" is presented in Section III.

In the second contribution in this section, Frederick Peterson and Jill Bley highlight the advantages of expanding one's clinical practice to include sex therapy and the promotion of sexual health. They examine the development of sex therapy as an expanding field of clinical practice.

The last two chapters address two areas of the intersection of clinical practice with the Internet. In the first of these two chapters, Anthony Ragusea provides tips for designing a mental health professional's website. It is written for practitioners who have little experience with web design and who are considering developing a web page for their practice. The author provides a useful worksheet for practitioners who are planning a website. In the second article, Paul Smiley and Leon VandeCreek describe some potential benefits of conducting online therapy, and they identify common problems with using this medium and propose some solutions to the problems.

Interventions for Bridging the Gaps in Minority Health

Tawanda M. Greer

The U.S. Census Bureau estimates that, by the year 2025, racial and ethnic minorities will account for at least 40% of the population in the United States (U.S. Department of Health and Human Services, 2001). To date, American residents speak at least 329 different languages, with 32 million Americans identifying English as a second language (Smith & Gonzales, 2000). The increased racial and cultural diversity in America raises concern about the existing disparities in utilization of all healthcare services by racial and ethnic minorities. Recent literature has documented the degree to which racial and ethnic minorities experience health declines and poor outcomes in comparison to Whites (e.g., Myers, Lewis, & Parker Dominguez, 2003; Williams & Rucker, 2000). Thus, a great challenge exists for healthcare professionals to ensure that, as the racial and ethnic population continues to grow, the existing gap in health disparities does not also continue to grow with similar proportion. This contribution has two primary objectives: (a) to discuss existing disparities in health and associated consequences among racial and ethnic minorities, and (b) to provide practical interventions as means for healthcare professionals to effectively address health concerns of racial and ethnic minorities within culturally relevant frameworks.

EXISTING HEALTH DISPARITIES

A plethora of literature exists documenting differences in physical and mental health outcomes between racial and ethnic minorities and Whites in America. White Americans have higher life expectancy rates and lower morbidity and comorbity of illnesses when compared to persons of color (e.g., Cohen, 2003). For example, when compared to Whites, African Americans are 1.4 times more likely to die of stroke, whereas two to four times the rate of diabetes can be found among Mexican Americans (Heisler et al., 2003). Heisler et al. (2003) also noted that Native Americans and Alaskan natives have higher death rates when compared to White Americans.

Poor physical, emotional, and psychological outcomes among persons of color have been linked to race, racism, and overall experiences of oppression. Overt and subtle racism and other forms of oppression remain entities in society that produce undercurrents of persistent stress for racial and ethnic minorities. The term "daily hassles" can be used to classify the degree of stress produced by oppression, especially subtle forms of racism and discrimination. In general, daily hassles stress produces more profound emotional, psychological, and physical impacts compared to events that do not happen as often (Kanner et al., 1981).

In one study, Klonoff, Landrine, and Ullman (1999) examined the relationship between pychiatric symptoms and experiences of racial discrimination, general stressors (e.g., getting married), and status variables (e.g., socioeconomic status [SES]) among African Americans. These researchers found that racial discrimination was the strongest predictor of psychiatric symptoms (e.g., anxiety, depression). General stress and gender were the next strongest predictors of psychiatric symptoms in this sample of African Americans. In another study, Ren, Amick, and Williams (1999) found that overall health disparities between Whites and African Americans were significantly explained by persistent racial discrimination among Blacks. Ren et al. (1999) reported that "experiences of discrimination due to race or low SES are significantly associated with . . . general health perceptions, mental health, and depression" (p. 162). It is also possible that racism and discrimination pose long-term effects which may contribute to overall health declines for African Americans of all ages (Ferrero & Farmer, 1996). Thus, given the widespread, systemic nature of racism and oppression, it is imperative that medical and mental health professionals consider its significance in their attempts to understand and address health disparities among racial and ethnic minorities.

ADDITIONAL FACTORS ASSOCIATED WITH HEALTH DISPARITIES

Although racism and other forms of oppression have been associated with health outcomes among persons of color, existing health disparities are also largely attributed to overall differences in health practices within the United States. Differences in treatments, referrals, and procedures serve to disadvantage persons of color in needed healthcare. Differences in health practices generally consist of diagnostic procedures, prescriptions for specific medications, perceived quality of medical treatment, access to transplants, pain management, access to outpatient and other referral services, and overall ability to afford medical care (e.g., Smedley, Stith, & Nelson, 2002). Cohen (2003) marked access to healthcare services as a primary predictor of the quality of health among racial and ethnic minorities. This author noted, "the issue of lack of insurance is an absolute indictment of our system, with as many as 42 million uninsured Americans, and is our single biggest problem in terms of healthcare disparities" (p. 1155). A recent publication by the Alliance for Health Reform (2004) reinforced this notion by noting that being uninsured or underinsured contributes to the lack of quality of care received and poor health outcomes for racial and ethnic minority populations.

However, the ability to afford healthcare, although it is a major problem in America, does not fully account for health disparities by race and ethnicity. A large body of literature exists which suggests that, even when persons of color are fully insured and/or can afford quality care, they still receive poorer quality of treatment by healthcare professionals compared to Whites (e.g., Alliance for Health Reform, 2004). This particular finding suggests that medical and mental health provider stereotypes, biases, prejudices, and discriminatory practices substantially contribute to existing health disparities. For instance, van Ryn and Burke (2000) found that physicians rated Black patients as more likely to engage in substance abuse, less likely to desire active lifestyles, less likely to comply with treatment recommendations for cardiac rehabilitation, and to be at high risk for low social support compared to White patients. Additionally, Black patients were rated by physicians as less intelligent and educated than Whites (van Ryn & Burke, 2000).

The problem with discrimination and biases is further exacerbated by the lack of representation of physicians, psychiatrists, dentists, and other healthcare professionals from various racial and ethnic backgrounds, especially African American, Native American, and Hispanic American. Other factors, such as gender and socioeconomic status, contribute to discriminatory practices in treatment. Therefore, healthcare professionals have the responsibility to engage in a process of self-reflection to determine the degree to which their practices are discriminatory in nature and, consequently, work toward minimizing biases and stereotypes in treatment.

Problems with healthcare management and administration have also been pinpointed as significant contributors to existing health disparities. Gatekeeping policies of managed care have been implicated as major sources of the poor quality of health among racial and ethnic minorities (e.g., U.S. Department of Health and Human Services, 2001; Williams & Rucker, 2000). Williams and Rucker (2000) noted that managed care often limits the number of referrals made by medical professionals who primarily treat underserved populations. Also, managed care generally seeks to encourage treatments and procedures that are low in cost. However, many racial and ethnic minorities tend to delay their efforts in acquiring medical services. Thus, many patients of color suffer from ailments that potentially have progressed to chronic conditions by the time they seek medical treatment (Williams & Rucker, 2000). Cost-containment practices serve to exclude many persons of color because their need for treatment potentially requires extensive medical attention, and thus increases the cost of care. "Red tape" and other administrative hassles with managed care pose challenges for patients seeking treatment through HMOs and other federally funded health plans (e.g., Medicaid, Medicare). For racial and ethnic minorities, administrative hassles become yet additional barriers with which to contend.

Additional problems with managed care can be found within the mental health profession. The U.S. Department of Health and Human Services (2001) noted that, in 1996, over $69 billion was spent on mental health services, with most of the spending occurring through Medicaid and Medicare. In spite of the large sum of money spent on mental health treatment from these sectors, the quality of care and management of services was perceived as less than favorable by many racial and ethnic minorities (U.S. Department of Health and Human Services, 2001). Additionally, several problems have arisen as managed care generally conceptualizes mental health treatment in the same vein as physical illnesses. Thus, coverage for some mental health services can be limited to three to five therapy sessions for disorders such as depression, anxiety, and other common psychological problems.

Factors among racial and ethnic minorities themselves also contribute to existing health disparities. Racial and ethnic minorities' experiences of racism and other forms of oppression are associated with mistrust of medical and mental health professionals. Therefore, as previously mentioned, many persons of color delay their efforts in addressing physical illnesses and mental health symptoms in an attempt to avoid potential discriminatory practices, in addition to other stressful hassles.

Avoidance behaviors also serve to ward off any stigma associated with some illnesses and problems (e.g., HIV/AIDS, alcohol addiction, mental disorders). Although cultural mistrust and avoidance behaviors influence help-seeking behaviors among racial and ethnic minorities, these problems are not insurmountable. Several research studies have demonstrated that awareness efforts and other forms of community education have assisted in minimizing delays in treatment (e.g., Jenkins et al., 2004) and, consequently, improving the overall quality of health among racial and ethnic minorities.

Additionally, many racial and ethnic minorities utilize English as a second language; thus, communication barriers potentially arise between themselves and healthcare professionals. Language barriers also prevent some persons of color from seeking treatment. The Alliance for Health Reform (2004) noted that it has been found that at least one-fifth of Spanish-speaking Latinos reported not seeking health treatment because of the underrepresentation of professionals of the same cultural and linguistic background. Furthermore, some racial and ethnic minorities are not astute at being assertive in acquiring needed information and answers from medical and mental health professionals. Many persons of color lack the necessary skills to advocate for themselves and their own well-being. These problems further exacerbate communication barriers in treatment.

Overall, a myriad of factors exist that are responsible for disparities in overall health outcomes among Whites and racial and ethnic minorities. It appears that both systemic and interpersonal changes (e.g., improvements in communication) are necessary in order to begin to effectively address the issues discussed. In the following section, practical interventions and techniques to effectively address existing health disparities will be discussed. Two case examples demonstrating some of the interventions will also be presented.

CULTURALLY RELEVANT INTERVENTIONS

In order to effectively address health disparities and poor health outcomes, medical and mental health professionals must adopt attitudes and behaviors that will facilitate multiculturally competent interventions in their work with persons of color. Anderson et al. (2003) discussed several strategies to improve the cultural competency of healthcare systems. Anderson et al. (2003) defined cultural competence as "a set of congruent behaviors, attitudes, and policies that come together in a system, agency, or among professionals and enable effective work in cross-cultural situations" (p. 68). This particular definition implies that, in order for cultural competence to be achieved, changes must occur among professionals as well as within systems.

A set of multicultural competency standards for practice and training purposes has been adopted within the profession of psychology (e.g., Sue, Arredondo, & McDavis, 1995). Many of these competencies address areas such as awareness of one's biases, prejudices, and stereotypes, as well as knowledge of history, cultural norms, and traditions of diverse populations. Multicultural competence also connotes that professionals incorporate societal realities and consequences associated with various characteristics of the individual (e.g., race, gender, and sexual orientation). Furthermore, the degree to which societal realities are related to presenting medical and/or mental health concerns is also a hallmark of culturally competent practice. The following sections will describe needed interventions among medical and mental health professionals.

Societal Forces

Health professionals must consider the societal experiences of persons of color as an intervention in working with racial and ethnic minorities. This task may lack some degree of feasibility for professionals who practice in settings with significant time constraints. However, it is imperative to engage in these efforts nonetheless. Assessment instruments are beneficial as means of acquiring information regarding societal experiences in a short period of time.

Many instruments that have been used to measure societal experiences of persons of color have been used significantly in research studies. However, such instruments can be effective in therapy sessions and other healthcare modalities. Additionally, measures that assess racial and other experiences can be incorporated as part of initial intake appointments prior to receiving medical and/or mental health treatment. For instance, Utsey (1999) developed The Index of Race-Related Stress-Brief Version (IRRS-B), which is a questionnaire that measures stress associated with racial experiences for African Americans. The IRRS-Brief Version consists of 22 Likert-type response items which measure dimensions of cultural racism (i.e., existing worldview that cultural values, traditions, and norms are inferior to the dominant group), institutional racism (i.e., racially discriminatory practices embedded within social institutions), and individual racism (i.e., personal experiences of racial prejudice in social interactions). The

IRRS-Brief Version (Utsey, 1999) can generally provide clinicians with in-depth substantive information regarding the degree to which African American patients/clients have experienced racism. This information can then be incorporated into further conceptualizations and interventions with African American clients/patients. Additional information on the IRRS-B (Utsey, 1999) and administrative instructions can be found in the "Assessment Instruments and Client Handouts" section of this publication (pp. 225-229).

Other measures can also be used to acquire information regarding cultural experiences of persons of color. Multidimensional measures generally capture several aspects of cultural identity formation and the degree of connectedness to one's cultural group(s). Examples of multidimensional tools include the Multigroup Ethnic Identity Measure (Phinney, 1992), the Multidimensional Inventory of Black Identity (Sellers et al., 1997), and some measures of various types of acculturation (e.g., Mendoza, 1989). The drawback of multidimensional measures is that some can be lengthy and time-consuming to administer. However, the wealth of information that is generated is highly beneficial for improving in-session dynamics and treatment planning. Qualitative approaches, however, can be used to compensate for limitations found in quantitative assessment tools (e.g., length). Qualitative approaches also enhance cultural sensitivity in working with racial and ethnic minorities, especially when clients' proficiency in English is limited. For example, open-ended questions (see p. 157) such as, "To what degree do you feel that racism and other forms of oppression are related to your physical and/or mental health concerns?" generate a wealth of information that clinicians can then consider in their conceptualizations, diagnoses, treatment plans, and interventions. Other qualitative cultural assessment methods include Dana's Cultural Assessment Model (1998) and Grieger and Ponterotto's (1995) Six-Step Applied Assessment Framework.

Communication Barriers

As mentioned previously, many persons of color within the United States utilize English as a second language. Thus, medical and mental health professionals must attempt to engage in effective dialogue in spite of potential language barriers. In cases in which a healthcare professional is linguistically different from the client/patient, this particular challenge can be met by including family members and significant others in treatment who speak the same language as the client/patient. In mental health and medical treatment, including family members and others may not be feasible in some cases due to issues of confidentiality and other circumstances. Thus, attempts to locate appropriate referral sources to colleagues and other professionals who are linguistically similar may be warranted in these cases.

In addition, communication barriers may also be alleviated by assisting clients/patients in advocating for themselves when interacting with healthcare professionals. As mentioned previously, cultural mistrust as well as a lack of knowledge of treatment modalities and other health-related information may limit some persons of color in asking questions and acquiring other needed information from healthcare professionals. Self-advocacy among racial and ethnic minorities can be facilitated in several ways. First, after gleaning an understanding of potential experiences of oppression within society, clinicians are then in a better position to engage clients/patients in dialogue about their concerns and apprehensions about treatment. The dialogue at this juncture can encompass a number of different issues, such as concerns about the race and ethnicity of the clinician, and the client's/patient's doubts about the clinician's ability to be empathic about presenting concerns, among other issues. Also, this dialogue serves as an opportunity for the clinician to build trust and rapport with the client/patient, and would inevitably improve communication and may lead to compliance with further treatment.

Second, clinicians can further empower clients/patients by ensuring their access to and understanding of needed health information. Specifically, healthcare agencies and treatment centers can have brochures and other printed information (e.g., descriptions of specific treatment modalities and procedures) translated and reprinted in different languages. Assessments, diagnoses, and treatments should be fully explained to clients/patients in a manner in which they become active participants in their treatment versus being uninformed participant-observers in the process. Lastly, it may also prove helpful for healthcare professionals to develop an aggregate list of Internet resources and other media sources that are relevant to medical and mental health concerns of persons of color.

EXAMPLE OF A THERAPEUTIC DIALOGUE

The following is an example of a dialogue between a psychologist (a 41-year-old, White, German male) and a 35-year-old, married, Native American female who was seeking mental health treatment for the first time in her life. Her presenting concerns consisted of symptoms of depression (e.g., hopelessness, insomnia, social withdrawal, and persistent sadness), substance abuse, and memory difficulties. The dialogue between the client and the psychologist occurred during the first session.

Psychologist: Tell me about the issues that have influenced your decision to seek therapy?

Client: Well, coming here was hard and I'm not sure where to start. I'm nervous about being here.

Psychologist: That's understandable. Lots of people have difficulty opening up in therapy, especially since I'm a complete stranger. You and I are also very different culturally. My being a White man may also make it difficult to talk.

Client: Yes, it does.

Psychologist: Would you like to tell me more about that?

Client: Well, my family does not think highly of White men or Whites in general. We're looked down upon or even ignored and forgotten. And then, so much has happened in the past between my group and Whites. We're still treated unfairly. It just makes me upset when I think about it.

Psychologist: It seems that that would be tough to deal with. It's unfortunate that there's so much negativity around race and culture in society. And you're right, there is a lot of history and painful things from the past that make it difficult for different racial groups to interact. It also seems that you personally have not had positive experiences with Whites. How might these issues impact our work together?

Client: It's hard to talk. I'm also not sure if you will understand what I'm really going through. I don't know if you can help me.

Psychologist: I can understand why you would feel that way. It's difficult for you to trust me. It will be hard for me to completely understand what it's like to be you because I'm limited in some ways by being a White man. However, I will try to understand enough for us to work together to address the problems that you have. I may also need to ask you questions sometimes about your culture and other experiences in your life just to make sure that you and I are communicating clearly. Would it be okay if I ask you questions sometimes about things that I don't know, like your culture and other issues about what it's like to be a Native American woman?

Client: Yes, that's fine. I would feel better if you asked instead of assuming.

Psychologist: Okay, I will ask when I'm not certain about some things. That makes me feel better also. This will probably not be the last time we have this conversation. We may need to revisit these issues from time to time as we continue to work together. Does that sound okay?

Client: Yes, I don't mind that. I'll be thinking about these things when I see you anyway. So, it would be good to talk about this.

Psychologist: I feel the same way. I'm glad we talked about this. Would it be okay now if we moved to talking more about you feeling depressed lately?

Significant Clinical Points from the Dialogue

This dialogue serves as a demonstration of the ways in which clinicians can begin to engage persons of color in treatment. In this example, the psychologist first acknowledges the client's apprehension in communicating about her presenting concerns by showing empathy as well as explicitly stating his hypothesis about obvious reasons for the client's apprehension: race, ethnicity, and gender. By mentioning these factors, the psychologist inherently provided the client with permission to respond as freely and openly as she desired. It is also important to note that the psychologist did not reflect back with any personal feelings about the client's response concerning Whites. We can assume that the psychologist indeed had a personal reaction. However, he chose to pursue the underlying meaning of the client's response. Due to historical experiences of oppression among her racial and ethnic group, as well as her personal experiences with Whites, she found it difficult to trust him as a psychologist who could assist her effectively. The psychologist then labeled the underlying meaning of her words by stating, "It's difficult for you to trust me." This particular statement clearly demonstrated empathy toward the client and the emotions that she conveyed in her response.

Additionally, the psychologist expressed genuineness in his dialogue with the client. He freely admitted to a very real limitation as a White man in society in fully understanding the client's experiences. This point is particularly important as any conveyance of "knowing what it's like to be in her shoes" would have been unrealistic and potentially damaging in his efforts to build trust. With the admission of his limitation, the psychologist was then able to solicit the client's permission to inquire about aspects of her life and culture that he would not be in a position to comprehend. The client's acceptance of this request enabled the psychologist to feel less pressured to be completely knowledgeable about the client's experiences. Also, this allowed the client to feel less anxious about their interactions because she felt more comfortable to convey her thoughts and feelings about her experiences, her culture, and issues of oppression.

Lastly, the psychologist normalized the difficulty of discussing oppression and cultural differences via indicating that their process of communicating will likely be influenced again by the differences between them. Therefore, there will be a need to revisit their discussion of race and culture, and experiences of oppression, throughout treatment. The psychologist's status as a White male in the United States will need to be further explored in subsequent sessions as privilege associated with his race and gender are also significant factors that will impact the process of therapy and the effectiveness of communication.

In sum, the therapeutic interventions demonstrated in the dialogue can be utilized to improve barriers of communication in working with racial and ethnic minorities. Healthcare professionals who engage in explicit discussions about race, gender, sexual orientation, and other cultural issues with racial and ethnic minorities are likely to improve trust and rapport. Furthermore, clinicians need to initiate discussions of culture and race at the beginning of the provision of services in order to ensure effective process and outcomes. A list of critical questions for clinicians in working with racial and ethnic minorities can be found on page 157 of this contribution. Healthcare professionals who refrain from engaging in such dialogues with racial and ethnic minorities must explore their own concerns and resistance to doing so. Consultation with other colleagues may also assist in alleviating anxieties and concerns in addressing race, oppression, and other cultural issues with clients/patients.

SYSTEMIC INTERVENTIONS

In the Alliance for Health Reform (2004) report, raising awareness among stakeholders, patients, employers, and the general society was an identified area of change regarding health disparities. Additionally, the U.S. Department of Health and Human Services (2001) proposed in *Healthy People 2010* goals to eliminate health disparities among African Americans, Native Americans, Alaska Natives, Asian Americans, Hispanic Americans, and Pacific Islanders. The *Healthy People 2010* plan is to decrease disparities in common illnesses and problems that affect racial and ethnic minorities such as cardiovascular diseases, diabetes, HIV/AIDS, breast and cervical cancer, and infant mortality. Community-based programming is an effective method to increase the level of awareness among racial and ethnic minorities regarding their own health. For instance, Jenkins et al. (2004), members of the Charleston and Georgetown Diabetes Coalition, documented the improvement of diabetes management among African Americans and Whites in selected South Carolina communities. This project was funded by the Centers for Disease Control and Prevention's (CDC) Racial and Ethnic Approaches to Community Health (REACH) 2010 program.

The Charleston and Georgetown Coalition, composed of several community organizations, engaged in a number of efforts for 2 years to reduce diabetes-related disparities among Blacks and Whites (270 participants). After an initial period of collecting baseline data and actively promoting change, the Coalition documented significantly lowered disparities among Blacks and Whites in the sample with African Americans showing improvements in diabetes management. Among African Americans, improvements were reported in cholesterol levels, blood pressure, foot exams, and other medical testing (e.g., kidney testing and eye exams). Jenkins et al. (2004) concluded, "after two years of program implementation, percentages of overall recommended testing for AAs [African Americans] compared favorably with percentages nationally for Medicare patients with diabetes and also for those in community plans" (p. 328).

Along with large-scale community-based projects, healthcare professionals can also avail themselves of other opportunities to increase awareness and improve health behaviors such as the implementation of educational programs (e.g., HIV/AIDs awareness, alcohol and substance use), blood drives, and depression and anxiety screenings. Overall, community-based efforts provide healthcare professionals opportunities to both effect change and also improve trust and rapport among racial and ethnic populations via consistent, personal interactions in communities. Community action is imperative as many racial and ethnic minorities do not frequent medical and mental health settings. Thus, it is vitally important that healthcare professionals choose to enter racial and ethnic minority communities in an effort to improve health outcomes, in addition to making effective changes within healthcare settings.

In addition to community interventions, diversity training among healthcare professionals should be an ongoing venture within healthcare settings. Diversity training should generally challenge healthcare professionals to become familiar with biases, stereotypes, and potentially discriminatory behaviors perpetuated against racial and ethnic minorities. In many instances, some healthcare professionals do not knowingly act upon prejudices nor have knowingly engaged in discriminatory practices with persons of color. However, "unintentional discrimination" can stem from differences in values and other variables (e.g., SES, gender) in cross-cultural interactions and may potentially lead to inappropriate conceptualizations, diagnoses, and interventions on the part of healthcare professionals. Thus, diversity training should also encompass consideration of personal backgrounds and values and the degree to which these variables may influence the provision of treatment to racial and ethnic minorities. Furthermore, instances in which healthcare professionals find themselves to be culturally similar to their clients/patients should also be explored in diversity training. Cultural similarity may pose an advantage in communication and general interactions with clients/patients due to shared traditions, language, and other experiences. Simultaneously, cultural similarity can lead to a form of "blindness" on the part of the healthcare professional in which important differences and other significant issues can be overlooked or minimized, thus greatly impacting conceptualization and treatment.

Administrative practices within healthcare settings also need to include programs to recruit and maintain employment of diverse healthcare professionals. Healthcare settings that lack the presence of culturally and linguistically diverse employees should consider evaluating their hiring practices to improve representation of professionals from diverse backgrounds. Many racial and ethnic minorities seek medical and mental health professionals who are racially and culturally similar to themselves (e.g., Alliance for Health Reform, 2004; Atkinson & Lowe, 1995). Therefore, by recruiting and hiring professionals from various racial and ethnic backgrounds, healthcare settings may experience a slight increase in utilization of services among racial and ethnic minorities, although other issues may continue to influence the process of seeking services (e.g., cultural mistrust).

In sum, addressing health disparities among racial and ethnic minorities is a complex and challenging process. However, healthcare professionals can assist in improving health outcomes via addressing issues among themselves (e.g., biases and stereotypes) and practice behaviors, as well as facilitating change within healthcare settings. Attempts should be made to raise awareness within society in general as insight potentially inspires action toward effective change. Above all, healthcare professionals have an inherent responsibility to improve the welfare of clients/patients served. Given existing health outcomes among many persons of color, culturally sensitive attitudes and interventions should be considered top priorities among medical and mental health professionals.

A CASE EXAMPLE OF CULTURALLY APPROPRIATE CONCEPTUALIZATION AND INTERVENTION

Joshua* (pseudonym) is a 42-year-old, single, Black, South African male who relocated and became a United States citizen 1 year after leaving South Africa. He enrolled in graduate studies after completing an undergraduate degree while living in his home country. He transferred his college credits to a university in the United States and subsequently earned a master's degree in Engineering. While living in America, Joshua acquired a job in his profession and developed friendships with fellow South Africans and colleagues. He resided in an apartment in a large urban city on the East Coast. His family members remained in South Africa; he rarely had phone contact with them, preferring to correspond by letters. Thus, he had not seen his mother, nor his three younger sisters, in the past year. When Joshua was 8 years old, his biological father died of an incurable illness.

Joshua presented at a local community mental health center complaining of disturbing dreams, insomnia, "night sweats," difficulty concentrating at work, and low motivation to arrive to work. He had also grown increasingly suspicious of others over the past year, which produced significant anxiety in social interactions. He reported having friends that he rarely visited due to increasing issues of trust and suspicion of others. During the initial intake session, Joshua exclaimed, "I feel as though I've grown sensitive to everybody and everything around me." He denied significant medical conditions and injuries. He also denied the use of alcohol and other substances.

---

* Names and characteristics in all case examples have been changed to protect privacy.

Joshua's assigned therapist was a younger African American female. During two sessions, his suspicions of his therapist became apparent. For the first 10 to 15 minutes of initial sessions, Joshua would question his therapist about whether she shared information about him to others in the agency, and, if so, what, if anything, they had done with the information shared about him. His therapist would revisit the discussion of confidentiality and explain other ethical obligations and agency policies regarding sharing of information throughout the provision of services. These discussions eventually served to slightly alleviate Joshua's suspicions. Initial attempts by his therapist to explore reasons associated with his seemingly unwarranted suspiciousness of others were thwarted by Joshua. Instead, Joshua spent the first two sessions in discussions that did not appear directly associated with his presenting concerns (e.g., his reasons for studying engineering).

In order to build trust and rapport, the therapist began to ask general, open-ended questions of Joshua concerning his experiences in South Africa (e.g., Tell me about what it was like to live in South Africa?). Joshua then began to describe many of his experiences as a soldier in the South African military during the time of apartheid. He reported serving in his country's military for 3 years as a means to survive extreme poverty experienced by him and his family. During that period, he witnessed violence committed against fellow Black South Africans and others. He had even seen many South Africans murdered during apartheid. Many of Joshua's immediate and extended family members had also been impacted by the hostility and violence of the time. Joshua described significant emotional pain that he experienced as some of his family members chose to engage in efforts to flee the country.

Joshua's involvement in the military also caused difficulty for him interpersonally. As a member of the military, he often was required to engage in hostile and occasionally violent acts toward his fellow Black South Africans. He lost many relationships due to his involvement in the military and eventually came to see himself as a traitor of his people. He expressed significant guilt and remorse for his involvement in the military. After a period of 3 years, Joshua decided to leave South Africa. He reported that he fled on foot late one night and hid in the woods for nearly a week. He had little food and water but he eventually was able to travel safely to a friend's home. Joshua reported that a friend, who was wealthy, assisted him by purchasing a plane ticket to Europe and assisted him with travel to an airport in a neighboring city outside of South Africa. Two weeks later, Joshua successfully arrived in Europe. He lived in Europe with a friend before relocating to the United States.

Therapy sessions with Joshua entailed exploring the relationship between his experiences in the South African military, apartheid, and his presenting mental health concerns. Joshua's therapist administered a personality inventory in order to measure symptoms associated with various psychiatric disturbances. Prior to administration, his therapist explained the significance of the assessment tool and also explained that the measure was normed on a predominantly White American sample. His therapist further explained that the results would be used qualitatively to assist in understanding his current mental health symptoms and would perhaps provide information about his current experience of being "overly sensitive" in his surroundings. The results of the personality assessment tool indicated that Joshua was experiencing symptoms associated with Postraumatic Stress Disorder (PTSD). The therapist then explained the meaning of PTSD in light of his experiences in South Africa. Joshua expressed significant relief about being able to place a label on his symptoms. He expressed relief that his symptoms would eventually subside with treatment by exclaiming, "I thought that something had happened to me in my life that made me permanently disturbed." Subsequently, the therapist and Joshua developed and implemented goals for treatment.

In spite of the therapist's past experience and competence in treating PTSD, she was unfamiliar with South African culture and treatment of mental health symptoms with individuals from this population. Thus, the therapist consulted other colleagues as well as existing literature to assist Joshua. In searching the literature, the therapist discovered several articles in which the psychological implications of apartheid were discussed. Many interventions discussed in the literature were cognitive behavioral in nature and consisted of "storytelling" and encouragement to refrain from overly structured and directive dynamics in session.

As part of treatment, Joshua's therapist engaged in efforts to empower him by allowing him to guide many discussions in sessions. This was a significant part of treatment given that Joshua had experienced a loss of power for several years while in South Africa. Thus, empowerment was achieved by allowing Joshua to share his story of painful experiences within a safe, empathic environment. By the 10th session, Joshua requested to use paper and markers to draw a picture of the continent of Africa. He expressed to his therapist that he needed to visually depict the sites of many of the travesties that he experienced. The visual depiction of the African continent was used by Joshua throughout therapy. The picture became a symbolic representation of his past and the pain from which he needed to recover.

Through the experience of storytelling, it became apparent to Joshua and to the therapist that, although he had significant loss of power due to apartheid and his involvement in the South African military, he yet held a significant amount of personal power which emanated from his view of himself as a male relating to a Black female therapist. Additionally, Joshua was the only male in his household in South Africa for several years; thus, he was unaccustomed to having less power in his interactions with women. Consequently, his therapist, on many occasions, engaged Joshua in discussions of gender role attitudes and stereotypes and the similarities and differences in gender roles in America and in South Africa. Moreover, the therapist emphasized the importance of a collaborative relationship in reaching treatment goals, as power conflicts would impede efforts to alleviate mental health symptoms. Afterward, Joshua was able to refocus his attention toward himself and his presenting concerns.

As Joshua continued to engage in processing his emotions regarding his past, many of his psychological disturbances began to dissipate. He began to report fewer experiences of insomnia and nightmares. He continued to complain, however, of problems in interacting with others. As he and the therapist explored his suspicion of others, it was revealed that Joshua was afraid that others would contact the South African government upon learning that he had fled from the military. In therapy, Joshua's core beliefs associated with his suspicion were challenged by assisting him in accepting the lack of evidence that others would report him to the South African government. Joshua eventually learned to challenge his own beliefs and assumptions about others in his interactions. He was also able to utilize his connection with his therapist as evidence of his ability to trust. Consequently, his suspiciousness and lack of trust in others were alleviated and he was able to enjoy existing friendships and to develop new relationships. Overall, Joshua's improvement was facilitated by explicit discussions of culture and oppressive experiences, in addition to processing gender and power dynamics in session. The therapist's efforts to consult colleagues and literature regarding South African populations and apartheid also facilitated insight and the alleviation of Joshua's mental health symptoms.

SUMMARY

Health disparities among racial and ethnic minorities remain a systemic and complex problem within the United States. Efforts to address these problems remain ongoing and have been spearheaded by agencies such as the Department of Health and Human Services and the CDC. Additional efforts to address health disparities must also continue among healthcare professionals. Healthcare settings are by no means immune from problems and issues that exist within the larger society (e.g., racism, discrimination, prejudice). Instead, healthcare settings are microcosms in which such problems are reflected and reinforced. Therefore, culturally competent healthcare settings are needed to minimize discriminatory practices in the provision of services to racial and ethnic minorities. Additionally, cultural competence among healthcare professionals is necessary in order to effectively meet the needs of the increasingly growing populations of persons of color. Failure to improve culturally sensitive practice would certainly prove to be a disservice to persons of color and, ultimately, would serve to continue the existing gap in health outcomes and utilization of health services by race and ethnicity.

Key Questions in Addressing Race and Cultural Issues With Racial and Ethnic Minorities

1. In what way(s) have you been discriminated against in the past and/or recently?

2. How did discriminatory experiences affect you (e.g., emotionally, socially, psychologically, economically)?

3. How do you perceive discriminatory experiences to be related to your current medical and/or mental health concerns?

4. What concerns do you have about seeking treatment to address your problems or symptoms?

5. What concerns do you have about me as your clinician (e.g., race and/or ethnicity, gender, cultural background, ability to appreciate presenting concerns or symptoms)?

6. A. What services, if any, do you utilize in your community to address your problems or symptoms?

    B. How have community services been of use to you?

7. What questions or concerns do you have about my recommendations for treatment, procedures, referrals, or diagnoses?

CONTRIBUTOR

Tawanda M. Greer, PhD, is an Assistant Professor in the Department of Psychology and Women's Studies at the University of South Carolina in Columbia, South Carolina. She received her doctorate degree in Counseling Psychology at Southern Illinois University at Carbondale in Carbondale, Illinois. Dr. Greer's areas of expertise include retention issues among African American college students, issues of race and racism, and multicultural counseling. Dr. Greer may be contacted at the Department of Psychology, Barnwell College, University of South Carolina, Columbia, SC 29208. E-mail: greertm@gwm.sc.edu

RESOURCES

Alliance for Health Reform. (2004). Closing the gap: Racial and ethnic disparities in healthcare. *Journal of the National Medical Association, 96*(4), 436-440.

Anderson, L. M., Scrimshaw, S. C., Fullilove, M. T., Fielding, J. E., Normand, J., & The Task Force on Community Preventive Services. (2003). Culturally competent healthcare systems: A systematic review. *American Journal of Preventive Medicine, 24*(3S), 68-79.

Atkinson, D. R., & Lowe, S. M. (1995). The role of ethnicity, cultural knowledge, and conventional techniques in counseling and psychotherapy. In J. G. Ponterotto, J. M. Casas, L. A. Suzuki, & C. M. Alexander (Eds.), *Handbook of Multicultural Counseling* (pp. 387-414). Thousand Oaks, CA: Sage.

Cohen, J. J. (2003). Disparities in healthcare: An overview. *Academic Emergency Medicine, 10*(11), 1155-1160.

Dana, R. H. (1998). *Understanding Cultural Identity in Intervention and Assessment.* Thousand Oaks, CA: Sage.

Ferrero, K. F., & Farmer, M. M. (1996). Double jeopardy to health hypothesis for African Americans: Analysis and critique. *Journal of Health and Social Behavior, 37,* 27-43.

Grieger, I., & Ponterotto, J. G. (1995). A framework for assessment in multicultural counseling. In J. G. Ponterotto, J. M. Casas, L. A. Suzuki, & C. M. Alexander (Eds.), *Handbook of Multicultural Counseling* (pp. 357-374). Thousand Oaks, CA: Sage.

Heisler, M., Blumenthal, D. S., Rust, G., & Dubois, A. M. (2003). The Second Annual Primary Care Conference-Programming to Eliminate Health Disparities among Ethnic Minority Populations: An introduction to proceedings. *Ethnicity and Disease, 13,* S31-S35.

Jenkins, C. J., McNary, S., Carlson, B. A., Givens King, M., Hossler, C. L., Magwood, G., Zheng, D., Hendrix, K., Shelton Beck, L., Linnen, F., Thomas, V., Powell, S., & Ma'at, I. (2004). Reducing disparities for African Americans with diabetes: Progress made by the REACH 2010 Charleston and Georgetown Diabetes Coalition. *Public Health Reports, 119,* 322-330.

Kanner, A. D., Coyne, J. C., Schaefer, C., & Lazarus, R. S. (1981). Comparison of two modes of stress management: Daily hassles and uplifts versus major life events. *Journal of Behavioral Medicine, 4,* 1-39.

Klonoff, E. A., Landrine, H., & Ullman, U. B. (1999). Racial discrimination and psychiatric symptoms among Blacks. *Cultural Diversity and Ethnic Minority Psychology, 5*(4), 329-339.

Mendoza, R. H. (1989). An empirical scale to measure type and degree of acculturation in Mexican-American adolescents and adults. *Journal of Cross-Cultural Psychology, 20,* 372-385.

Myers, H. F., Lewis, T. T., & Parker Dominguez, T. P. (2003). Stress, coping, and minority health: Biopsychosocial perspective on ethnic health disparities. In G. Bernal, J. E. Trimble, A. K. Burlew, & F. T .L. Leong (Eds.), *Handbook of Racial and Ethnic Minority Psychology* (pp. 377-400). Thousand Oaks, CA: Sage.

Phinney, J. S. (1992). The Multigroup Ethnic Identity Measure: A new scale for use with diverse groups. *Journal of Adolescent Research, 7,* 156-176.

Ren, X. S., Amick, B. C., & Williams, D. R. (1999). Racial/ethnic disparities in health: The interplay between discrimination and socioeconomic status. *Ethnicity and Disease, 9*(2), 151-165.

Sellers, R., Rowley, S., Chavous, T., Shelton, J. N., & Smith, M. (1997). Multidimensional Inventory of Black Identity: A preliminary investigation of reliability and construct validity. *Journal of Personality and Social Psychology, 73,* 805-815.

Smedley, B. D., Stith, A. Y., & Nelson, A. R. (2002). *Unequal Treatment: Confronting Racial and Ethnic Disparities in Healthcare.* Washington, DC: National Academy Press.

Smith, S., & Gonzales, V. (2000). All health plans need culturally and linguistically appropriate materials. *Healthplan, 41,* 45-48.

Sue, D. W., Arredondo, P., & McDavis, R. J. (1995). Multicultural counseling competencies and standards: A call to the profession. In J. G. Ponterotto, J. M. Casas, L. A. Suzuki, & C. M. Alexander (Eds.), *Handbook of Multicultural Counseling* (pp. 624-640). Thousand Oaks, CA: Sage.

U.S. Department of Health and Human Services. (2001). *Mental Health: Culture, Race, and Ethnicity–A Supplement to Mental Health: A Report of the Surgeon General.* Rockville, MD: Author.

Utsey, S. O. (1999). Development and validation of a short form of the Index of Race-Related Stress (IRRS)-Brief Version. *The Journal of Measurement and Evaluation in Counseling and Development, 32*(3), 149-167.

van Ryn, M., & Burke, J. (2000). The effect of patient race and socioeconomic status on physicians' perceptions of patients. *Social Science and Medicine, 50,* 813-828.

Williams, D. R., & Rucker, T. D. (2000). Understanding and addressing racial disparities in healthcare. *Healthcare Financing Review, 21*(4), 75-91.

The Development of a Sexual Health Component In Your Practice

Frederick L. Peterson, Jr. and Jill W. Bley

This contribution highlights the advantages of expanding one's clinical practice to include sex therapy and the promotion of sexual health. In doing so, the development of sex therapy as a new field of clinical practice is examined, as well as its relationship to other mental health professions. Sexual health definitions and concepts are introduced that might be new to most mental health professionals.

Currently, all mental health disciplines are being challenged to expand their professional practice by promoting sexual health and developing skills in sex therapy. Each of the mental health professions has unique contributions to make in resolving sexual health problems on individual as well as global levels. Former U.S. Surgeon General Dr. David Satcher emphasized the public health need when he implored mental health professionals with this warning: "We as a nation must address the significant public health challenges regarding the sexual health of our citizens" (U.S. Department of Health & Human Services, Public Health Service, Office of the Surgeon General, 2001, p. 1).

To the practitioner, one of the benefits of providing sex therapy is a positive increase in referrals. Most importantly to the client, he or she will be treated with a more holistic approach. Mental health professionals are trained to pay attention to both the mental (psychological, emotional) and physical (somatic) manifestations of mental health issues. Very few have been trained to pay attention to, much less treat, the sexual problems that may affect their clients' minds and bodies.

Recent studies indicate that an alarming number of people suffer from some type of sexual dysfunction. Bartlik and Goldberg (cited in Leiblum & Rosen, 2000) found that "a significant proportion of women in all age groups are affected by female sexual arousal disorder" (p. 86). They estimated that one in five premenopausal women and two in five postmenopausal women suffer from this disorder. Women who come to therapy with this problem are usually baffled about what might be causing it. Similarly, untrained therapists are also baffled, not only about what might be the cause of the problem, but also what to do about it.

Consider the case of a 39-year-old woman* who tells the therapist that she used to enjoy sex, but since having three children, giving up her career so that she can stay home with them, and being the primary parent because her husband travels for his job two or three days a week, finds that she is having difficulty "really getting into it lately." An untrained therapist would probably decide that the problem is that she is overworked and perhaps resentful about giving up her career and decide to try to help her find ways to reduce her workload and let go of her resentments.

However, further exploration of this woman's problem revealed that, although she said that she enjoyed sex in the past, the truth was that when she was younger and free of these

---

* Names and identifying characteristics in all case examples have been changed to protect privacy.

pressures she rarely had orgasm and she wasn't sure if she lubricated because she always used a lubricant. She did enjoy her sexual experiences because she felt some emotional satisfaction. Her history revealed that she never masturbated, knew very little about how her body functioned sexually, and her first sexual experience was a date rape. Untrained therapists rarely feel comfortable asking questions about and exploring these sensitive, highly private, and personal areas.

A trained sexuality therapist takes a thorough sexual history that elicits this kind of information. Then the therapist presents a treatment plan to the patient that includes education about date rape and treatment of the issues related to the rape. The treatment plan also educates her about female sexual response and about the importance of self-exploration in learning to focus her full attention on sexual pleasure and teaching her body how to have orgasm.

Men also suffer in large numbers with sexual arousal disorders. In the National Health and Social Life Survey (a representative sample of men ages 18 to 59), Lauman et al. (1994) found that 10.4% of men reported being unable to achieve or maintain erection during the past year (complete erection dysfunction). Feldman et al. (1994) reported in The Massachusetts Male Aging Study (a community-based survey of men between the ages of 40 and 70 years) that 52% of respondents had some degree of erectile difficulty.

A male patient complained to his therapist that when he was young he was a "real stud," able to perform all night. His wife was just as interested in sex as he was. Lately, he has been a real disappointment to her and to himself. He often has no erection, and when he does have one, he frequently loses it when he tries to have intercourse. He has no problem with his erection when he masturbates or when he fantasizes about a female coworker. He is thinking about having an affair to find out if he has an erection problem or has just lost interest in his wife.

Untrained therapists may make the mistake of focusing on whether he is interested in his wife. Some might refer him to a physician for medication to enhance his erectile capability, and some may even advise him to have the affair to test his virility. A trained sexuality therapist would take a history of the problem and try to learn everything possible about what was happening when the problem began.

This man needed education about male sexuality and the myths that surround erectile functioning. The history revealed that the problem started about 4 years prior when he was laid off from his job for a year and his wife's income had to support them. He felt ashamed and depressed about not fulfilling his responsibilities as a provider. His sense of "impotence" worsened when, one night when he was very tired, he tried to have sex with his wife because he thought she wanted it. He lost his erection before he could penetrate her. After that he began to worry that he was letting her down as a provider not only of money but also of sex. These concerns created "performance anxiety" that persisted even after he was functioning again as a financial provider. Performance anxiety is a common cause of erectile dysfunction. Providing this man with medication would have masked the real problem. Supporting his belief that he needed to test his virility outside the marriage might have ruined an otherwise good marriage.

Even though arousal disorders are more likely to get the attention of the media and medical researchers, low sexual desire is the most common presenting complaint of clients in sex therapy clinics (Pridal & LoPiccolo, cited in Leiblum & Rosen, 2000). Among sexuality professionals, desire disorders have become the main focus of attention and concern. Not only are they the most prevalent problem, they are also the most difficult to understand and treat. The treatment protocols used successfully to treat arousal and orgasm disorders are generally ineffective in resolving desire disorders.

A common presentation of a desire phase disorder is one partner in a relationship insisting that the other partner, who does not want sex very often, needs help. However, like most couples' issues, the problem is rarely just the problem of the one who does not want sex. In fact, low sexual desire is such a complicated issue that it is difficult to think of one case that might elucidate the many facets and nuances of this highly distressing disorder. Causes range from childhood emotional, physical, and/or sexual abuse to adult trauma to intense or subtle anger between the partners. Treatment requires that the therapist have skills in ferreting out, from the couple's family, social, sexual, and relationship histories, information that will shed light on the origins of the underlying cause or causes.

What exactly is sexual health and sex therapy? How do consumers find a qualified heath care professional to address concerns of a sexual nature, such as the sexual dysfunctions described previously, a sexual compulsive behavior, or a sexual disorder such as dyspareunia (sexual pain)? How do mental health professionals train to be sex therapists? This contribution aims to answer these questions, provide the reader with a greater understanding of the many "players" in sex therapy (individuals as well as organizations), and give a new perspective on the unique place sex therapy plays in the health care delivery system.

WHAT ARE SEXUAL HEALTH, SEXOLOGY, AND SEX THERAPY?

The World Health Organization (WHO) has been evolving the concepts and definitions of sexuality and sexology. At a regional conference, the Pan American Health Organization, in collaboration with the World Association of Sexology (WAS), updated concepts and definitions and published them (WHO, 2001).

The basic concept of sexuality refers to the core dimension of being human, which includes sex, gender, sexual and gender identity, sexual orientation, eroticism, emotional attachment/love, and reproduction. Sexuality is experienced or expressed in thoughts, fantasies, desires, beliefs, attitudes, values, activities, practices, roles, and relationships. Sexuality is a result of the interplay of biological, psychological, socioeconomic, cultural, ethical, and religious/spiritual factors (WHO, 2001).

Sexual health is a closely related concept. Sexual health is considered the ongoing process of physical, psychological, and sociocultural well-being related to sexuality. It has also been more specifically defined as the integration of the physical, emotional, intellectual, and social aspects of being sexual, in ways that are positively enriching and enhance personality, communication, and love (WHO, 2001). For health care professionals, the promotion of sexual health includes specialists in fertility/infertility, the prevention of sexually transmitted infections (especially HIV/AIDS), and sexology (WHO, 2001).

Sexology is defined as a professional practice informed by interdisciplinary science, focused upon all aspects of sexuality, and traditionally inclusive of three main areas of activity: sex education, research sexology, and clinical sexology. These three aspects of sexology are divided into subspecialties. There are differences in practice between those who specialize in sex education for K-12 students and those who teach graduate students in professional programs such as medicine or psychology. Sex research is often divided into focus areas (e.g., "at-risk" sexual behaviors, women's sexual arousal) and the populations studied (e.g., adolescents, postmenopausal women).

Similarly, clinical sexology is divided into four subspecialties: sexual medicine, sexual surgery, sexual counseling, and sexual psychotherapy (WHO, 2001). Sexual medicine is provided by primary care physicians, endocrinologists, psychiatrists, and other subspecialists. Sexual surgery is provided by urologists, gynecologists, and plastic/cosmetic surgery specialists.

The last two divisions of clinical sexology, sexual counseling and sexual therapy, are the specialty services in which mental health clinicians are being trained and are expanding their clinical practices. Although there is more similarity than dissimilarity, the basic differences between sex counseling and sex therapy are in the level of training of the provider (sex therapists more often have doctoral degrees) and the more stringent standards employed for certification at the sex therapy level (American Association of Sex Educators, Counselors and Therapists [AASECT], 2003).

A CONSUMER WEB SEARCH FOR SEX THERAPISTS*

If individuals want to know what type of professional they should consult regarding a sexual concern, and have Internet access and experience, they can search the Web for the American Psychological Association (APA) website (www.apa.org). There they will find APA guidelines for selecting a qualified mental health professional.

APA has a fairly user-friendly website, which allows an individual to search for the keywords "sex therapy." Over 100 matches will be found, with a broad range of everything from sexual orientation policies to sexual health associated with having cancer. On the APA website is a section entitled "Find a Psychologist," which can help the individual find the kind of sex therapy expertise he or she seeks. However, APA's referral system is via phone service. Therefore, the individual has to call APA to find the closest APA member who provides the kind of sex therapy that is desired.

Other potential resources include the websites for the American Psychiatric Association, the Society for the Scientific Study of Sexuality (SSSS) (www.sexscience.org), and the American Association of Sex Educators, Counselors and Therapists (AASECT) (www.aasect.org). The website of the American Psychiatric Association does not provide a format for finding a sex therapist. The Society for the Scientific Study of Sexuality (SSSS) website gives valuable information about sexuality research but no information about how to find a sexuality therapist.

The AASECT website is a sophisticated information center on par with the American Psychological Association, although AASECT gives you a greater search option for finding a sex therapist. On a map of the United States, you click on the state you want and a list of certified sex educators, counselors, and therapists is generated. A detailed summary of the sex therapist's qualifications and practice information is also provided. AASECT describes itself as "a not-for-profit, interdisciplinary professional organization" whose members include physicians, nurses, social workers, psychologists, clergy, attorneys, sociologists, family planning specialists, and therapists of various types. AASECT's interests are to "promote the understanding of human sexuality and healthy sexual behavior." AASECT is the national accrediting body for people who wish to call themselves "sex therapists, sex educators, or sex counselors." The site provides information on the certification standards, which help the public understand the different levels of expertise reflected in the different levels of certification.

A BRIEF INTRODUCTION TO SEXOLOGY

German physician Iwan Bloch, in his text *The Sexual Life of Our Time* (1907/2001) first proposed sexology in 1907. It was just 6 years later that Albert Moll established the International Society for Sex Research, while the first Institute for Sexology was established in Berlin by Magnus Hirshfeld (who also edited the first *Journal of Sexology*). Other milestone events included the Jewish exodus from Germany, which spread the German sexological intelligentsia across the globe. As part of this movement, Hans Lehfeldt came to New York to practice

---

* Although all websites cited in this contribution were correct at the time of publication, they are subject to change at any time.

gynecology; in 1957 he helped establish the Society for the Scientific Study of Sexuality (SSSS). Physician Mary Calderone established the Sexuality Information and Education Council of the United States (SIECUS) in 1964. Three years later, attorney Judith Schriller established the American Association for Sex Educators, Counselors and Therapists (AASECT). In 1978, the World Association of Sexology (WAS) was established in Rome.

In America, over the last 50 years, there have been tremendous changes in sexual attitudes and behaviors on a societal level. To name a few, consider the sexual revolution of the 60s, the women's movement to reverse the repression of female sexuality, the gay rights liberation movement, the people-with-disability movement culminating in the Americans With Disabilities Act, the sex education movement in public schools, and the increased acceptance of premarital sex and cohabitation (to the level where both are considered as a norm by the younger generation). These incredible cultural changes have been fueled in large part by ground-breaking sex research that shocked the sensibilities of many Americans but also corrected many commonly held sexual myths. In other words, the American zietgeist has shifted in the last 50 years to allow a more informed and permissive sexual culture.

Medical historian Edward Brecher, in his 1979 publication *The Sex Researchers*, stated:

Three times during my lifetime the publication of sex research findings has rocked the sexual complacency of our culture:

1948:   *Sexual Behavior in the Human Male,* by Alfred C. Kinsey, Wardell B. Pomeroy, and Clyde E. Martin,

1953:   *Sexual Behavior in the Human Female,* by Alfred C. Kinsey, Wardell B. Pomeroy, Clyde E. Martin, and Paul H. Gebhard,

1966:   *Human Sexual Response,* by William H. Masters and Virginia E. Johnson. (p. xiii)

Perhaps the most well-recognized contributor to sex research is Dr. Alfred Kinsey, who was a biology professor at Indiana University and is famous for the ground-breaking "Kinsey reports," *Sexual Behavior in the Human Male* (1948) and *Sexual Behavior in the Human Female* (1953). Numerous changes in how Americans perceive sex were facilitated by Kinsey, including greater understanding of the incredible diversity in sexual behaviors, which are now considered within a typical range of sexual activity. The remarkable contributions of Alfred Kinsey and the impact he made in American culture are captured in the Fox Films' 2005 release *Kinsey*.

The other key American researchers were William Masters and Virginia Johnson, who were considered the pioneer sex researchers of the physiology of sexuality. Using a sample of about 800 subjects, Masters and Johnson observed and measured over 10,000 orgasms under laboratory conditions between 1954 and 1966 (Brecher, 1979; Masters, Johnson, & Kolodny, 1995). Essentially, all contemporary sex therapy is historically rooted in the Masters and Johnson research (Lieblum & Rosen, 2000).

HOW TO BECOME A COMPETENT SEX THERAPIST

Few training opportunities in the specialty area of sex therapy are available to professionals who have completed graduate school, postdoctoral internships, and licensing. The website for AASECT (www.aasect.org) has a page titled "How to become a Sexuality Educator, Counselor or Therapist." Because most graduate programs in counseling, psychology, or social work typically do not offer courses in human sexuality as part of their curriculum, this information is helpful. However, three programs are listed on this site that offer degrees "focused in a concentrated and specialized manner on clinical and educational services in the field of human sexuality." They are the Institute for Advanced Study of Human Sexuality located in San Francisco, Maimonides University located in southern Florida, and Widener University located in Philadelphia.

The Society for the Scientific Study of Sexuality (SSSS) (www.sexscience.org) provides information about sexuality education on a page titled "Educational Opportunities in Human Sexuality: A Sourcebook." This page also provides information about graduate programs that offer training in sex therapy, counseling, education, and research. There are 44 programs listed.

Many mental health providers may not want to go back to graduate school or complete another internship program in order to gain the knowledge base of sexual science, acquire training in sex therapy, and build a sex therapy component to their clinical practice. Accessing the resources to accomplish postlicensing certification as a sex therapist can be daunting. However, certification as a sex counselor is less stringent.

The first step one should take is to go to www.aasect.org/certification.asp. That site will inform the reader regarding everything that is needed to prepare for certification as a sex counselor or therapist. AASECT uses the P-LI-SS-IT model to differentiate between the training needed to be a sex counselor as opposed to a sex therapist. The P-LI-SS-IT model proposes four steps to certification within sex therapy. Sex counselors are trained to perform the first three steps (P-LI-SS), and sex therapists are trained to do all four steps (P-LI-SS-IT). The acronym stands for the following: P – Permission for the client to talk about sexual concerns; LI – Limited Information, which means that the therapist corrects any myths or misinformation; SS – Specific Suggestions are made by the therapist to aid clients in understanding their sexual problems and in developing goals and solutions for the problems; and IT – Intensive Therapy (Annon, 1976).

Requirements for sex counselor and sex therapist certification are listed on the AASECT site:

1. One must possess state certification or a license to practice in a related field, such as psychology, social work, medicine, and so on. Academic and work requirements are similar to those of most state licensing/certification boards.

2. There is a requirement for sexuality education of 60 clock hours for a sex counselor and 90 clock hours for a sex therapist. This sexuality education requirement covers general knowledge in core areas of human sexuality which may be gained through academic courses and training workshops. AASECT has made it possible for people who are already practicing professionals to complete this general knowledge of human sexuality requirement by providing a number of training workshops throughout the year. Other organizations such as SSSS, the Society for Sex Therapy and Research (SSTAR), and the American Association for Marriage and Family Therapy (AAMFT) also provide general knowledge training workshops related to human sexuality. AASECT usually accepts continuing education (CE) credits from these organizations. They also will provide CE accreditation to certain training and/or treatment facilities for training workshops that they may present to the professional community on topics related to sexuality.

3. One must complete AASECT requirements in clinical training. Certification as a sex counselor requires that the mental health professional has completed a minimum of 60 clock hours of training in how to do counseling with clients. Although a portion of these hours in counseling training may be in general counseling, at least 30 hours must be in sex counseling. Those hours may be obtained through credit courses, tutorials, workshops, practicum experiences, and so forth. There are six core areas of

training listed. For sex therapists, this step requires 60 clock hours of training in how to do therapy with clients whose diagnoses include psychosexual disorders described in the current edition of the *Diagnostic and Statistical Manual of Mental Disorders* of the American Psychiatric Association (*DSM-IV-TR*; American Psychiatric Association, 2000). This training may also be obtained through similar courses and workshops. There are seven core areas of training listed for certification at the sex therapist level. The rules for training allow for the possibility that persons may design their own learning and training experiences. If practitioners choose to design their own program, they need to submit a written plan for approval to the AASECT Certification Committee for either counselors or therapists.

4. Applicants must also complete a minimum of 12 clock hours of Attitudes/Values Training. These training experiences are described as structural group experiences consisting of a process-oriented exploration of the applicant's own feelings, attitudes, values, and beliefs regarding human sexuality and sexual behavior. AASECT strongly recommends that this experience occur early in the applicant's training for it to be most beneficial and regularly offers this training at AASECT's annual conferences.

5. Anyone interested in this training needs to pay special attention to the supervision requirements that are listed on the AASECT website. Since clinical competency is demonstrated in the actual performance of skills and application of knowledge, supervised clinical work is the crux of certification. The applicant must complete a minimum of 100 hours of supervised sex counseling for sex counselor certification, and 250 hours of supervised clinical treatment of clients who present with sexual concerns for sex therapist certification.

6. Face-to-face supervision for a minimum of 30 hours for sex counselors and 50 hours for sex therapists is an important requirement. Supervision can be individual or group, but group supervision cannot constitute more that 50% of the required hours. The supervisor must submit a supervision contract/plan to the appropriate AASECT Certification Committee for approval before the supervision begins. Sex counselors may receive their supervision from an AASECT Certified Sex Counselor or Therapist, or an AASECT Certified Supervisor. Sex therapists must receive their supervision from an AASECT Certified Supervisor. However, if a Certified Supervisor is not available, supervision may be arranged (with approval from AASECT) by a Certified Sex Therapist who has experience in supervision of clinical work. (See Table 1 on page 166 for a summary and comparison of certification requirements.)

Faced with this lengthy process, many psychotherapists opt to treat sexual problems only within special populations, such as men with erection dysfunction, women with genital pain syndrome, or men and women with sexual compulsivity issues. It is possible for a psychotherapist who has not been trained as a sex therapist to successfully treat some individuals who present with sexual concerns.

The reason that the training process takes a long time and is very intensive is because there is a lot to learn. Unfortunately, most sex therapists have seen clients who have previously spent a significant amount of time and money trying to correct a sexual problem with a therapist who, although well intentioned, did not have enough knowledge and/or skill in this specialized field. Many of these clients felt that they were hopeless cases because they had "failed" in previous therapy. Some report that they are not able to convince their partner to try again with another therapist because the partner is so angry or depressed because the initial therapy didn't help them. If psychotherapists choose to practice without the specialized training, it is very important that they understand their limitations, explain these limitations to the client, and be prepared to refer to a sex therapist if it becomes clear that they are not able to help the client.

TABLE 1: American Association of Sex Educators, Counselors and Therapists Summary and Comparison of Certification Requirements

Requirement	Sex Counselor	Sex Therapist
Membership	Yes	Yes
Code of Ethics	Yes	Yes
Academic and Professional Experience	BA + 2 years (minimum)	MA + 2 years or Doc. + 1 year
General Eligibility	Clinical license not required	State license required
Human Sexuality Education	60 clock hours	90 clock hours
Sex Counseling or Sex Therapy Training	60 clock hours (30 general/30 sex)	60 clock hours (30 general/30 sex)
Sexual Attitudes and Values Training Experience	12 clock hours	12 clock hours
Clinical Training or Professional Experience	100 hours of supervised sex counseling	250 hours of supervised sex therapy
Supervision	30 hours (6 months minimum)	50 hours (50% group, 6 months >) (15 years experience = 25 hours)
Application Process	$250 and documentation	$250 and documentation

DISCUSSION

None of the single-discipline professional societies (such as APA, American Counseling Association, or National Association of Social Workers) appear to have associated with the field of sexual health and sex therapy. The age-old taboo associated with the topic of sexuality (and mental health professionals' discomfort with it as a legitimate subject of scholarly study) still may exert influence, albeit to a lesser degree, as it did over 100 years ago when G. Stanley Hall (APA's first president) censored his sex research as a result of professional criticism. Hall was accused of having prurient interests because of his "excessive focus on sex," and contemporary psychologist E. L. Thorndike even called him a "mad man" (D. P. Schultz & S. E. Schultz, 2000).

Sexual health and sex therapy are not under the wing of any traditional discipline or professional society but rather represent interdisciplinary fields. Hence, interdisciplinary societies appear to be "home" to mental health professionals engaged in the subspecialities of sexology: sex education, sex research, and clinical sexology. Accordingly, the organization of the field of sexology is split three ways: SIECUS for sex education, SSSS for sex research, and AASECT for clinical sexologists of varied disciplines.

The new interdisciplinary field of sexual health is exploding with relevance and synergy. Worldwide, approximately 20 million people have died from the AIDS pandemic. In the United States the deaths of 501,669 persons were attributed to AIDS from 1998 to 2002. Among males, male-to-male sexual contact accounted for 249,198 of those deaths. Heterosexual contact was the cause of the deaths of 20,820. Among women, heterosexual contact was implicated in 34,661 deaths (Centers for Disease Control and Prevention, 2004). AIDS is not the only sexually transmitted infection that kills. Another one million die annually from other sexually transmitted infections – tragically multiplying our need for our understanding of "at-risk decision making" and sex behavior related to prevention of transmission (WHO, 2001). Sexual medicine's expanding understanding of specific mechanisms of sexual function has led to a revolution in sexual pharmacology and movement to primary care physicians for first-line treatment of erection dysfunction (Peterson, 2000). The development of feminist scholarship has illuminated the recognition of sexual violence as a serious threat to women's and children's health worldwide. Other problems related to sexual health (such as the movement for equal rights for sexual minorities and challenges in the field of reproductive health) bring attention to the shortage of sexual health professionals that can effectively aid in the resolution of these global challenges.

After 100 years of maturity for both professions of psychiatry and psychology, psychiatrists and psychologists are generally perceived today as having expertise in human behavior and behavior change through psychopharmacology and psychotherapy, respectively. Even though individual members are personally doing important work in these areas, it does not appear that their national associations are committed to supporting their members in developing expertise in human sexuality, overcoming their feelings of discomfort, and innovating community interventions for changing sexual behavior of "at-risk populations" related to these pressing global problems.

Few mental health practitioners have the opportunity to make their contribution, due to a lack of opportunity to undertake three important steps: master the knowledge base of sexual science, gain learning experiences to overcome personal discomfort and biases related to sexuality, and build and apply clinical skills in sexual health to assist others to resolve personal challenges to sexual worth and satisfaction. The challenge to all mental health disciplines is to expand efforts and resources devoted to promoting sexual health and developing skills in clinical sexology for those engaged in specific undergraduate curricula, professional training programs, and postgraduate education. Although these types of professional supports are not widely available today from professional graduate programs and societies, mental health professionals are encouraged to personally overcome the obstacles. This contribution promotes mental health practitioners expanding their own knowledge and skills in this critical area of human welfare. In doing so, we then define sexual health as an important component of the delivery of mental health care as well as health care.

CONTRIBUTORS

Frederick L. Peterson, Jr., PsyD, is a health psychologist at the Veterans Healthcare System of Ohio, Dayton Campus, where he coordinates a Sexual Health Clinic and the Smoking Cessation Programs. Dr. Peterson is the Co-Director of the Psychology Internship Program. He completed postdoctorate training as a Clinical Fellow at the Masters and Johnson Institute. Research interests include sex therapy, tobacco use treatment, and the effects of masculinity-related personality factors on health. He holds four academic appointments at Wright State University, including the School of Professional Psychology and the School of Medicine (Psychiatry). Dr. Peterson may be contacted at Sexual Health Clinic, VA Medical Center, Dayton, OH 45428. E-mail: docpete100@aol.com

Jill W. Bley, PhD, is a clinical psychologist. She is certified by the American Association of Sex Educators, Counselors and Therapists as both a sex therapist and a supervisor. She taught sex therapy to graduate students in clinical psychology at the University of Cincinnati. During that time she trained and supervised many students. Dr. Bley wrote a syndicated column, "Speaking of Sex," which appeared in some downtown newspapers. Her columns addressed the diverse issues related to human sexuality. She is a founder of Women Helping Women/Rape Crisis Center and a Sex Therapy Clinic, both in Cincinnati. She has lectured extensively on topics of sexuality. Dr. Bley is a Volunteer Associate Professor in the Department of Psychiatry University of Cincinnati Medical Center. Dr. Bley can be reached at 750 Red Bud Avenue, Cincinnati, OH 45229. E-mail: drjillbley@cinci.rr.com

RESOURCES

Cited Resources

American Association of Sex Educators, Counselors and Therapists. (2003). *Standards for Certification*. Retrieved June 30, 2004, from http://www.aasect.org

American Psychiatric Association. (2000). *Diagnostic and Statistical Manual of Mental Disorders* (*DSM-IV-TR*; 4th ed. text rev.). Washington, DC: Author.

Annon, J. S. (1976). *Behavioral Treatment of Sexual Problems: Brief Therapy*. New York: Harper & Row.

Bartlik, B., & Goldberg, J. (2000). Female sexual arousal disorder. In S. Leiblum & R. Rosen (Eds.), *Principles and Practices of Sex Therapy* (3rd ed., pp. 85-117). New York: Guilford.

Bloch, I. (2001). *The Sexual Life of Our Time*. (Original work published 1907) In World Health Organization *Promotion of Sexual Health: Recommendations for Action*. Proceedings from a regional consultation convened by Pan American Health Organization and the World Health Organization in collaboration with the World Association for Sexology, Antigua Guatemala, Guatemala.

Brecher, E. M. (1979). *The Sex Researchers* (Expanded Edition). San Francisco, CA: Specific Press.

Centers for Disease Control and Prevention. (2004). *HIV/AIDS Surveillance Report* (Vol. 14). Atlanta, GA: Author.

Condon, W. (2005). *Kinsey* [Film]. Los Angeles: Fox Searchlight Films

Feldman, H. E., Goldstein, I., Hatzichristov, D., Krane, R., & McKinlay, R. (1994). Impotence and its medical and psychosocial correlates: Results of the Massachusetts Male Aging Study. *Journal of Urology, 151*, 54-61.

Kinsey, A., Pomeroy, W., & Martin, C. (1948). *Sexual Behavior in the Human Male*. Philadelphia: W. B. Saunders.

Kinsey, A., Pomeroy, W., Martin, C., & Gebhard, P. (1953). *Sexual Behavior in the Human Female*. Philadelphia: W. B. Saunders.

Lauman, E., Gagnon, J., Michael, R., & Michaels, S. (1994). The Social Organization of Sexuality. *Sexuality Practices in the United States*. Chicago: University of Chicago Press.

Leiblum, S. R., & Rosen, R. C. (2000). *Principles and Practice of Sex Therapy* (3rd ed.). New York: Guilford.

Masters, W. H., & Johnson, V. E. (1966). *Human Sexual Response*. New York: Brown.

Masters, W. H., Johnson, V. E., & Kolodny, R. C. (1995). *Human Sexuality* (5th ed.). New York: HarperCollins College Publishers.

Peterson, F. L. (2000). The assessment and treatment of erection dysfunction. In L. VandeCreek & T. L. Jackson (Eds.), *Innovations in Clinical Practice: A Source Book* (pp. 57-71). Sarasota, FL: Professional Resource Press.

Pridal, C., & LoPiccolo, J. (2000). Multi-element treatment of desire disorders: Integration of cognitive, behavioral, and systemic therapy. In S. Leiblum & R. Rosen (Eds.), *Principles and Practice of Sex Therapy* (3rd ed., 57-82). New York: Guilford.

Schultz, D. P., & Schultz, S. E. (2000). *A History of Modern Psychology* (7th ed.). New York: Harcourt College Publishers.

U.S. Department of Health & Human Services, Public Health Service, Office of the Surgeon General. (2001, July 9). *The Surgeon General's Call to Action to Promote Sexual Health and Responsible Sexual Behavior* (DHHS Publication No. HE1.2:2001040313).Washington, DC: U.S. Government Printing Office.

World Health Organization. (2001). *Promotion of Sexual Health: Recommendations for Action*. Proceedings from a regional consultation convened by Pan American Health Organization and the World Health Organization in collaboration with the World Association for Sexology, Antigua Guatemala, Guatemala.

Additional Resources

Society for the Scientific Study of Sexuality. (2003). *Educational Opportunities in Human Sexuality: A Sourcebook*. Retrieved June 30, 2004, from www.sexscience.org

Strong, B., Devault, C., Sayad, B. W., & Yarber, W. (2002). *Human Sexuality: Diversity in Contemporary America* (4th ed.). New York: McGraw-Hill.

Designing a Mental Health Professional's Website: Practical and Ethical Issues*

Anthony Ragusea

No one knows exactly how many mental health professionals have websites. Many sites vanish overnight and others suddenly appear, and it is difficult to tell how many sites are run by legitimate and licensed professionals. Even fewer sites could be considered "models" of both ethical and consumer-friendly website design. There is no wave of public outcry at present to indicate that unethical behavior on the Internet is an epidemic in the mental health field, but this does not excuse therapists from seeking to attain a higher level of professionalism on the Internet. Some therapists may put little thought into a website design. Others may desire to have a website that is ethical, user-friendly, and good for business, but do not know how to achieve such high standards. Resources exist for these professionals, but it may take more time to find them than the clinician is willing to spend.

A recent article in the newsletter *Psychotherapy Finances* ("Quick and Easy," 2003) noted that "a growing portion of the public just assumes that *any legitimate professional has a Web site*" (p. 4). The article evaluated a few Internet service providers and Web hosts in terms of features and ease of creating a simple website, but did not discuss what a therapist would want to put on the site. Practitioners use websites for different reasons. Most use them as online analogies to "Yellow Pages" advertisements. Some use them as places to post articles, opinions, or mental health information. Online therapists may even use them to host online support groups or communicate with clients via e-mail. This contribution provides an outline of some of the most important elements that therapists should consider incorporating into the design of their websites. These elements include visual aesthetics, the intended purpose of the site, budget, and specific content that most, if not all, sites should include. This contribution will focus largely on the practical considerations and challenges of designing a website, and to a lesser degree the ethical issues that may be involved. The intended audience of this contribution is therapists who have little or no experience with web design and who are interested in starting a website; however, this contribution is not intended to be a comprehensive resource.

WEBSITE VOCABULARY

Numerous books are available on the basics of website construction, such as *Building a Web Site for Dummies* (D. A. Crowder & R. Crowder, 2000). A brief course on website vocabulary is still in order for those therapists reading this contribution who have little background in web design. Many of these terms can be defined more precisely and comprehensively, but for the purposes of this discussion they will be defined in the simplest terms that will be most useful to therapists.

---

* Although all websites cited in this contribution were correct at the time of publication, they are subject to change at any time.

WWW

This acronym stands for "World Wide Web." When most people refer to the "Web," they are referring to a network of computers across the globe or "servers" that store and transmit web pages to "client" web browsers. The World Wide Web is often interchangeably referred to as the Internet, though they are technically different. To make things more complicated, an "internet" (lower case i) refers only to any two or more networks that are connected together and share resources.

Client

This term refers to the person who is requesting to view a web page. Client software must exist on one computer that contacts and obtains data from a "server" computer. When a person is surfing the Web, the web browser being used is a piece of client software.

Server

In web design, the "server" typically refers to a specialized computer on which are stored all of the files related to a web page. When a person with a web browser types in the address for a web page, a specific server responds to the request by transmitting all the text and images to the person's browser for display. When designing a website, all of the files related to the site must be moved or "uploaded" onto a server before other people surfing the Web can access them.

HTTP

This acronym stands for "HyperText Transfer Protocol" and is a software protocol for transferring "hypertext" files across the Internet. The protocol requires an HTTP client program on one end and an HTTP server program on the other end. The average user does not need to know anything about HTTP, except that every website on the Internet has an address that starts with "http://."

FTP

This acronym stands for "File Transfer Protocol" and refers to the most common method for retrieving and sending files to and from a server. There are many FTP programs available. Novice designers need to know that an FTP program is necessary to transfer all files related to their website off of their home computer and onto a server. The FTP program will require the user to know the FTP address for the site (e.g., ftp://ftp.mysite.com) and the username and password for gaining access.

HTML

This acronym stands for "HyperText Markup Language." HTML is the language in which most websites are written. Beginning designers may not need to know how to write in HTML, because many programs will write the code automatically. This is particularly true of companies that market to amateur website designers like Yahoo! and America Online, which provide their own software tools that make website design as simple as point-and-click. Simplicity comes at the expense of greater options, though, and the flexibility to add more advanced features. A file that uses the suffix ".html" is basically a text document; it contains no images, no colors, only code. An .html file can be likened to a map that contains directions to all the parts of the web page. It has directions on how all those parts are arranged on the page and where they are located on the server.

Hit

Every time a user visits a website, that visit is referred to as a "hit." Programs are available that tally the number of hits to a website.

WYSIWYG

This acronym stands for "what you see is what you get." Software that allows the user to design web pages without programming in HTML is referred to as WYSIWYG software. Such software allows the user to design pages more intuitively, so that the user chooses the colors, places the images where desired, and organizes the page to look just as it would on the Internet. The necessary code is written automatically and invisibly to the user. Most programs, including expensive high-end software such as Macromedia's Dreamweaver and Adobe's GoLive, allow for designing websites in this manner.

Compression

Image files tend to be very large and require compression before they are appropriate to be uploaded to a server. Compression refers to removing some of the data from a file in order to make it smaller. Many people still use dial-up modems to access the Internet, so it is best to make all of the image files on websites as small as possible. Two of the most common compression formats for images on the Web are "GIF" and "JPEG."

GIF

The "Graphic Interchange Format" is a common compression format and file suffix for pictures. It works best on images with little complexity and few colors.

JPEG

This acronym stands for "Joint Photographic Experts Group." This is a common compression format and file suffix for pictures. It works best on photographs.

HOSTING A WEB PAGE

Hiring a professional web designer can be expensive. The advantage of hiring a professional is that almost all of the work described in this contribution will likely be handled by the designer. If you choose to hire a professional, be very clear when reviewing the contract about who owns the site. There is anecdotal evidence of companies that have designed and hosted sites for therapists only to take control of the site in an attempt to hijack the therapist's business. If the therapist chooses to be the primary designer of the website, one of the first decisions to be made is who will host the web page. A host is the company (or more accurately, the server) that will house the web page and make it available for people to view on the Internet. Individuals can host their own website provided they have the right equipment and access to the Internet. The therapist usually can move the website to a different host at any time if he or she wishes.

The therapist also will want to think about where he or she will find the tools to design a web page. Many professional hosts will also provide programs that the customer can use to design a website. The *Psychotherapy Finances* article cited previously ("Quick and Easy," 2003) tested several services that provide easy-to-use, WYSIWYG tools to quickly design a simple website. These services included America Online (www.aol.com), Earthlink (www.earthlink.net), Yahoo! (www.yahoo.com), and GoDaddy (www.godaddy.com). Using the first two services may be most convenient for the therapist who does not already have Internet access, as America Online and Earthlink are both Internet Service Providers (more on this distinction below). There are also plenty of web design software packages available for purchase, such as Microsoft's FrontPage, Adobe's GoLive, and Macromedia's Dreamweaver. Evaluating these various services and programs is beyond the scope of this contribution.

Understanding the difference between an Internet Service Provider (ISP) and a Web host is important. An ISP will provide the customer with access to the Internet and probably some simple tools for setting up a web page. A Web host may also provide site-building tools, but a host does not provide access to the Internet. Hiring a host can instead be thought of as renting office space on the Internet, while an ISP sells the car to get to the office. The ISP may also provide a small office as an incentive to buy the car, but the host will focus on selling enormous luxury offices tailored to the customer's needs. The decision about which to choose depends on the therapist's needs: Does the therapist need a lot of space to accommodate a large site? Does the therapist want the ability to create an online store? Does the therapist care if the website is required to have advertising on it? How much does the therapist want to pay? These are only some of the questions to be answered.

Some people with relatively new computers can use their home computer as a server and thus as a host for their own website, but this system is often not practical. The computer would need to stay turned on 24 hours a day and remain perpetually connected to the Internet in order for other people to connect to the website whenever they want. A professional Web host will provide more sophisticated servers to house the website, servers that are almost always "up" (i.e., turned on and functioning properly), that can accommodate more visitors if the site becomes popular, and can support advanced features such as ecommerce (the ability to buy and sell items directly through the website). An ISP also will not likely provide a large amount of space for the website without additional fees, while a Web host is more likely to provide a large amount of space to accommodate pictures, movies, or a large number of pages.

When researching Web hosts, remember that it is often a case of "You get what you pay for." Hosts offer a wide range of fees. Beware of a fee that looks too good to be true! The host may charge low fees but require advertisements to be posted on the website, use substandard equipment that frequently "goes down" (i.e., malfunctions), or provide a limited range of services. Customer support may be poor. A host that charges more is more likely to take greater precautions to protect its customers' data, though do not expect the company to openly share with the public all of the steps it takes.

There are literally dozens of websites that offer rankings of different web hosting companies. Different sites may use different criteria for ranking (e.g., customer support, reliability, cost), and do not assume that the rankings are scientific or even objective. A good idea would be to look at several lists of rankings and look for hosting companies that appear on multiple lists, and then investigate those companies personally. To find rankings, simply do a search for "web hosts" using your favorite Internet search engine (e.g., www.google.com or www.altavista.com).

One additional factor that may influence the choice of ISP or Web host is the domain name of the website. The domain name or URL (Universal Resource Locator) is the address that is typed into a web browser, and it can be long and awkward (e.g., http://telosnet.com/oz-saje-counseling/saje.html). Some people prefer a brief, personalized domain name (e.g., www.drsmith.com), though these come at a price. Most Web hosts and some ISPs offer a domain registration service for a monthly or yearly fee. Registering a personalized domain name with a particular company does not obligate the customer to stay with that company, as the domain name is usually considered the property of the customer (pay attention to the fine print in the contract) and can be "forwarded" to a different hosting company for a fee. In other words, if the therapist is dissatisfied, it is possible to move a website from one host to another and not lose the personalized domain name. However, a domain name that is provided by the host (e.g., www.geocities.com/mysite) cannot be transferred to a different company.

Personalized domain names may or may not be worth the extra cost. Some people think that a personalized domain name earns its value by helping the therapist's website look professional or by being easier for potential customers to remember. Others argue that a domain name that mentions the business of the site (e.g., www.mytherapist.com) will increase the site's "visibility" to search engines. Visibility will be discussed in greater detail below. If the therapist does not plan to make the website a major element in his or her business model, then the extra cost may not be justified.

Picking the perfect domain name can be difficult. The name should be short, easy to remember, and hard to misspell. The suffix (e.g., .com, .net, or .org) is another choice to be made. Most people assume that a website ends in .com, which may make the difference between a successful hit and a frustrated potential customer who decides that figuring out the correct suffix isn't worth the effort. However, some therapists may object to a .com suffix on principle, especially if the web page is intended to be a health information site rather than a commercial site. For more tips on picking a domain name and other tips on web design, visit http://www.wannabewebster.com.

PRINCIPLES OF DESIGN

Regardless of the purpose of the site, if a therapist wishes to create a successful website that attracts customers and he or she does not wish to hire a web design company, then certain principles of design should be taken into consideration. In general, there should be overall consistency in the design with some variation to prevent boredom, the site should successfully convey an intended message, and the design should support the message. It is important for the designer to consider the intended audience of the site and shape the site around the audience. The website for a therapist who is looking to attract geriatric clients may look very different from that of a therapist who specializes in adolescent issues. There are many books and college courses available on website design, but there are also sites on the Internet that will provide some free advice. Visit the following website for an introduction to good website design: http://www.wdvl.com/Authoring/Design/Pages/index.html.

Color

Many therapists are at least superficially aware of the relationship between color and emotion. Red can be associated with power or anger, for example; softer colors may help some persons feel calm or relaxed. For a slightly more advanced discussion of color theory, visit the following website: http://www.colormatters.com/colortheory.html. In general, the color scheme chosen should support the intended "feel" of the site. Many clinicians who advertise their practice choose to use pastels or bright colors to help visitors feel soothed or comfortable, but this is not a requirement. Some people make a mistake in selecting pastel-colored text to complement a pastel-colored background. Although a general principle of good design is that the colors, fonts, and images selected should all come together to express a consistent theme, low contrast between the foreground and the background can be straining on the eyes. People who have difficulty seeing may even find reading low-contrast text to be impossible. Thus, if there is a decision to use colored fonts, then there should be a high degree of contrast between the text and the background. In general, choosing an image or pattern as the background of the page (such as your company logo) is a bad idea because it makes the text more difficult to read.

Complexity

As computers became more prevalent in offices and in homes, many believed that traditional books would be abandoned for a new invention called the digital book or "e-book."

Businesses would throw out their old photocopiers and printers and publish all of their documents electronically. The belief was that people would want to throw away their heavy, easily torn, impractical paper books, and read everything off of computer screens. These prophecies have so far turned out to be false, for a number of reasons. One reason has been that most people find it difficult or unpleasant to read lengthy texts on a computer screen. A computer monitor is immobile unless it is on a laptop, which forces the reader to sit more or less in the same position and makes lengthy reading uncomfortable. Amateur web designers need to keep in mind that it is possible to overburden visitors with text. There is no way to tell how much text is too much, and every viewer's tastes will be different. However, the Internet has created an expectation for speed. Most people spend very little time on any one site; they want the information they are looking for and then they leave. Most people do not "browse" the Internet the way people browse through a library. Therapists should keep this issue in mind when designing their site.

In addition, websites with a high degree of visual complexity can be overstimulating for viewers. This means that "eye-catching" websites with lots of colors, advertisements, text, music, and animations can actually be off-putting. There is no rule of thumb to know what is too complex and what is not. A good suggestion for therapists is to spend a little time surfing the Web looking at sites owned by large companies and organizations. These groups have the money to hire experienced professionals who are more likely to know when "enough is enough."

Interactivity

Interactivity refers to the exchange of information between a website and its users, and is the greatest advantage of the Internet (Huang, 2003). The exchange is two-way, and can take many forms. Examples include the user clicking on a hyperlink or "button" which connects the user to another page or site, the ability for the user to post opinions or comments onto the site, and the ability to make purchases through the site. Huang (2003) noted that sites that possess a high degree of interactivity give users a sense that they are in control of their experience on the website and in the kinds of information they receive. Users also feel that moving around within the site takes little effort, that the site is quick and responsive, and that it is personalized to the user's needs. In addition, the site implicitly communicates an awareness that its audience is human by presenting information through multiple media (e.g., audio, video, text) and by appealing to the human senses of sight, hearing, and touch.

In a study of what attributes play the greatest role in making the experience of a website a satisfying one for users, Huang (2003) discovered that interactivity is the most critical. Other attributes considered included novelty, aesthetics, and complexity. Findings suggested that the novelty of a site is important to initially attract users, but that interactivity is what keeps users from leaving. Similar conclusions about the importance of interactivity for user satisfaction were found by Teo et al. (2003).

Increasing interactivity within a website can be easy to achieve. Haring (2000) suggests five features that can be added to any website that supports forms, that is, pages that collect information and return it to the server (often called Common Gateway Interface [CGI] scripts or programs). These features include sweepstakes, quizzes, polls/surveys, scavenger hunts, and guestbooks. Sweepstakes do not need to involve large prizes, but to get the most "bang for the buck," the owner of a website needs to spend some time advertising the contest throughout the website as well as across the Internet in general. Quizzes can be tailored to the purpose of the website, so a therapist might design an easy quiz that focuses on mental health issues, the answers for which may be found throughout the website. Polls and surveys benefit the therapist by collecting valuable information about the opinions of customers, and they help users feel that their views are important to the therapist. Scavenger hunts, like quizzes, may encourage users to explore the website for information or pictures and thus increase users' sense of involvement in the site, except scavenger hunts come with a prize at the end. Guestbooks are forms where a user can identify himself or herself and provide positive or negative comments about the site, which can be beneficial to both the therapist and the user.

The general goal of interactivity is to avoid causing users to feel that the website is a passive recipient, something to browse, rather than an active participant that reaches out and engages the user. Part of achieving this goal is imbuing the website with a certain degree of novelty. The site should not remind users of every other site they have visited while in search of a therapist. Therapists are encouraged, then, to avoid strict formality and indulge their creative impulses, while at the same time communicating a high degree of professionalism. This can be a difficult balancing act. Filling a site with contests and entertainment can be a turn-off to visitors who do not equate "entertaining" with "professional." A good idea would be to formally or informally survey a group of people about their experiences and impressions while navigating the proposed website before it is officially opened to the public. A therapist's website should always be constructed based on a consideration of the intended audience's needs and desires.

Conveying a Message

Designing a website involves balancing the needs of the audience or customers with the needs of the therapist. A visitor comes to a site with certain wants and expectations, which the therapist will either meet or fail to meet. For example, the visitor may be looking for specific information, or a particular product or service. The visitor may be looking for a therapist with certain personality characteristics, of a certain demographic, or with certain competencies. The therapist, by contrast, may be looking for clients with particular characteristics or problems, needs to provide information and services in an ethical and professional manner, and needs to obtain informed consent when necessary. A good rule of thumb when designing a website is for the therapist to think carefully about what he or she wants to communicate about himself or herself, both personally and professionally, and then seek to accurately convey those messages through all aspects of the website. This will help to meet the needs of both the therapist and the client.

The message of the therapist can be conveyed through words, pictures, sounds, and colors. Therapists should pay attention to the implicit and perhaps unintended messages within the site. For example, a therapist may choose not to put a picture of himself or herself on the site. The therapist may want to stop and think about what message it sends to a visitor that there is or is not a picture of the therapist on the site. Is that message consistent with the message the therapist wishes to convey? Because the Internet affords therapists with an enormous amount of flexibility in conveying messages that brochures and advertisements cannot provide, a visitor implicitly assumes that the therapist's website will convey everything that the therapist wishes to convey just as it is intended to be conveyed. A reader looking for a therapist in the Yellow Pages recognizes that only limited information can be conveyed through a tiny advertisement and that the therapist may not be able to put everything into the ad that he or she wants. A web page is more of a blank slate, an "open mike." What does the therapist want to say?

Accessibility

Accessibility is a general term that may refer to making a website easier for anyone to use, from people with slow computers to people with physical handicaps, or it may be used to refer only to people with disabilities. For the purposes of this discussion, accessibility refers to making websites easier to use for people with disabilities.

People with a wide variety of physical limitations surf the Internet every day, with varying degrees of difficulty. Some have hearing limitations, some have visual impairments, some have motor limitations, and some have cognitive limitations. Specific examples include people who are partially blind, deaf, dyslexic, or who have cerebral palsy. The kinds of changes that might be made to a therapist's website to optimize accessibility varies widely depending on the content of the site. Changes might range from giving a user control over slowing down or stopping the movement of text in order to provide more time to read, to minimizing flashing colors that could induce an epileptic seizure.

Software designers are increasingly sensitive to accessibility issues. Apple Computer, for example, currently includes accessibility options as a standard feature of its operating system software. These optional adjustments include oversized text for the visually impaired, replacing auditory alerts with screen flashes for the hearing impaired, and modifications in how the mouse and keyboard respond for people with motor difficulties. For those interested in making their website more accessible to people with physical handicaps, one of the most comprehensive resources available belongs to the World Wide Web Consortium (W3C), an organization that publishes guidelines and standards for virtually all aspects of website construction. Most of the W3C guidelines are far too technical to be useful to the amateur designer, but their Web Content Accessibility Guidelines 2.0 (available at http://www.w3.org/WAI/) are generally easy to understand. Understandability does not equal ease of implementation, unfortunately, and therapists should be aware that full compliance with these suggested guidelines is likely to cost extra in terms of time and effort. Because the guidelines are lengthy and detailed, a concise summary cannot be presented here and the reader is thus referred to the original document.

One simplistic yet effective strategy for maximizing accessibility is to design sites that are simple and clear. Content should be easy to find, text should be easy to read, and the site should be easy to navigate. The simpler and clearer the site is, the easier it will be to explore for people with limitations.

THE BUSINESS CARD WEBSITE

Most therapists do not provide services online but rather work out of a traditional brick-and-mortar building. These therapists are likely to be interested in using the Internet only as a cheap and easy way to advertise their services; their websites are digital business cards. A web page can display more information in a more attractive manner than even a full-page advertisement in the Yellow Pages, at a fraction of the cost. Creating a website through a large company such as America Online or Yahoo! can cost as little as nothing, but, as previously discussed, the address for the site may be long and awkward. Spending a little more money can provide the therapist with a custom-made web address and additional server space to create a larger site.

The layout and content of a "business card" website can vary greatly, but these websites are likely to have similar elements. These might include (a) the name and credentials of the therapist, (b) a business address and phone number, (c) a description of the services provided by the therapist or the therapist's company, (d) a picture of the therapist and/or the therapist's office, and possibly (e) the policies of the therapist, written just as a client would see them in the office. There are no standards or requirements for the content of a therapist's website, provided that the content is consistent with the ethical standards of the therapist's profession. For example, Standard 5.01 of the American Psychological Association's *Ethical Principles of Psychologists and Code of Conduct* (2002) requires that psychologists avoid using false or deceptive statements in advertising.

One of the downsides of advertising on the Internet is that far fewer people are likely to come across a web page than they are a Yellow Pages advertisement. This is because most people surfing the Web are likely to use a search engine and perform a search using a generic word or phrase (e.g., "therapists" or "therapists in [state of residence]") which is likely to result in many thousands of websites being retrieved. The chances of any one therapist's website appearing as one of the top 10 or 20 search engine results is very small unless the search engine query is more specific (e.g., "Dr. Smith, psychologist" or "The Wellness Center") or if the therapist takes additional steps to try to increase the site's "visibility" to the search engine. "Visibility" or "positioning" refers to the odds that a given site will be listed at or near the top of the displayed results from a search engine query. Search engines such as Google or Yahoo! are complicated and may appear to work in mysterious ways. Only the companies that own them know exactly how the engines decide which sites get top priority. Having a site that is linked to many other sites increases its search engine visibility, but it is difficult to achieve this kind of popularity. Also, incorporating certain "keywords" and "metatags" into the site can increase visibility. Therapists can hire companies who will guarantee increased visibility across many search engines, though often for a sizeable fee. It is also possible to pay directly the companies that own the search engines to increase positioning, but this can also be very expensive. There is always the "old-fashioned" way of drumming up public awareness of a website, of course, which includes advertising the site on listservs, bulletin boards, flyers, and so on.

In summary, the therapist should take into account the following variables when considering how much effort to put into creating a "business card" website:

1. *The therapist's business model.* Does the therapist intend to draw a large number of clients from the Internet, or does the therapist merely want a source of free advertising that may draw only a few, if any, clients? Does the therapist often provide services to populations that are likely to see the website (e.g., people who have access to computers), or does the therapist provide services to a specialized population that is not likely to be Internet-savvy? Does the therapist wish to attract clients from a wide geographic area or from the local population?

2. *The therapist's budget.* How much money is the therapist willing to spend on a website? Will the therapist develop a simple site himself or herself, or will he or she hire a professional web design company? Is an easy-to-remember site address a priority, even if it comes at a higher price? Is the therapist prepared to spend time and money to increase the site's "visibility" on the Internet?

THE ONLINE THERAPIST'S WEBSITE

Some mental health professionals are intrigued by the potential of online therapy. These therapists likely view the Internet not only as a new form of advertisement but also as a place to provide innovative services to populations that may otherwise not seek out traditional face-to-face therapy. The online therapist may wish to practice entirely through electronic means (i.e., e-mail, chat rooms, or video teleconferencing) or to supplement his or her face-to-face practice. This decision should greatly influence the design of the website.

Two options are available for the online therapist: (a) The site can alert the customer to the availability of online services and the therapist can arrange provision of those services separate from the website; or (b) the site can be designed as a portal for the provision of online services. An example of the first option would be a site that is similar in purpose and design to the "business card website" described above, with the therapist then arranging e-mail transactions or online chats using other software programs or third-party services. An example of the second option would be a website that both serves to advertise the availability of therapy using online chat rooms or e-mail, and offers the ability for the client to pay for and join a live chat session or send an e-mail on the same website.

The second option is analogous to how many businesses now are choosing to offer customer services. Many businesses now offer answers to "Frequently Asked Questions" (FAQs) on their websites, and in the event that the FAQs are not sufficiently helpful, the customer can then type and submit his or her question to a customer service representative directly through the website, or even join a chat session with a live representative without ever leaving the website or needing to use or download additional software. Few online therapists offer this option, partly because designing such a site is beyond the technical abilities of most therapists. However, companies are available that provide mental health services online and directly through the company's website (e.g., www.find-a-therapist.com). The advantages of this option are convenience for the client and greater security. The client does not necessarily need additional software, only a web browser, and the client can access the therapist's services from almost any computer with a web browser and a connection to the Internet. Because the therapist has full control over how the client accesses services, there can be a greater degree of consistency in terms of security. For example, the therapist's website can be designed to support encryption of all information sent between the client and the therapist, instead of the therapist having to deal with the fact that some clients use chat or e-mail programs that support encryption while others do not. The primary disadvantage to this option is greater cost for the therapist.

The advantages of the first option include convenience for the therapist and lower cost. The therapist can design a simple site at little or no expense, arrange for payment of services through a third party, and provide the services using whatever software the therapist wishes. An example of a model for this business design follows:

> A potential client visits a therapist's website. → Potential client is interested in the services offered and wishes to pay for a certain number of e-mail transactions at the advertised cost. → Potential client clicks a "button" on the website that directs him or her to a third-party website, where he or she becomes a client by purchasing the therapy package using his or her credit card. → The third party notifies the therapist that he or she has a new customer, confirms that the client has paid for the services, and provides a name, number, and e-mail address. → The therapist contacts the client by phone or by e-mail using the therapist's preferred e-mail program and address. → The client responds by phone or by e-mail, using his or her preferred e-mail program and address.

The disadvantage to allowing both the therapist and the client to use their preferred e-mail programs is that if security is a concern it becomes harder to ensure security when the therapist cannot control the program the client uses and how he or she uses it. Most clients probably will not be concerned about the security of the transmissions, either because they are unaware of the security limitations or because they already feel comfortable using e-mail and chat rooms. The burden then falls on the therapist to ensure security to the best of his or her ability and to educate clients about how breaches in security occur online. The American Psychological Association's *Ethical Principles of Psychologists and Code of Conduct* (2002), standard 4.02c, specifically instructs therapists who "offer services, products, or information via electronic transmission" to discuss limits of confidentiality with clients. Even if the program being used is not chosen by the therapist, the therapist can still urge the client to take simple precautions to help protect confidentiality. These steps might include (a) not storing therapy-related e-mails or chat sessions on the client's computer if there is a possibility that others might read them; (b) not communicating with the therapist at all if the client is at work, as the employer would have the right to read those communications; and (c) sending e-mails with ambiguous subject lines that do not indicate that they are therapy related (e.g., "I have a question"). The therapist may also urge or even require that the client use software that increases security, such as firewall software (to help prevent stored e-mails from being stolen off the client's computer) and e-mail software that supports encrypted e-mails (many programs do not). The higher the security standards the therapist imposes on the client, regardless of the fact that the standards are in the client's best interest, the greater the risk that the client will not be willing or able to meet them.

Payment for services in this model can be arranged through any number of companies, but one of the companies most commonly used by online therapists is PayPal (www.paypal.com). PayPal offers free sign-up and a number of options for collecting payments, is easy to use, and has earned its success largely through its enormous popularity with users of the online auction company Ebay (www.ebay.com). PayPal does require customers to create an account before purchases can be made. Creating an account involves providing PayPal with a confirmed credit card number that PayPal then stores on its own secure servers. This makes the process of paying for online services more difficult for potential clients who do not already have PayPal accounts. Although an online therapist could create a website where credit card information is supplied through the therapist's website, the therapist must have a website that is hosted by a company that provides support for ecommerce transactions, a service most web hosting companies offer but one that typically costs more money. PayPal claims to have over 40 million customers and is considered by most to be safe and secure, though recently some customer information was obtained by scam artists. The perpetrators obtained e-mail addresses, mailing addresses, and transaction data for a small percentage of customers by tricking retailers who used PayPal into giving them the information. The scam worked by sending retailers fake e-mails that appeared to come from PayPal, thus bypassing PayPal's security features (Musgrove, 2004).

Whatever the method for payment collection the therapist chooses, the most important factor must be the security of the transmission. When a client enters his or her credit card information on a website and sends that information to the company's servers, there is always a risk that that information could be intercepted in transmission. Once the information reaches its destination and is stored on the host server, the information also becomes vulnerable to piracy. Although it is impossible to fully guarantee security at either point, reasonable steps to ensure security can and should be taken. In transmission, data can be secured through encryption, a process that changes the data into meaningless gibberish until it reaches its destination and is reconstituted to its useful state. Therapists who collect money electronically have a responsibility to ensure that either their website or the third party that collects the money uses encrypted data transmission.

Financial or other client-identifying information must ultimately be stored somewhere, whether on a computer that the therapist controls or on a server that a web host or Internet Service Provider (ISP) controls. If the storage place is not under the therapist's direct control, it becomes more difficult for the therapist to ensure security. Although many companies use multiple techniques to prevent the loss or piracy of their customers' personal information, these techniques are often unknown to the therapist and the client, and it may be very difficult for the therapist to find out what steps the company takes. The Web host or ISP should, however, be able to speak at least in general terms about the security of its servers. Beyond that, the therapist may have to rely on faith that the company is telling the truth and that the security measures it describes are in fact sufficient.

This dilemma raises a question about the extent of a therapist's legal responsibility for electronic financial and personal health information that is stolen either through transmission or storage. Although the Health Insurance Portability and Accountability Act (HIPAA) provides standards of security when transmitting client information to and from insurance companies, no standards exist for other situations. Many private practitioners accept credit cards as means of payment for services; if that information were to be intercepted in transmission from the therapist's office to the credit card company, the therapist would not be considered liable but the credit card company would. Similarly, if a therapist uses a third-party company like PayPal to collect fees, it is the company's responsibility then to ensure security to the extent possible.

THE NEED FOR "DOTCOMSENSE"

Creating content for a website can be challenging and fun. A new website may seem like a blank canvas, but there is a lot of information that a therapist's website should have. Just as a therapist's office has specific information available such as the therapist's prices, policies, and qualifications, a website should probably have equivalent kinds of information. Every website is different, however, and there are no "rules" about what information a therapist is required to post. A responsible therapist should seriously consider following most if not all of the recommendations that will be discussed, but a therapist may also have perfectly good reasons for not following some of the recommendations.

There is currently a great debate in the field of mental health about whether or not online therapy is ethical. Some have asked whether online therapy is ethical at all, ethical only in certain circumstances or with certain populations, or if it is even as effective as therapy done face-to-face. The ethical issues that confront online therapists are largely separate from those faced by therapists who simply want to create a website that advertises their face-to-face services. For a more thorough discussion of these issues, the reader is referred to Ragusea and VandeCreek (2003).

There are many organizations that have published guidelines regarding health information websites and/or the provision of online therapy. These organizations include the Health On the Net Foundation, Health Internet Ethics, the American Accreditation HealthCare/Commission, the American Medical Association, the Internet Healthcare Coalition, the National Board for Certified Counselors, the American Medical Informatics Association, the International Society for Mental Health Online, and the American Counseling Association. All of these guidelines are available on the respective websites of these organizations. These organizations have noted that the online therapist faces unique ethical challenges in the areas of (a) anonymity/confidentiality, (b) informed consent, (c) duty to protect, (d) advertising, and (e) the competent provision of services.

These issues will be briefly summarized here. Clients can maintain their anonymity online much more easily than they can in traditional face-to-face therapy. Although some have lauded this fact as one of the advantages of online therapy, it can also create risks for the therapist. Confidentiality may not necessarily be more difficult to guarantee in cyberspace, but the nature of technology allows for breaches in confidentiality that are different from those faced in traditional office-based therapy. Online therapists need to educate themselves about how information can be lost or stolen from computers.

Because online therapy is a new practice, many experts advocate acknowledging the experimental nature of online therapy in the informed consent form. In addition, the limitations of nonvisual, computer-based treatment should be acknowledged along with the advantages.

The duty to protect can become complicated when the client is not in the same room as the therapist, and may very well not even be in the same state. Online therapists would be well advised to locate emergency resources near the client's locale early on in treatment.

Advertising is a common way to help cover the overhead costs of a website, but advertising online can mislead visitors into thinking that the therapist has endorsed those sites. And finally, providing services online competently requires sophisticated knowledge about the technology being used as well as the differences in how people communicate online. Therapists interested in providing online therapy should seek further education either through literature or through seminars and workshops.

There is some information that all therapists should incorporate into their website. In 2000 the American Psychological Association (APA) published *Dotcomsense: Common Sense Ways to Protect Your Privacy and Assess Online Mental Health Information* (APA, 2000). This brochure was created by APA to help educate the public on what to look for when seeking quality information or services on the Internet. The brochure encouraged consumers to investigate the credibility of mental health sites and to seek additional information when in doubt. Unfortunately, publication of this useful brochure was later terminated and it is no longer accessible.

Despite its brief existence, *Dotcomsense* contained important recommendations that are still relevant today. The authors of the brochure also recognized that there is an enormous need to educate the public about how to safely obtain health care information and services on the Internet. It is difficult to know who to trust on the Internet. Health care providers have an obligation to act as lighthouses in the fog of cyberspace, guiding people to safe harbors. This begs the question, what does a lighthouse look like in cyberspace? In brief, therapists must educate the public on what health care looks like on the Internet and then exemplify those behaviors or characteristics. Here is a summary of the suggestions that *Dotcomsense* offered:

1. Any site that collects personal information should have a page for "disclaimers" and a "privacy policy." Consumers are warned to be cautious of sites that do not display such policies. The policy should explain how the information is used, and offer an opportunity for the consumer to opt out of arrangements if the information is sold or used to solicit further business from the consumer.

2. Ownership of the site should be clearly identified. Credibility is lost when a service-oriented site is used by its owners to sell another product, or when the financial support of another company influences the content of the information provided. Advertisements should be clearly separated from health information. If links to other sites are paid for by other companies, this arrangement should be clear to the consumer.

3. Explicit description of the purposes and goals of the site should be available to the consumer on the site.

4. Information that can change over time should be clearly dated, so that consumers know when it was last updated. (It may be inferred from this suggestion that the owner of the website has a responsibility to keep information on the site updated on a regular basis.)

5. Sources of information should be explicitly displayed. This means that images, text, and assessment instruments need to be attributed to their authors and copyright laws need to be respected.

6. The website should provide a way for consumers to contact the administrators of the site to provide feedback.

CONCLUSION

This contribution has attempted to introduce technologically unsophisticated therapists to the language and possibilities of web design and the Internet. Some may feel even more overwhelmed now at the end than they did at the beginning. For the undaunted, learning how to design sophisticated web pages can be very time-consuming but can result in more professional, unique, and aesthetically pleasing sites. Fortunately, the simple template-based web design tools that some companies provide and that are described in *Psychotherapy Finances* ("Quick and Easy," 2003) will still produce acceptable results and require virtually no expertise in web design. Please note the worksheet that has been included in this contribution on pages 183 and 184. The worksheet is designed to encourage thoughtful planning as one considers building a website. It does not include all of the issues and decisions that will be made, but does include many that have been discussed in this contribution.

Web design can be fun and the product can be very rewarding, but hopefully this contribution has highlighted some of the serious responsibilities a professional has to keep in mind. It is becoming cliché to describe the Internet as full of possibilities as well as dangers. The therapists reading this contribution should remember that it is very easy for people to masquerade as professionals on the Internet. Therapists should strive to make it simple for the public to distinguish between legitimate professionals and imposters. It is not enough to simply have good intentions. Transparency and accountability are necessary but not sufficient elements. For example, while some therapists choose to post their license number, others are concerned that doing so is as risky as posting one's social security number. However, even if one posts a license number, how does a consumer know that it is a legitimate number? There is currently no independent service that will verify a therapist's credentials and provide a digital "badge" for display on the website, though such a service would be welcomed. A service did exist called Credential Check, but it closed due to financial reasons (Holmes, n.d.).

Websites allow therapists to express their ideas and personalities to the public through an affordable and flexible medium. Therapists can use a website as a tool, a service, an introduction, an advertisement, or a business. Websites can reveal as much, or as little, about the therapist as he or she chooses. A site can, depending on the quality of the design and content, serve to engage or frustrate, educate or obfuscate. This contribution has touched on some of the ways therapists can design high quality websites, but no single paper can be a complete tutorial. Many people have tinkered with website design, so valuable resources may be nearer than one may think. Interested therapists should seek to educate themselves through classes, books, consultation, and experimentation. Technological ignorance can be overcome. The Internet is a large world, and therapists should not fear claiming a little of its territory for themselves.

Planning a Website: Worksheet

Before you make any commitments about your website, think about some of the important decisions that need to be made! Use this worksheet as a guide.

Purpose

What is the purpose of my site (e.g., information? online therapy? business card?)?

_____

_____

Who is my audience (e.g., adults? teens? locals? busy travelers? other professionals?)?

_____

_____

What are my criteria for a successful site (e.g., attract a certain number of visitors, generate a certain amount of profit)?

_____

_____

Budget

How much am I willing to spend upfront (e.g., design costs, buying a domain)? _____

How much am I willing to spend to maintain the site on a monthly/yearly basis? _____

Hosting a Website

Do I want full control over my site's address (URL)?   ❑ Yes   ❑ No

Do I anticipate needing a lot of server space?   ❑ Yes   ❑ No

Do I plan to sell products/services through my site?   ❑ Yes   ❑ No

How much flexibility do I need over the services I pay for? _____

_____

The previous answers should influence the following decision: Should I
use an Internet Service Provider or a professional Web host to host my site?   ❑ Yes   ❑ No

Design

If I were to have full control over my domain name, what name would I want (e.g., www.mysite.com)?

_____

_____

How is the name consistent with my site's goals/audience/purpose? _____

In considering my site's overall "look," what qualities do I want it to have (e.g., colorful, conservative, playful, informative, interactive, multimedia)?

_____

_____

How can I help make my site more accessible to people with physical and cognitive limitations, or people from different cultures?

_____

_____

Content

Will my site be advertisement-supported? ❑ Yes ❑ No

Do I have a page on my site for policies/informed consent? ❑ Yes ❑ No

Do I provide a method for visitors to contact me and/or provide feedback? ❑ Yes ❑ No

What kinds of content do I wish to provide (e.g., psychoeducation, therapy, bulletin boards, self-administered tests, etc.)?

_____

_____

How do I plan to help visitors trust that I am a legitimate professional providing legitimate information/services?

_____

_____

Is the content on my site, or, are the services I provide
on my site, consistent with the ethical standards of my profession? ❑ Yes ❑ No

CONTRIBUTOR

Anthony Ragusea, PsyD, is currently a psychology resident at Care Center for Mental Health in Key West, Florida. He recently completed his doctorate in clinical psychology from Wright State University in Dayton, Ohio. His interest in psychology and the Internet began with his doctoral dissertation on the ethics of online therapy. Mr. Ragusea may be contacted at 3930 S. Roosevelt Boulevard, W112, Key West, FL 33040. E-mail: anthony@ragusea.com

RESOURCES

American Psychological Association. (2000). *Dotcomsense: Common Sense Ways to Protect Your Privacy and Assess Online Mental Health Information.* Washington, DC: Author.

American Psychological Association. (2002). Ethical principles of psychologists and code of conduct. *American Psychologist, 57*(12), 1060-1073.

Crowder, D. A., & Crowder, R. (2000). *Building a Web Site for Dummies.* Foster City, CA: IDG Books Worldwide.

Haring, R. (2000). Entertain me! A guide to website interactivity. Retrieved March 13, 2004, from http://www.webpronews.com/archives/100500.html

Holmes, L. (n.d.). Can you verify the credentials of your cybershrink? Retrieved April 13, 2004, from http://mentalhealth.about.com/library/weekly/aa060997.htm

Huang, M. (2003). Designing website attributes to induce experiential encounters. *Computers in Human Behavior, 19*, 425-442.

Musgrove, M. (2004, March 16). PayPal warns its customers to safeguard personal data. *The Washington Post*, p. E05.

Quick and easy ways to get your practice on the Web. (2003, December). *Psychotherapy Finances, 29*(12), 4-5.

Ragusea, A., & VandeCreek, L. (2003). Suggestions for the ethical practice of online therapy. *Psychotherapy: Theory, Research, Practice, Training, 40*(1/2), 94-102.

Teo, H., Oh, L., Liu, C., & Wei, K. (2003). An empirical study of the effects of interactivity on web user attitude. *International Journal of Human-Computer Studies, 58*(3), 281-305.

Problems and Solutions With Online Therapy

Paul A. Smiley and Leon VandeCreek

The popularization of the Internet has changed the way our society functions, and people seem to be benefiting from it. The Internet provides a seemingly endless amount of information to its users, and mental health professionals are beginning to offer services to clients through it. Online therapy is a potential niche market for those clinicians electing to provide services to clients through different modalities via the Internet. For the purposes of this contribution, online therapy will be defined as therapy conducted via e-mail, chat rooms, or interactive video.

Online therapy is a new mode of treatment through which professionals can provide mental health services to clients. Relatively limited research has been published on its treatment outcomes, but recently some support has been reported for the effectiveness of online therapy. For example, Day and Schneider (2002) found no statistically significant difference in outcome variables between face-to-face therapy and real time video conferencing. Zetterqvist et al. (2003) found that providing stress management techniques to people online was an effective method for stress relief. Additionally, Lange, Van de Ven, and Schrieken (2003) described outcomes of their protocol-driven Internet treatment of people with posttraumatic stress and grief. They concluded that online treatment was effective in reducing avoidance behaviors and symptoms of depression. Ruskin et al. (2004) compared treatment outcomes of people with depressive disorders who were treated through in-person therapy with those treated through telepsychiatry, where treatment was conducted via computer video. They concluded that telepsychiatry had the same treatment outcomes as in-person therapy, including levels of patient adherence and satisfaction. McCrone et al. (2004) concluded that people with depression and anxiety showed more improvement in their depressive symptoms through computerized Cognitive Behavioral Therapy programs compared to a matched population who received traditional face-to-face therapy. No additional published studies were found that addressed the efficacy of online therapy. Some online therapy websites post client testimonials supporting the effectiveness of online therapy, but the validity of such claims remains questionable. The purpose of this contribution is to describe some potential benefits of online therapy, identify common problems with online therapy, and propose solutions of such problems to professionals looking to provide mental health services online.

BENEFITS OF ONLINE THERAPY

Despite the limited amount of published empirical support for treatment outcomes of online therapy, clinicians should recognize the many benefits it offers to both themselves and their clients when juxtaposed with more traditional forms of face-to-face therapy.

Convenience and Accessibility

One benefit of online therapy is that it is convenient and allows greater outreach of mental health care services to traditionally underserved populations, such as people who live in rural areas and people with restrictive physical disabilities. For example, online therapy may be a preferred alternative to face-to-face therapy for people who are deaf or hard of hearing (Zelvin & Speyer, 2004). Online therapy can also be utilized by people who relocate to a different country where language barriers may prevent them from seeking local mental health resources (Rochlen, Zack, & Speyer, 2004). Some online services such as e-mail do not even require an advance appointment, because clients can contact their therapists whenever they have computer access (Manhal-Baugus, 2001; New Freedom Commission on Mental Health, 2003).

Decreased Stigmatization

A second benefit of online therapy for at least a small number of clients is that it allows for more anonymity in therapy. Increased levels of anonymity could benefit people who feel shame or are afraid of being stigmatized by seeking in-person services (Ragusea & VandeCreek, 2003). Online therapy reportedly helps to eliminate the stigma and embarrassment that has prevented some people from seeking mental health services in the past (Freeny, 2001). Suler (2004) reported that increased anonymity creates a disinhibition effect, where people feel less vulnerable about discussing personal aspects of their life.

Written or Spoken Communication

Not only does online therapy create an opportunity to provide mental health services to more people, but it carries the additional benefit of allowing both the client and therapist to reflect on topics discussed in previous correspondence (Manhal-Baugus, 2001), a benefit that Suler (2004) referred to as the *zone of reflection*. The act of writing provides additional benefits for the client, such as allowing time for self-reflection and ownership of the therapeutic process (Rochlen et al., 2004). Zelvin and Speyer (2004) contended that some people are more accessible and authentic through writing. Writing is considered a therapeutic process itself, with effects similar to journaling, from which many clients generally benefit (Murphy & Mitchell, 1998). Furthermore, unlike face-to-face therapy, online therapy allows time for the clinician to identify and explore a client's concerns without the awkwardness or need to think on one's feet (Grohol, 1999).

Some people may also be less inhibited describing their situations in writing compared to verbally articulating them in face-to-face therapy. With online therapy, some people may have reduced anxiety about hearing themselves tell personal and/or possibly embarrassing life stories, and they do not have to worry about facing the visible expected reactions of others (e.g., shock, disbelief, disappointment, etc.) when listening to their presenting problems (Suler, 2004).

Available Resources

A final benefit is that during a therapy session, a therapist may choose to provide a client with additional resources or references to read or complete before the next session. Through online therapy, a clinician can quickly provide clients with relevant resources by sending links to websites, video clips, documents, and assessment tools. With face-to-face therapy, in contrast, clinicians are limited to what they physically possess in their office (Rochlen et al., 2004).

POTENTIAL PROBLEMS AND SOLUTIONS

Professionals need to be aware of many potential problems associated with online therapy and should contemplate how to overcome them before providing services online. We identify common problems with online therapy and propose solutions for professionals looking to provide mental health services online. As will become apparent, online therapy poses several risks that cannot be fully offset.

Validating Professional Credentials

One general problem with online therapy is that it lacks a mechanism for assuring the identity of professionals providing online therapy. People claiming to be licensed clinicians are not currently required to verify their credentials prior to providing online therapy (King & Poulos, 1999). Therefore, nothing prevents nonprofessionals from declaring themselves to be licensed clinicians and providing therapy to unsuspecting clientele. Huang and Alessi (1996) contended that poorly informed clients with a history of mental illness may become easy targets for such fraudulent online clinicians. Ideally, this type of fraud and misrepresentation would not happen, but it is important for licensed clinicians considering the provision of online therapy to be aware of this potential dilemma clients may face, and should consider how to effectively advertise themselves in a truthful and attractive manner.

Potential clients may feel more trustworthy of online clinicians who provide standard credentials that describe a professional's qualifications. Recommended credentials include one's license number and a listing of professional degrees and board certifications, including the institutions from which they were earned. Other suggestions include listing one's office location and phone number, and a message encouraging potential clients to call the office for verification. These are basic credentials listed by face-to-face therapists in their offices, and these should be provided by online therapists as well. In addition, online clinicians can apply for online certification seals from the Better Business Bureau Online (www.bbbonline.org)* to verify that the information provided on their website is valid and accurate. Upon passing inspection, the clinician's website will receive a posted certification that helps users identify reliable and trustworthy online businesses.

Client Anonymity

The increased level of anonymity created through online therapy creates potential problems not only for clients, but for therapists as well. Compared to face-to-face therapy, online therapy provides less verification of client identity, as another individual may be impersonating the client during an online therapy session (Ragusea & VandeCreek, 2003; Rochlen et al., 2004). There will always be some degree of uncertainty regarding the true identity of the person for whom the therapist is providing services. However, this uncertainty is increased with the anonymity afforded by the Internet. To help reduce this problem, Ragusea and VandeCreek (2003) recommend creating a password during the initial session that is known only to the therapist and client, and which is exchanged at the beginning of each session to confirm their identities to each other.

A second problem caused by increased client anonymity is that online clinicians need to verify whether the client has shared an accurate identity or not. One reason this is important is to confirm that clients are over 18 years old before providing services (Fisher & Fried, 2003). Among many reasons, this is critical because most states have mental health care laws regulating the amount of services minors are able to receive without their parents' consent. If the client is not at least 18 years of age, the clinician should obtain parental permission before proceeding with therapy (Ragusea & VandeCreek, 2003). This verification process may prove difficult, as there is an increased risk for identity falsification on the part of the client, as previously discussed (Ragusea & VandeCreek, 2003; Rochlen et al., 2004). Age verification programs are

---

* Although all websites cited in this contribution were correct at the time of publication, they are subject to change at any time.

still in the developmental stages; however, online therapists should consider utilizing services offered at an online consumer authentication service: http://idresponse.com. This website claims to use technology (patent pending) to verify consumers' age and shipping address. Ragusea (2005) also suggested asking clients to mail or fax additional forms of identification to the office, such as a copy of a social security card, driver's license, or birth certificate.

A third potential problem for online therapy created by increased client anonymity is the risk of dual relationships (Kraus, 2004). Dual relationships are issues for all mental health professionals. For example, it is unethical for psychologists to be in a professional role with a client with whom a preexisting nontherapeutic relationship exists (American Psychological Association, 2002, Standard 3.05a). Online therapists will generally experience greater difficulty clearly identifying who their clients are and consequently deciding whether to engage in a therapeutic relationship with them. Therefore, increased client anonymity creates a greater opportunity for online clinicians to mistakenly accept a client based on the identifying information the client has provided, without knowing for certain if a previous nontherapeutic relationship was already in existence. This problem could be avoided by verifying the client's accurate identity through methods mentioned previously. This would allow clinicians more information on which to base their professional decision of whether or not to engage in a therapeutic relationship with this prospective client.

Reduction/Loss of Nonverbal Communication

Potentially the greatest concern associated with online therapy is the complete loss of nonverbal forms of communication. Transferring from face-to-face communication to only written communication provides many limitations. Without nonverbal cues, communications from the client to the clinician and vice versa have a greater chance of being misunderstood (Grohol, 1999; Koocher & Morray, 2000). For example, sarcasm in writing is difficult to recognize, and failing to recognize it could lead to serious misunderstandings, particularly for people with mental disorders (Manhal-Baugus, 2001; Ragusea & VandeCreek, 2003). Clients with poor ego strength or paranoid tendencies may misinterpret written information because they do not have access to the reassuring visual and auditory cues from the clinician (Rochlen et al., 2004). Koocher and Keith-Spiegel (1998) noted that specific aspects of nonverbal communications absent from online therapy include voice, pitch, and tone of voice, the absence of which likely increases the potential for errors and problems. Missing such nonverbal cues may also limit highly experiential therapeutic approaches that strongly rely on "in the moment" nonverbal cues (Alleman, 2002).

Without explicit nonverbal communication, online therapy will be more difficult than face-to-face therapy, but it is not impossible. Rapport can be established through empathy, as the client feels listened to and respected by the therapist paying close attention to what is being typed (Stofle & Chechele, 2004). It is also recommended for professionals to take extra care in the syntax of information delivered to the client to reduce the likelihood of misinterpretations. Substitutes for some nonverbals can be the use of emoticons (i.e., ☺ ☹), acronyms (LOL for "laugh out loud"), and changing fonts, case, or style (Ragusea & VandeCreek, 2003; Suler, 2004). Furthermore, Suler (2004) suggested using parenthetical expressions (e.g., sigh, feeling unsure here) to convey body language or nonvocal thoughts and feelings. One can also use notations to indicate a pause in thinking (such as ellipsis) which can also mimic face-to-face communication patterns of speech (Suler, 2004). Technological hardware can also assist with the reduction or loss of nonverbal communication: Video- and still cameras can be hooked up to computers, and images can be transferred between clinician and client to aid in communication. If this option is not possible for either party, the clinician can request that a recent photograph of the client be mailed to his or her office to help the clinician visualize the person with whom he or she is providing services. Additional recommendations are discussed in the next section.

Mental Status Assessments

It is also difficult for clinicians to accurately assess a client's mental status without utilizing additional sources of information, such as visual, auditory, or olfactory information typically used in more traditional assessment therapy settings (Fenichel, 2000). For example, clinicians providing online therapy would not be able to detect the smell of alcohol on a client who denies having had anything to drink, or the nonverbal body cues that suggest a client is anxious about a particular issue (Grohol, 1999).

There are no quick solutions to this dilemma, but skills can be developed to reduce the potential loss. Similar to how a person who is blind may learn to rely more on a keen sense of hearing, online clinicians will benefit from developing a more keen sense for analyzing written expressions. Analyzing the words people use in communication can tell much about an individual's personality (Groom & Pennebaker, 2002). For example, Pennebaker, Mehl, and Niederhoffer (2003) contended that analyzing particles of speech (i.e., pronouns, articles, prepositions, conjunctives, and auxiliary verbs) can provide insight into emotional states, social identity, and cognitive styles. Online clinicians can invest in computer programs such as Linguistic Inquiry and Word Count (LIWC; Pennebaker, Francis, & Booth, 2001), which can help to identify individual differences in language content and style.

Timing of Responses

Online therapy such as with e-mail does not always involve synchronous responses, and a client may misinterpret a delay in the therapist's response, which could increase a client's anxiety or other thoughts related to his or her pathology (Suler, 2002). To prevent this problem, it is recommended that professionals clearly inform clients when e-mails will be read and how long it will typically take for a response. For example, clinicians could say, "E-mail will be checked every evening by 6:00 p.m., and you can expect to get a response within 14 to 18 hours." Clinicians should also set their own boundaries with respect to clients who request an immediate response.

Collection of Fees

Online clinicians need to be clear about their fees, particularly if there are additional fees for time spent reading and writing e-mails. Insurance plans may cover some costs for traditional mental health services, but most do not yet cover Internet therapy (Kraus, 2004; Neubauer, 2004). Therefore, the costs for online therapy will mostly be paid on a fee-for-service basis. Most clinicians who work with fee-for-service arrangements require fees to be paid in full prior to or at the end of each session, and online therapists can, too. Services such as PayPal (www.paypal.com) allow individuals to securely, easily, and quickly send and receive payments online. For example, a client's PayPal account could be linked to a credit card, and the clinician's account could be linked to a bank account into which funds are directly deposited. Ironically, this online service also requires the verification of an anonymous client's identification, and its user agreement states that it uses a combination of many unidentified techniques to reduce the likelihood of someone falsifying his or her identifying information, but that it is still unable to guarantee any user's identity.

Suitability for Online Therapy

Another potential problem for online therapy is that this modality of treatment may not be suitable for all people. Before engaging in online therapy, the clinician needs to consider his or her and the client's level of computer skills. More basic computer skills like maintaining sufficient spelling and grammar are important, as are being a reasonably good writer and typist (Ragusea, 2005; Stofle, 2001; Zack, 2002; Zelvin & Speyer, 2004). Ragusea (2005) also suggested that clients should have prior Internet experience, such as e-mailing or participating in chat rooms. Grohol (1999) and Suler (2001) recommended screening potential clients for online therapy, as it is important for clients to be relatively proficient and comfortable with reading and writing, as well as able to communicate at comparable levels of comprehension. Suler (2001) listed many recommended screening topics and specific questions to ask, including:

1. How might the person's computer skills, knowledge, platform, and Internet access affect the therapy?

   • Does the person demonstrate adequate knowledge of his or her computer system and Internet technology?
   • Is the person's computer system compatible with that of the clinician?
   • What kind of Internet access does the person have?

2. How knowledgeable is the person about online communication and relationships?

   • What experience does the person have with communicating online?
   • If the person has online relationships or belongs to online groups, what have these social activities been like?
   • In what settings did these relationships develop and for how long?

3. How well is the person suited for the reading and writing involved in text communication?

   • Does the person like reading and writing?
   • What kinds of experiences has the person had with reading and writing?
   • Are there any known physical or cognitive problems that will limit the ability to read and write?
   • How well can the person type?

Additionally, online clinicians should have more advanced computer technological skills, such as being able to troubleshoot on the spot by answering clients' questions related to specialized software complications that may arise (Ragusea, 2005). Furthermore, clinicians may need to know how to use encryption software and be able to provide technical support for clients on how to use similar software to help maintain confidentiality while transmitting information online (Ragusea & VandeCreek, 2003). The International Society for Mental Health Online (2001) listed additional practical and emotional skills for clinicians, such as fast typing; comfort using Internet modalities (e.g., instant messenger, e-mail, chat rooms); ability to receive, store, and protect communications with clients; comfort describing one's own and others' feelings in text; ability to make effective therapeutic interventions using text only; and an awareness of how clients perceive therapists online.

Confidentiality

Issues around confidentiality are a prime concern for all clinicians, but those providing online therapy need to take extra precautions, because there is an increased threat to clients' privacy and confidentiality (Zack, 2004). Safeguards can be installed to help increase privacy and confidentiality, such as firewalls, intruder detection systems, and virus detection software, but no combination of these devices can guarantee privacy and confidentiality (Ragusea & VandeCreek, 2003). Encrypting e-mails is another way to increase the security of confidential communications (Ragusea, 2005), and at the very least, Zack (2004) recommended utilizing a basic computer password required at startup.

Keeping conversations private and confidential from computer hackers is one threat, but one should also be concerned about the information saved on the client's computer. Online therapy creates more of a paper trail on the client's end, which creates additional opportunities for confidential information to be exposed. This can be particularly dangerous for clients experiencing domestic violence, as their perpetrators may gain access to e-mails or other documents of private communications with the client's therapist (Ragusea & VandeCreek, 2003). As previously discussed, it is recommended that clinicians and clients mutually decide on e-mail subject headings that will discourage other people from reading private communications by making them less "catchy" and more mundane and vague. Ragusea and VandeCreek (2003) suggested using more ambiguous lines, such as "Regarding the assistance you requested" to reduce the temptation of others reading the private communication. Ragusea (2005) also suggested creating a separate e-mail account for therapy to avoid the risk of others viewing confidential communications.

Crisis Situations

Another problem relates to the limitations of online therapy in a crisis situation. In such an event, a clinician would have less control over the situation when conducting online therapy compared with more traditional forms of therapy. For example, if a client is suicidal, a clinician providing face-to-face therapy can take reasonable steps to alert other persons who can assist in providing protective care or can ensure the client is safely transported and admitted into a hospital. However, with online therapy, a client can "log off" or become nonresponsive in e-mail correspondence and cut off the clinician from further interventions. This would reduce the clinician's ability to ensure that the client receives the necessary assistance. Murphy and Mitchell (1998) recommended that online therapists obtain direct contact information from clients to be used in an emergency, such as a phone number or street address where the Internet is being accessed (a way to verify the location of the Internet connection is described in the next section). Clinicians should also be aware of local resources available for clients to be referred, but understand that local emergency or crisis intervention services may be difficult to arrange, particularly from out-of-town, state, or country (Koocher & Morray, 2000). We suggest that online clinicians screen clients carefully to identify those who may pose special crisis intervention needs.

Licensure and Other Legal Requirements

A current problem for online therapists relates to licensure requirements. For example, states require clinicians to be licensed in the state in which the services are being provided. In the case of online therapy, however, it is not clear whether licensure boards consider that the therapy is being provided where the therapist is located or where the client receives the services. This lack of clarity creates a problem for online professionals, because clients could reside in a state other than where the professional is licensed to practice. From one perspective, it could be argued that because the primary purpose of professional licensure is to protect the public, the provider should be licensed in the state where the client resides and the provider should be held to the laws and regulations of that state. From a different perspective, one could argue that when face-to-face services are provided, the client comes to the office of the provider, wherever the office is located. Some clients cross state lines to see their provider of choice. Online therapists could argue that clients are coming to their offices as well, except that clients do so through the Internet. Until state licensure boards, or the courts, provide clarification on this issue, online therapists should at least be alert to the uncertainty of the legality of providing services in states in which they are not licensed. Additionally, Kraus (2004) stated that most malpractice insurance policies are only valid within the scope of the professional's license and therefore may not be valid if one provides online services to an individual residing in a state in which he or she is not licensed to practice. Kraus also recommended that online clinicians become licensed in more states to expand the scope of their practice.

Some state licensure boards permit clinicians to practice for a limited number of days (e.g., 30 days) in their state without being licensed there, if the clinician is licensed in another state. These exceptions to licensure were created to facilitate the process of obtaining a license in the new state and to permit clinicians to practice in an emergency or other unusual circumstances. Clinicians are encouraged to contact the licensure boards where their online therapy clients reside to inquire about obtaining limited permission to practice with clients who reside in that state.

Clinicians also need to be knowledgeable about other laws in states where clients reside, and practice according to these laws. For example, all states have mandatory child abuse reporting laws, but there are sufficient differences across states and by profession that online clinicians should become familiar with the laws in the states in which the clients reside. Greater differences are found in legal mandates to report the abuse of elderly, handicapped, disabled, or dependent adults. States also differ in what measures need to be taken to protect third parties from harm (Koocher & Morray, 2000). We and others (e.g., Fisher & Fried, 2003) recommend that clinicians become knowledgeable about laws relating to duty to warn or protect and other mandatory disclosures in the client's state. Fortunately, this information is now available online in most states.

As noted earlier, it is a good idea for online clinicians to take steps to verify the client's identity and location at the beginning of therapy. Clinicians can confirm the client's computer location by verifying the Internet Protocol (IP) address from the computer where the last contact was made. An IP address is a unique number assigned to every computer connection to the Internet. Consequently, the IP address will change when the client accesses the Internet from a new location, such as would occur when the client travels and accesses the Internet from a hotel or library. Clients can automatically find their computer's IP address by going to the following website: http://www.lawrencegoetz.com/programs/ipinfo/. Online clinicians can then enter the client's IP address at the following site to confirm the computer's location: http://www.geobytes.com/IpLocator.htm?GetLocation. This website also provides a detailed map and lists nearby cities, which may aid the clinician in finding local resources for the client.

Summary of Recommended Suggestions To Consider for Online Therapy

We summarize our suggestions for clinicians who are considering e-therapy with the following list of things to consider:

1. Provide standard credentials on a website, including one's license number, listing of professional degrees, board certifications and institutions from which they were earned, office location, phone number, and a message encouraging potential clients to call the office for verification. Clinicians can also certify information on their website by contacting the Better Business Bureau Online (www.bbbonline.org).
2. Create a mutually agreed-upon password with clients to exchange at the commencement of each session to verify their identities to each other. Clinicians should also verify their clients' age by using an online authentication service (http://idresponse.com)

or by requesting clients to mail or fax copies of a driver's license or birth certificate to their office.

3. Become proficient in expressing thoughts and feelings nonverbally through a computer by using emoticons (☺ ☹), acronyms (LOL for "laugh out loud"), changing fonts, case, or style, and ellipses.

4. Consider investing in computer software and hardware to aid online therapy. Programs such as Linguistic Inquiry and Word Count can help to analyze and interpret written language content and style. Firewalls, intruder detection systems, and virus detection software can help increase confidentiality of online communications. Video- and still cameras can provide additional nonverbal information to the clinician about the client.

5. Let clients know when to expect responses to e-mails.

6. Collect fees for services through PayPal (www.paypal.com) or other sites that allow clients to securely, easily, and quickly submit payments online.

7. Assess one's suitability for online therapy, and screen potential clients for their suitability for online therapy. Clients should have basic computer skills, and clinicians should be able to provide a minimal level of computer technical support to their clients if requested.

8. Increase confidentiality through the use of software and hardware options as previously mentioned, but also by creating less "catchy" e-mail subject headings and encrypting online communications.

9. Obtain clients' phone numbers and verify their location by obtaining their computer's IP address. This will provide the clinician with a more direct method of contacting the client and referring him or her to local resources in a crisis situation. Additionally, identifying a client's location may minimize legal issues for clinicians who want to provide services only to clients residing in states in which they are licensed to practice.

CONCLUSION

As our society continues to push into a more computer-assisted world, where there is a demand for services to be faster with more convenient access, online therapy may expand into a more utilized niche market for clinicians. Online therapy generates several benefits for professionals; however, many potential problems need to be addressed to help prevent clinicians from getting into ethical or legal problems. An area of future research is to further investigate how cultural variables interact with online therapy, as currently there is limited research in this area. The Internet provides great opportunity for a new forum for mental health care services, but clinicians who want to engage in online therapy should be cautious of heightened risks associated with this potential niche market. Few, if any, legal cases involving online therapy exist that can be used to help set precedents. This contribution may help to fill this void and prepare clinicians for potential problems and issues to consider prior to engaging in online therapy.

CONTRIBUTORS

Paul A. Smiley, BS, is a doctoral student in clinical psychology. His areas of interest include health psychology and technological advancements for mental health treatment. Mr. Smiley may be contacted at the School of Professional Psychology, 117 Health Sciences Building, Wright State University, 3640 Colonel Glenn Highway, Dayton, OH 45435-0001. E-mail: smiley.5@wright.edu

Leon VandeCreek, PhD, is a licensed psychologist who is the past dean and current Professor in the School of Professional Psychology at Wright State University in Dayton, Ohio. He has been awarded the Diplomate in Clinical Psychology and he is a Fellow of several divisions of the American Psychological Association. His interests include professional training and ethical/legal issues related to professional education and practice. Dr. VandeCreek has served as President of the Pennsylvania Psychological Association, Chair of the APA Insurance Trust, Chair of the Board of Educational Affairs of the APA, and Treasurer of the Ohio Psychological Association. In 2005 he served as President of the Division of Psychotherapy of the APA. He has authored and coauthored about 150 professional presentations and publications, including 15 books. Since 1992, he has served as Senior Editor of the *Innovations in Clinical Practice: A Source Book* series, published by Professional Resource Press. Dr. VandeCreek can be reached at the Ellis Human Development Institute, 9 N. Edwin C. Moses Boulevard, Dayton, OH 45407. E-mail: leon.vandecreek@wright.edu

RESOURCES

Cited Resources

Alleman, J. (2002). Online counseling: The Internet and mental health treatment. *Psychotherapy: Theory, Research, Practice, Training, 39*, 199-209.

American Psychological Association. (2002). Ethical principles of psychologists and code of conduct. *American Psychologist, 57*(12), 1060-1073. Available from the APA website: http://www.apa.org/ethics

Day, S., & Schneider, P. (2002). Psychotherapy using distance technology: A comparison of face-to-face, video, and audio treatment. *Journal of Counseling Psychology, 49*, 499-503.

Fenichel, M. (2000). *Online Psychotherapy: Technical Difficulties, Formulations, and Processes.* Retrieved November 3, 2004, from http://www.fenichel.com/technical.shtml

Fisher, C., & Fried, A. (2003). Internet-mediated psychological services and the American Psychological Association Ethics Code. *Psychotherapy: Theory, Research, Practice, Training, 40*(1-2), 103-111.

Freeny, M. (2001). Better than being there. *Psychotherapy Networker 25*(2), 31-39.

Grohol, J. (1999, May 14). *Best Practices in E-therapy: Definition and Scope of E-therapy.* Retrieved November 3, 2004, from http://psychcentral.com/best/best3.htm

Groom, C., & Pennebaker, J. (2002). Words. *Journal of Research in Personality, 36*(6), 615-621.

Huang, M., & Alessi, N. (1996). The Internet and the future of psychiatry. *American Journal of Psychiatry, 153*(7), 861-869.

International Society for Mental Health Online. (2001). *Myths and Realities of Online Clinical Work.* Retrieved January 22, 2005, from http://www.fenichel.com/myths/

King, S. A., & Poulos, S. T. (1999). Ethical guidelines for on-line therapy. In J. Fink (Ed.), *How to Use Computers and Cyberspace in the Clinical Practice of Psychotherapy* (pp. 121-132). Lanham, MD: Jason Aronson.

Koocher, G. P., & Keith-Spiegel, P. (1998). *Ethics in Psychology: Professional Standards and Cases* (2nd ed.). New York: Oxford University Press.

Koocher, G. P., & Morray, E. (2000). Regulation of telepsychology: A survey of state attorneys general. *Professional Psychology: Research and Practice, 31*(5), 503-508.

Kraus, R. (2004). Ethical and legal considerations for providers of mental health services online. In R. Kraus, J. Zack, & G. Stricker (Eds.), *Online Counseling: A Handbook for Mental Health Professionals* (pp. 123-144). San Diego, CA: Elsevier Academic Press.

Lange, A., Van de Ven, J., & Schrieken, B. (2003). Interapy: Treatment of post-traumatic stress via the Internet. *Cognitive Behaviour Therapy, 32*(3), 110-124.

Manhal-Baugus, M. (2001). E-therapy: Practical, ethical, and legal issues. *CyberPsychology and Behavior, 4*(5), 551-563.

McCrone, P., Knapp, M., Proudfoot, J., Ryden, C., Cavanagh, K., Shapiro, D., Ilson, S., Gray, J., Goldberg, D., Mann, A., Marks, I., Everitt, B., & Tylee, A. (2004). Cost-effectiveness of computerized cognitive-behavioural therapy for anxiety and depression in primary care: Randomized controlled trial. *British Journal of Psychiatry, 185*, 55-62.

Murphy, L., & Mitchell, D. (1998). When writing helps to heal: E-mail as therapy. *British Journal of Guidance and Counseling, 26*, 25-32.

Neubauer, D. (2004). *Is Online Therapy for You?* Retrieved January 23, 2005, from http://www.healthatoz.com/healthatoz/Atoz/dc/cen/ment/info/onlinetherapy.jsp

New Freedom Commission on Mental Health. (2003). *Achieving the Promise: Transforming Mental Health Care in America.* Final Report (DHHS Publication No. SMA-03-3832). Rockville, MD: Author.

Pennebaker, J., Francis, M., & Booth, R. (2001). *Linguistic Inquiry and Word Count: LIWC.* Mahwah, NJ: Erlbaum.

Pennebaker, J., Mehl, M., & Niederhoffer, K. (2003). Psychological aspects of natural language use: Our words, our selves. *Annual Review of Psychology, 54*, 547-577.

Ragusea, A. (2005). Suggestions for the ethical practice of online psychotherapy. Unpublished doctoral dissertation, Wright State University, Dayton, Ohio.

Ragusea, A., & VandeCreek, L. (2003). Suggestions for the ethical practice of online psychotherapy. *Psychotherapy: Theory, Research, Practice, Training, 40*(1-2), 94-102.

Rochlen, A., Zack, J., & Speyer, C. (2004). Online therapy: Review of relevant definitions, debates, and current empirical support. *Journal of Clinical Psychology, 60*(3), 269-283.

Ruskin, P., Silver-Aylaian, M., Kling, M., Reed, S., Bradham, D., Hebel, R., Barrett, D., Knowles, F., & Hauser, P. (2004). Treatment outcomes in depression: Comparison of remote treatment through telepsychiatry to in-person treatment. *American Journal of Psychiatry, 161*(8), 1471-1476.

Stofle, G. (2001). *Choosing an Online Therapist.* Harrisburg, PA: White Hat Communications.

Stofle, G., & Chechele, P. (2004). In-session skills. In R. Kraus, J. Zack, & G. Stricker (Eds.), *Online Counseling: A Handbook for Mental Health Professionals* (pp. 181-196). San Diego, CA: Elsevier Academic Press.

Suler, J. (2001). Assessing a person's suitability for online therapy: The ISMHO clinical case study group. *CyberPsychology and Behavior, 4*(6), 675-679.

Suler, J. (2002). The basic psychological features of cyberspace. In *The Psychology of Cyberspace*. Retrieved November 4, 2004, from http://www.rider.edu/~suler/psycyber/basicfeat.html

Suler, J. (2004). The psychology of text relationships. In R. Kraus, J. Zack, & G. Stricker (Eds.), *Online Counseling: A Handbook for Mental Health Professionals* (pp. 19-50). San Diego, CA: Elsevier Academic Press.

Zack, J. (2002). Online counseling: The future for practicing psychologists? *National Psychologist, 11*, 6B-8B.

Zack, J. (2004). Technology of online counseling. In R. Kraus, J. Zack, & G. Stricker (Eds.), *Online Counseling: A Handbook for Mental Health Professionals* (pp. 93-121). San Diego, CA: Elsevier Academic Press.

Zelvin, E., & Speyer, C. (2004). Treatment strategies and skills for conducting counseling online. In R. Kraus, J. Zack, & G. Stricker (Eds.), *Online Counseling: A Handbook for Mental Health Professionals* (pp. 163-180). San Diego, CA: Elsevier Academic Press.

Zetterqvist, K., Maanmies, J., Strom, L., & Andersson, G. (2003). Randomized controlled trial of Internet-based stress management. *Cognitive Behaviour Therapy, 32*(3), 151-160.

Additional Resources

http://www.fenichel.com/OnlineTherapy.shtml
http://webpages.charter.net/stormking/ethguide.html
Kraus, R., Zack, J., & Stricker, G. (2004). *Online Counseling: A Handbook for Mental Health Professionals.* San Diego, CA: Elsevier Academic Press.

Introduction to Section III: Assessment Instruments and Client Handouts

This section of *Innovations* includes instruments and handouts that practitioners can use to collect and organize information. Although some of the items included here have been formally developed and normed, others were designed for informal application and should not be used as formal instruments or for making specific diagnoses.

The value of forms and instruments depends upon their appropriate application by the clinicians who use them. It is important to emphasize that these forms are not necessarily designed to generate the types of inferences often associated with more formalized tests that have a long history of use. Readers should recognize the potential as well as the stated limitations of these materials and use them in accordance with accepted ethical principles and practice standards. It is assumed that anyone who uses these instruments will have a general clinical knowledge of the areas being evaluated.

Given the limitations noted previously, we have attempted to ensure that the materials that follow include sufficient information to allow readers to evaluate their appropriate application. Certain basic information and instructions have been included with each contribution, and the Resources sections contain references to more detailed materials and studies. Readers who wish to use these materials are advised to obtain the additional resources. If there is a desire to use the material for research purposes, most authors would appreciate being contacted so that data may be shared.

Four instruments are included in this section. The first one, the "Quality of Life Rating (QOLR) Instrument" was compiled by Jeffery Allen and describes a self-report instrument that was developed by Gust for use with rehabilitation populations. The questions of the QOLR have been shown to load on five domains: self-esteem and well-being, interpersonal attachment, economics or basic needs, avocational, and spiritual. The instrument can be used with adults between the ages of 18 and 65. This instrument is a companion piece to the chapter by Jeremy Bottoms and Jeffery Allen that was included in Section I.

The second instrument is entitled "Adolescent Suicide Assessment Protocol-20" and has been created by William Fremouw, Julia Strunk, Elizabeth Tyner, and Robert (Bob) Musick. The authors present a suicide assessment protocol for use by mental health workers, along with a rationale and guidelines for use of the instrument. It is intended to be used to provide an initial objective assessment of adolescent suicide risk.

The third instrument, compiled by Tawanda Greer, is "The Index of Race-Related Stress—Brief Version (IRRS-B)." It was created by Utsey in 1999, and is a 22-item measure designed to capture experiences of race-related stress among African American adults that are related to their encounters of racism. The instrument was developed based on the theoretical notions of daily hassles and stress and persistent, everyday experiences of racism.

The final instrument, "Eating Behaviors and Body Image Test for Preadolescent Girls" was created by Candy and Fee in 1998 and was compiled for this volume by Eve Wolf. It is a 42-item self-report questionnaire developed to measure body image satisfaction and eating behaviors and disturbances in preadolescent girls. The instrument yields two factors. Factor one measures restrictive eating behaviors and body image dissatisfaction and factor two assesses binge eating.

In addition to the four instruments presented here, several contributions in Sections I and II include brief screening and assessment devices that have been identified in the section introductions.

This section also includes six client handouts. The first handout provides questions and answers on how to cope with a serious illness. The remaining five handouts address eating disorders in children and adolescents and are designed to be given to children and their parents.

Quality of Life Rating (QOLR) Instrument*

Jeffery B. Allen

SCALE DESCRIPTION

The Quality of Life Rating (QOLR) is a 20-item self-report instrument developed by Gust (1982) for use in rehabilitation populations. Huebner et al. (1998) assessed the psychometric properties of the instrument. The instrument uses a 5-point scale for each item to measure a patient's perceived quality of life, where 5 means *quality is excellent: no improvement necessary* and 1 means *quality is extremely poor: I need to make changes as soon as possible* (Huebner et al. 1998). The questions of the QOLR have been shown through factor analysis to load on five domains: Self-Esteem and Well-Being, Interpersonal Attachment, Economics or Basic Needs, Avocational, and Spiritual.

SCALE DEVELOPMENT

The QOLR demonstrated good reliability with a Cronbach alpha of 0.87, the test-retest coefficient of stability was 0.74, and adequate concurrent validity was established with a correlation coefficient between the total score of the QOLR and the Satisfaction With Life Survey (SWLS) at 0.69 (Huebner et al., 1998). Although generalizability of the results of the Huebner et al. study may be reduced due to the homogeneity of their sample, the QOLR is a good generic measure of QOL, sensitive to change, and practical to use.

SCALE ADMINISTRATION

The QOLR is appropriate for use with adults between the ages of 18 and 65. Along with normative information on college-aged individuals without medical/rehabilitation related conditions, the scale has also been applied to clients in treatment for psychological problems, and individuals undergoing inpatient rehabilitation for spinal cord injury, head trauma, and stroke. Finally, the scale has been used with geriatric patients during rehabilitation for a variety of orthopedic injuries or diseases. Along with an overall score for the QOLR, five factor scores can be generated: Self-Esteem and Well-Being, Interpersonal Attachment, Economics or Basic Needs, Avocational, and Spiritual. A calculation sheet is provided in this document.

* Reprinted with the permission of Aspen Publishers, from R. A. Heubner, J. B. Allen, T. H. Inman, R. Gust, and S. G. Turpin, "Quality of Life Rating: Psychometric Properties and Theoretical Comparisons," *Journal of Rehabilitation Outcomes Measurement, 2*(5), 8-16, 1998.

SCORING AND INTERPRETATION

Scoring and interpretation of the QOLR is relatively simple, with total scores ranging from 20 to 100 points. Among 384 undergraduate students, the total score on the QOLR was determined to have a mean of 73.99 and a standard deviation of 10.11 (Huebner et al., 1998). The QOLR can be used at the beginning of treatment, and may aid the tracking of progress if readministered at critical intervals throughout treatment.

Quality of Life

Summary Sheet

Client: _____   Date Administered: _____

_____	Total Score	Mean of Items 1-20
_____	Self-Esteem/Well-Being	Mean of scores for Items 10, 15, 17, 18, and 20
_____	Spiritual	Item 5 score
_____	Interpersonal Attachment	Mean of scores for Items 3, 12, and 17
_____	Avocational	Mean of scores for Items 1 and 4
_____	Economics or Basic Needs	Mean of scores for Items 7 and 9

---

5 = Excellent   4 = Very Good   3 = Satisfactory   2 = Not Too Good   1 = Extremely Poor

---

Self-Rating of Life Quality

Your Name: _____   Today's Date: _____

Our Quality of Life is related to our values, desires, and beliefs, plus our perception of ourselves and our world. Use the key scale statements below to rate your present quality of life on the following items.

> 5 = Quality is excellent: no improvement is necessary.
> 4 = Quality is very good: better than I expect.
> 3 = Quality is satisfactory: average compared with my expectations.
> 2 = Quality is not too good: I would like to plan changes.
> 1 = Quality is extremely poor: I need to make changes as soon as possible.

Place a score (between 1 and 5) in the blank before each item below.

_____   1. Recreation activities

_____   2. Social/Friendly relationships

_____   3. Close/Intimate relationships

_____   4. Hobbies

_____   5. Spiritual activities/Belief in meaning of life

_____   6. Volunteer activities

_____   7. Financial conditions

_____   8. Learning/Education/Training activities

_____   9. Work/Career activity

_____   10. Emotional balance

_____   11. Transportation availability

_____   12. Sexual adjustment/Relationship

_____   13. Family involvement and support

_____   14. My physical/bodily condition

_____   15. Liking/Loving of myself

_____   16. Housing/Living conditions

_____   17. Receiving affection

_____   18. Control of my life and my future

_____   19. Amount of stress/tension/pressure (5 = no stress; 1 = severe stress)

_____   20. Overall, I view my life quality as: _____

SCORING

	Total	*Mean*
QOL Total (Sum Items 1-20):	_____	_____
Self-Esteem/Well-Being (Sum Items 10, 15, 17, 18, and 20):	_____	_____
Spiritual (Sum Item 5):	_____	_____
Interpersonal Attachment (Sum Items 3, 12, and 17):	_____	_____
Avocational (Sum Items 1 and 4):	_____	_____
Economics/Basic Needs (Sum Items 7 and 9):	_____	_____

NORMATIVE COMPARISONS (*N* = 384)		
Scale Item	**Mean**	**SD**
Recreation Activities	3.52	.91
Social Relationships	3.89	.97
Intimate Relationships	3.69	1.25
Hobbies	3.50	.99
Spiritual Activities	3.44	1.16
Volunteer Activities	2.66	1.09
Financial Conditions	3.11	1.03
Learning Activities	3.74	0.90
Work/Career Activity	3.23	1.05
Emotional Balance	3.59	1.04
Transportation Availability	3.84	1.26
Sexual Adjustment	3.68	1.15
Family Involvement	4.22	1.00
Physical/Bodily Condition	3.55	1.04
Liking Myself	3.74	1.03
Housing/Living Conditions	3.85	0.93
Receiving Affection	3.96	1.03
Control of Life and Future	3.96	0.96
Amount of Stress	2.83	0.92
Overall Life Quality	3.88	0.76

CONTRIBUTOR

Jeffery B. Allen, PhD, ABPP-CN, is board certified in Clinical Neuropsychology by the American Board of Professional Psychology. He is currently a Professor in the School of Professional Psychology at Wright State University and teaches courses in physiological psychology and clinical neuropsychology. Dr Allen completed a postdoctoral fellowship at the Rehabilitation Institute of Michigan in Detroit. He is widely published in the areas of neuropsychology, head injuries, and memory and recently completed the text, *A General Practitioner's Guide to Neuropsychological Assessment* (American Psychological Association, in press). Dr. Allen's interests include neurobehavioral disorders, quality of life in medical populations, cognitive and neuropsychological assessment, and outcome measurement in rehabilitation. Dr. Allen can be reached at SOPP, Wright State University, 3640 Colonel Glenn Highway, Dayton, OH 45435-0001. E-mail: jeffery.allen@wright.edu

RESOURCES

Gust, T. (1982). *Quality of Life Rating*. Unpublished instrument.

Huebner, R. A., Allen, J. B., Inman, T. H., Gust, R., & Turpin, S. G. (1998). Quality of life rating: Psychometric properties and theoretical comparisons. *Journal of Rehabilitation Outcomes Measurement, 2*(5), 8-16.

Adolescent Suicide Assessment Protocol-20

William Fremouw, Julia M. Strunk,
Elizabeth A. Tyner, and Robert (Bob) Musick

Youth suicide is the third leading cause of death, behind accidents and homicide, among young people from 15 to 24 years old (Centers for Disease Control [CDC], 1995). Adolescent suicide is increasing at an alarming rate. From 1980 to 1992, completed suicides by adolescents increased over 28%. Fortunately, this rate has slightly decreased from 1994 to 2000 but is still 10.4 suicides per 100,000 among 15- to 24-year-olds (Miniño et al., 2002). In 2001, 3,409 males and 562 females between the ages of 15 and 24 committed suicide (Anderson & Smith, 2003).

Young males and females complete suicide at a comparable rate between the ages of 10 and 14. However, teenage boys ages 15-19 commit suicide 3.6 times more often than teenage girls. This gender difference further increases through ages 20 to 24. Although more boys complete suicide, girls have a much higher rate of attempting suicide (CDC, 1995).

In just 1 year, almost 3 million teenagers in the United States attempted or seriously considered suicide (Substance Abuse and Mental Health Services Administration, 2002). Bell and Clark (1998) estimate that there are 15 to 20 nonfatal suicide attempts for each adolescent who commits suicide. Attempting suicide is one of the strongest predictors of completed suicide. The CDC (1998) reported that 10.3% of white female adolescents and 3.2% of white male adolescents attempted suicide, with 2.6% and 1.5%, respectively, requiring medical attention for this attempt.

Litman (1990) defined any suicide contemplation, attempt, and completion as forming a suicide zone of risk. Although the exact classification of suicidal behaviors remains a challenging area for researchers (O'Carroll et al., 1996), the identification of adolescents who are in this zone of risk is the essential task of the clinician. The second task is to respond appropriately to reduce this risk (Rudd & Joiner, 1998).

The purpose of this contribution is to describe a suicide assessment protocol for use by mental health intake workers, hotline workers, school counselors, and other gatekeepers who interact with adolescents who may be in the suicide zone of risk. Goldston (2003) reviewed over 50 suicide assessment instruments ranging from four-item questionnaires to multilevel intensive clinical assessments. Most of these instruments require an adolescent to complete extensive written measures of ideation, mood, and history and to cooperate with an in-depth clinical interview. Unfortunately, there is not a "gold standard" assessment procedure for the initial screening of adolescents who may be at risk for suicide that can be used easily by professionals conducting intake interviews.

This contribution presents the rationale and guidelines for a brief, user-friendly, structured clinical interview called the Adolescent Suicide Assessment Protocol-20 (ASAP-20). It is intended for use by mental health workers and/or school counselors to provide an initial objective assessment of adolescent suicidal risk. The ASAP-20 is organized based on a risk assessment model. An adolescent will be classified as either low, medium, or high risk upon completion of the assessment. If an individual is classified as medium or high risk for suicide, then a more intensive evaluation should be conducted with prevention and treatment interventions implemented immediately.

RISK ASSESSMENT AND GUIDED CLINCIAL INTERVIEW

Historically, risk assessment has been conducted by two distinctive procedures: (a) the unstructured clinical judgment or (b) the actuarial risk assessment database procedure. McNiel et al. (2002) reviewed the risk assessment procedures. The authors criticized unstructured clinical interviews and also examined the limitations of actuarially based assessments. They identified the guided clinical interview as an innovative synthesis of the unaided clinical judgment and pure actuarial prediction methods. This approach has been used in other areas of clinical-forensic assessments such as competency to stand trial. A structured or semistructured clinical interview is developed based on research findings from actuarial and/or clinical research. McNiel and colleagues (2002) conclude that guided clinical assessments can perform equal to or even better than some actuarial predictions.

The ASAP-20 is modeled after the HCR-20 guided clinical interview developed by Webster et al. (1995), which assesses future risk of violence by forensic or psychiatric inpatients. A 20-item guided interview was developed and organized into three domains: historical, clinical, and risk management. Their manual provided a research rationale and coding instructions for each item. HCR-20 is not a test; instead it is presented as a guide to the assessment of violence for mental health professionals. This instrument guides the interviewer to assess the most relevant areas, based on empirical research, prior to coming to a clinical judgment about an individual's level of risk for violence. Douglas and Webster (1999) reported that prisoners with high HCR-20 scores above the median were associated with four times the rate of violence than prisoners who scored below the median. In a follow-up study of civilly committed psychiatric patients 2 years after discharge, Douglas et al. (1999) reported that scores above the median on the HCR-20 had rates of violence more than six times that of the group that scored below the median.

RATIONALE FOR THE ASAP-20

The ASAP-20 was developed from a careful review of the adolescent suicide risk literature to identify both static and dynamic factors associated with both adolescent attempted and completed suicides. In 1990, Fremouw, DePerczel, and Ellis wrote *Suicide Risk Assessment and Response Guidelines*, which identified and addressed risk factors of both adults and adolescents. The authors identified demographic factors, historical factors, and current clinical factors which were relevant to the assessment of suicidal risk. The book provided treatment guidelines for individuals at different levels of suicidal risk. The assessment of contextual factors, such as availability of weapons, was not included in this work. This empirical review of adolescent literature served as the starting point for the development of the ASAP-20. ASAP-20 items were generated based on this work, current research summarized in Spirito and Overholser (2003), and empirical articles such as the New York State Psychological Adolescent Autopsy Study of 120 suicides completed by individuals under 20 years of age and 147 control subjects (Gould et al., 1996) and the Pittsburgh Psychological Autopsy Study of 67 adolescent suicide victims and 67 control participants (Brent et al., 1988; Brent et al, 1993).

Twenty-four items were generated based on the literature review. These items were piloted with mental health intake workers who evaluated 100 adolescents using the preliminary scale and coding guidelines. Based on these data, items were eliminated or refined to be more sensitive and helpful. ASAP-20 presents the 20 items most discriminating of ratings of low, medium, and high risk of suicide by mental health professionals of adolescents who are presenting for initial evaluation.

ASAP-20 is organized into four domains: *Historical, Clinical, Contextual,* and *Protective. Historical* items include a history of prior suicide attempts or history of family suicide attempts/completions. *Clinical* items consist of the presence of hopelessness, depression, or anger, and *specific* clinical items such as current suicidal ideation and communication of suicidal wishes. *Contextual* or environmental factors include recent losses, access to firearms, or the absence of family and peer support. *Protective* factors are the presence of current treatment and reasons for living. Protective factors are an emerging area in the risk assessment literature. In general, protective factors are those variables that reduce the likelihood of violence or suicide by reducing the negative impact of the risk factors. Eggert, Thompson, and Herting (1994) included the assessment of protective factors such as social support, self-esteem, and spirituality in their model of adolescent suicide risk.

Although courts do not expect mental health professionals to perfectly predict future behavior, courts do expect mental health professionals to demonstrate reasonable care and judgment in their predictions and clinical decision making (Fremouw et al., 1990). The use of a guided clinical instrument such as the ASAP-20 would ensure that a professional is conducting a thorough clinical assessment prior to concluding the risk level of the respondent. In short, it is just good clinical practice to use such an instrument and should become the "best practice" for mental health intake workers to guarantee a minimum level of thoroughness in these important evaluations.

ASAP-20 MANUAL

The following sections describe the empirical basis, coding guidelines, and suggested questions for the 20 items. The ASAP-20 protocol is on pages 221 to 222. The scoring ranges from 0 to 3 and the endpoints are defined in the coding guidelines. The clinician must use judgment for the intermediate levels of each item, such as mild or moderate ratings.

Historical Factors

Historical factors in adolescent suicide risk assessment include past experiences that are static, or unchangeable, at the time of assessment. Previous experiences, especially of suicide or violence, are strong predictors of future risk (Fremouw et al., 1990).

1. History of Suicide Attempts

Fremouw et al. (1990) state that "the history of an individual's prior suicide attempts is the most significant historical factor that must be considered in assessing current suicide risk" (p. 39). Research indicates that 25% to 33% of adolescents who completed suicide made prior attempts. Furthermore, boys who have a history of prior suicide attempts are especially at risk (30-fold increase) and girls are slightly less at risk (3-fold increase) of completing suicide (Gould & Kramer, 2001). A suicide attempt is defined as an intentional, self-harming act with greater than zero probability of death (O'Carroll et al., 1996).

Coding Guidelines / Suggested Questions

1. Have you ever tried to kill yourself?
2. Describe what you did.

Any suicide attempt significantly raises the risk of future suicide behavior and death.

Coding: 0 = No previous suicide attempt(s)
               (scores of 1 and 2 are not used)
            3 = Suicide attempt(s)

2. History of Physical/Sexual Abuse

According to Brent (2001), "ongoing physical or sexual abuse is a particularly ominous precipitant" (p. 109) for suicidal behavior. The risk of suicide becomes greater as the length and frequency of the abuse increases (Kaplan, 1996) and may be more likely to result in completed suicide (Brent, 2001).

Coding Guidelines / Suggested Questions

1. Have you ever been physically or sexually abused?
2. If so: When did the abuse occur?
3. If so: How often did the abuse occur?

The rating of physical and sexual abuse of the adolescent should involve three dimensions: frequency, duration, and intensity. A high number of occurrences of the abuse will increase the risk of suicide attempt. Additionally, ongoing abuse qualifies as a higher risk factor than abuse that has ceased. Finally, high-intensity abuse will predict a more severe risk for the adolescent.

Coding: 0 = No history of physical and/or sexual abuse
            1 = History of mild physical and/or sexual abuse
            2 = History of moderate physical and/or sexual abuse
            3 = History of severe physical and/or sexual abuse

3. History of Antisocial Behaviors

Adolescents displaying antisocial behaviors have an increased risk of suicide attempts. The risk is particularly high if these individuals have encounters with the law (Marttunen et al., 1998). Data from the New York Psychological Autopsy Study revealed that the rate of suicide in boys with antisocial behavior is 35 per 100,000, as compared to a base rate of 11 per 100,000; and for girls with antisocial behavior the risk is 7 per 100,000 (Gould et al., 1992).

Coding Guidelines / Suggested Questions

1. Have you ever been in any fights at school/in neighborhood? Describe.
2. Have you ever been arrested or placed in jail? Explain.
3. Have you ever been on probation or had any legal conflicts? Explain.

Consider the frequency and seriousness of the antisocial behavior when scoring.

Coding: 0 = No history of antisocial behavior
            1 = History of mild antisocial behavior
            2 = History of moderate antisocial behavior
            3 = History of severe antisocial behavior with legal conflicts

4. History of Family Suicide Attempts/Completions

Numerous studies have found that suicidal behavior in family members significantly increases the risk for adolescents attempting or completing suicide (Goldman & Beardslee, 1999; Gould & Kramer, 2001). Gould et al. (1992) report that in the New York Psychological

Autopsy Study, "approximately 40% of the suicide completers had a first- or second-degree relative who had previously attempted or committed suicide" (p. 138). Although genetic factors or general family dysfunction may contribute to this pattern of suicidal behavior, Gould and Kramer (2001) report that family histories "increase suicide risk even when studies have controlled for poor parent-child relationships and parental psychopathology" (p. 9).

Coding Guidelines / Suggested Questions

1. Have any of your close family members ever attempted suicide?
2. Have any of your close family members ever completed suicide?

"Family" should include relatives outside the immediate family unit, such as grandparents. Due to the prevalence of extended families living in the same household, aunts, uncles, and cousins should also be considered if interaction with the adolescent is frequent and significant to him or her. Score 3 if either attempts or completions have occurred.

Coding: 0 = No history of family suicide attempts or completions
(scores of 1 and 2 are not used)
3 = History of family suicide attempts or completions

Clinical Factors

Clinical items address the current psychological condition of an individual. These factors are dynamic, or changeable, and represent potential areas for change and treatment. Regardless of an individual's history, suicide risk assessment should include an examination of the client's current clinical state, including specific thoughts or plans of suicide.

5. Depression

Brent et al. (1993) state that in the Pittsburgh Psychological Autopsy Study, "affective disorder, most specifically, major depression, was the single most significant risk factor for completed suicide in adolescents" (p. 524). Other research has revealed that among suicide attempters, depression is the most prevalent psychological disorder (Brent, 2001; Gould & Kramer, 2001). The New York Psychological Autopsy Study found that 61% of the suicide completers met criteria for mood disorder and 52% for major depressive disorder (Shaffer et al., 1996). The Pittsburgh Psychological Autopsy Study found depressive disorders in 49% of suicide completers (Brent et al., 1993). Although these studies examined suicide completers, studies of suicide attempters reveal even higher estimates of the prevalence of mood disorders. Pfeffer et al. (1991; cited in Wolfsdorf et al., 2003) found mood disorders in 80% of adolescents who had attempted suicide following hospitalization.

Coding Guidelines / Suggested Questions

1. Do you feel depressed or sad?
2. Have there been any changes in sleeping/eating?
3. Have you lost interest in previously enjoyable activities?

In addition to direct inquiries about depressed mood and feelings of hopelessness, several symptoms of depression seen in adolescents can be addressed when rating this item. Disturbances in sleep and eating patterns are characterized by reversal of normal sleep patterns (retiring early or rising early) and loss of interest in food and eating. Adolescents often appear complacent or lethargic and become socially withdrawn when depressed. The cognitive components of depression include feelings of worthlessness, self-condemnation, impaired self-defense, and pronounced self-deprecation (Fremouw et al., 1990). Questions about feeling in control of the future and the likelihood of making future plans can address the hopelessness component (see next item).

Coding: 0 = No depression
1 = Mild levels of depression
2 = Moderate levels of depression
3 = Severe levels of depression

6. Hopelessness

One aspect of depression is the cognitive state of hopelessness, which Fremouw et al. (1990) state is "especially indicative of suicide risk" (p. 65). As a construct, hopelessness includes "feelings of despair, lack of control, and pessimism about the future" (Fremouw et al., 1990, p. 66). Hopelessness is a dominant characteristic of adolescent suicide attempters (Brent, 2001; Esposito et al., 2003) and should be considered as an indication of the severity of depression and increased risk of suicide (Fremouw et al., 1990). In the New York Psychological Autopsy Study, 44% of boys and 35% of girls who met criteria for an Axis 1 disorder expressed hopelessness, with mood disorder being the most common criterion met (Shaffer et al., 1996).

Coding Guidelines / Suggested Questions

1.   How do you feel about your future: okay, slightly negative, discouraged, or clearly hopeless?
2.   What are your future plans: next week? next year?

In scoring hopelessness, answering that the future is okay and that he or she has plans for this weekend, next week, or next year would indicate a score of 0. Feeling that the future is slightly negative or discouraging indicates a score of 1. Feeling that the future is bleak indicates a score of 2, and feeling completely hopeless about the future indicates a score of 3.

Coding: 0 = No hopelessness
1 = Mild levels of hopelessness
2 = Moderate levels of hopelessness
3 = Severe levels of hopelessness

7. Anger

Anger is prevalent in most adolescents, and many studies demonstrate that anger is correlated significantly with adolescent suicide, especially in noninstitutionalized adolescents who have attempted suicide (Wolfsdorf et al., 2003). The emotion of anger can be externalized and displayed as aggression. Conversely, anger can be internalized and manifested as depression (Myers et al., 1991). This emotion is a risk factor, as Negron et al. (1997) suggest that adolescent suicide "may function as an outlet for their anger" (p. 1517).

Coding Guidelines / Suggested Questions

1.   How often do you feel angry or lose your temper?
2.   Would people describe you as "hot-headed"?
3.   Have you ever threatened or assaulted anyone when you were angry?

Some characteristics of anger are resistance and lack of self-control. Some behavioral indicators of anger are temper tantrums and making threats or assaults. Score 1 if there are some less serious characteristics or displays of anger. Score 2 if the adolescent frequently expresses anger. Score 3 if there are physical manifestations of anger such as threats and assaults.

Coding: 0 = No anger
1 = Mild anger
2 = Moderate anger
3 = Severe anger

8. Impulsivity

Research consistently recognizes impulsivity as a psychological characteristic that is highly correlated with adolescent suicidal behavior. In a study examining adolescent suicidal inpatients, nonsuicidal inpatients, and high school controls, Kashden et al. (1993) found suicidal inpatients to be more impulsive than both groups. The authors suggest that impulsivity may cause problem-solving deficits in suicidal adolescents. Poor problem-solving skills do not allow for thorough evaluation of suicidal acts, including their potential lethal consequences (Brent, 2001). Furthermore, research by Horesh et al. (1999) demonstrates that impulsivity is a stronger risk factor for adolescent suicide for males than females.

Coding Guidelines / Suggested Questions

1. Do you act on whim/do things without thinking first?
2. Are you impatient?
3. Have you been told that you have ADHD?

Impulsivity may be manifested as a personality trait or as a behavior. Impulsive behavior may be difficult to define as it overlaps with other suicidal behaviors such as aggression and violence. Some indicators of impulsivity are impatience, acting without thinking, becoming easily frustrated, and lack of ability to plan ahead. Additionally, a clinical diagnosis of ADHD indicates an increased risk.

Score 1 if there are less serious impulsive characteristics or behavior. Score 2 if the individual has some impulsivity in one setting (e.g., school, home, or work). Score 3 if the individual has encountered multiple problems across settings because of impulsivity. Also, a previous or current prescription of medication for ADHD indicates a severe risk.

Coding: 0 = No impulsivity
1 = Mild impulsivity
2 = Moderate impulsivity
3 = Severe impulsivity

9. Substance Abuse

Substance abuse is a strong risk factor for suicide (Brent, 2001). Fremouw et al. (1990) state that "chronic and excessive use of such substances substantially increases the risk of self-destructive behaviors" (p. 67). Gould and Kramer (2001) suggest that substance abuse is the most significant difference between those who actually attempt suicide and those with suicidal ideation. Suicide completions are the result of a combination of factors; however, studies have found that the most deadly combinations involve an element of substance abuse. Shaffer et al. (1996) report in the New York Psychological Autopsy Study that 42 of the 119 suicide completers had a diagnosis of substance abuse, 39 of which were male, indicating that substance abuse is a more significant risk factor for males than females. In the Pittsburgh Psychological Autopsy

Study (Brent et al., 1993), substance abuse was found to be a significant risk factor as well, particularly when comorbid with an affective disorder. Of the 67 suicide completers in this study, 27 were estimated to have a substance abuse diagnosis.

Coding Guidelines / Suggested Questions

1. How often do you indulge in alcohol and/or drugs?
2. How often are you intoxicated?
3. What type(s) of drug do you use?
4. What is your "drug of choice"?

Substance abuse involves illicit and prescription drugs, as well as alcohol and toxins (fuel, paint, glue). Toxin use is indicative of severe abuse. A score of 1 may be given for occasional, recreational drug use or experimentation. When abuse is moderate and causes some impairment or problems, a score of 2 should be given. A score of 3 indicates regular abuse and/or addiction with serious impairment or problems, such as arrests for underage drinking, drug treatment, or school/family problems.

Coding: 0 = No substance abuse
1 = Mild substance abuse
2 = Moderate substance abuse
3 = Severe substance abuse

10-12. Suicidal Ideation Items

Overholser and Spirito (2003) state that "suicidal ideation is an important precursor to attempted suicide" (p. 19). Although not all adolescents who think about suicide actually attempt it, most of those who do attempt or complete suicide have ideation in the preceding days or weeks before (Brent et al., 1993; Overholser & Spirito, 2003). Levels of severity range from mere thoughts of dying to wishing one were dead to creating an active plan, and frequency can range from occasional thoughts to those that are persistent and intrusive (Brent, 2001). In the Pittsburgh Psychological Autopsy Study (Brent et al., 1993), 77% of suicide victims had suicidal ideation and a plan within a week of death. This same study found that "past suicidal ideation with a plan was at least as strongly associated with completed suicide as was a past attempt" (p. 526). Andrews and Lewinsohn (1992; cited in Overholser & Spirito, 2003) report that 90% of a community sample of suicide attempters had suicidal ideation before the attempt.

Coding Guidelines / Suggested Questions

See ASAP-20 items 10 (frequency), 11 (specificity of plan), and 12 (intention) in the instrument on page 221.

Contextual Factors

Contextual factors are external to the individual and can significantly raise or lower the probability of suicidal behavior. These factors can be static or dynamic.

13. Recent Losses

Interpersonal loss and conflict with peers or family may trigger adolescent suicide (Overholser & Spirito, 2003). Interpersonal loss is operationalized as death of a loved one; the abandonment, divorce, or separation of a parent; or a breakup from a romantic relationship. Conflict refers to turmoil in a peer, significant other, or family relationship (Fremouw et al.,

1990; Goldman & Beardslee, 1999; Overholser & Spirito, 2003). Furthermore, for adolescents younger than 16 years old, interpersonal loss or conflict involving a parent is especially impacting. Regarding adolescents aged 16 or older, interpersonal loss or conflict of a significant other is a predominant trigger in suicide. In some cases of recent losses, adolescent suicide functions as a motivational factor. That is, suicide might be perceived as a means to eliminate suffering from a recent loss. Conflict may lead to an anticipation of a serious loss, which could, in turn, result in suicide. Additionally, adolescents may believe that suicide could provide a reunion with a deceased loved one (Goldman & Beardslee, 1999).

Coding Guidelines / Suggested Questions

1. Have you recently had conflict with a peer, significant other, or parent?
2. Have your parents divorced or separated recently?
3. Have you recently lost someone due to a breakup or a move?
4. Did someone you were close to recently die?

The rating of severity must consider the individual's perception of the magnitude of the loss. The more recent the loss, the higher the potential impact will be for the individual. Multiple losses also increase the risk of suicide. Also consider unfulfilled goals and dreams or recent disappointments, as these items may be just as potent as losses or conflict.

Coding: 0 = No recent losses
1 = Recent loss of minor magnitude
2 = Recent loss of moderate magnitude
3 = Recent loss of severe magnitude

14. Firearm Access

Adolescents select a method of suicide based on convenience and availability (Overholser & Spirito, 2003). Not surprisingly then, the use of firearms is the most frequent method for suicide (Gould & Kramer, 2001; McKeown et al., 1998). Therefore, access to firearms greatly increases the risk of suicide. In fact, households that contain firearms are the strongest situational predictive factor of committing suicide, especially for adolescents who have made previous suicide attempts (McKeown et al., 1998). Specifically, an unlocked, loaded handgun in the home poses the greatest risk (Brent, 2001).

Coding Guidelines / Suggested Questions

1. Are there any firearms in your home?
2. Do you have access to any firearms anywhere else (e.g., friend's house)?
3. If yes to 1 and/or 2: Are they locked up? If no: Can you gain access to them?

Score 0 if the individual has no access to firearms. Score 1 if the individual could potentially gain access through relatives, friends, neighbors, and so on. Direct access indicates the presence of firearms in the individual's immediate environment. Restricted access, a score of 2, refers to a locked gun cabinet or trigger lock. Unrestricted access, a score of 3, indicates immediate accessibility to unlocked, loaded firearms.

Coding: 0 = No firearm access
1 = Indirect firearm access
2 = Direct, restricted firearm access
3 = Direct, unrestricted firearm access

15. Family Dysfunction

Fremouw et al. (1990) state that "foremost among contributing environmental factors [for suicide risk] is the child's family system" (p. 62). Parents of children who attempt or commit suicide have significantly high rates of mood disorders (primarily depression), substance abuse, and psychopathology (Brent, 2001; Gould & Kramer, 2001). A 1994 study by Brent and colleagues, which show that not only genetic factors, but also environmental components of parental depression impact adolescent suicide risk. Both the New York and Pittsburgh Psychological Autopsy Studies of completed adolescent suicides report problems in parent-child relationships (Gould et al., 1996; Brent et al., 1993). Divorce or unstable family relationships, inappropriate family boundaries, absent or ineffective discipline, lack of emotional support, physical or sexual abuse, poverty, and family illness are all components of familial distress that impact an adolescent's ability to effectively cope with emotional problems and/or life stressors (Brent, 2001; Goldman & Beardslee, 1999; Gould & Kramer, 2001). For adolescents, Goldman and Beardslee (1999) suggest that suicidal behaviors could "generally be seen as both embedded in and a response to the family's distress or dysfunction" (p. 425).

Coding Guidelines / Suggested Questions

1. Do you communicate with your family?
2. Does anyone living with you suffer from depression, substance abuse, or other psychopathology?
3. How stable do you think your home life is/has been?
4. Is your family supportive?

Support, stability, and psychopathology are three factors to consider in a global assessment of family functioning. A score of 0 indicates minimal to no family problems. A score of 1 suggests occasional family disturbances not involving external involvement. A score of 2 indicates more serious problems such as abuse, illness, separation, and instability. A score of 3 indicates severe dysfunction with chronic problems such as abandonment, homelessness, and chaos.

Coding: 0 = No family dysfunction
1 = Mild family dysfunction
2 = Moderate family dysfunction
3 = Severe family dysfunction

16. Peer Problems

Prinstein (2003) states that "interpersonal factors, and specifically difficulties in peer functioning, have frequently been cited as precipitants to adolescents' suicidal behavior" (p. 191). Although peer problems encompass a wide area of concerns and minimal research has focused on this specific area, several studies have found relationships between suicidal behavior and social isolation, sexual orientation, and peer rejection. In the New York Psychological Autopsy Study, Gould et al. (1996) report that adolescents who did not attend school or go to work, indicating social isolation, were at a significantly higher risk for suicide. Because homosexuality often leads to social isolation and/or victimization by peers, rates of depression and substance abuse are high in this group, both of which increase suicide risk for adolescents regardless of sexual orientation (Brent, 2001; Goldman & Beardslee, 1999). Prinstein (2003) reports findings that "low levels of close friendship support and high levels of perceived peer rejection were significantly associated with more severe suicidal ideation" (p. 202).

Coding Guidelines / Suggested Questions

1. Do you have friends?
2. Do you feel like you have support from your friends?
3. Have you been bullied or rejected by peers?
4. Do you attend school? Go to work?

If an adolescent reports problems with a friend or boyfriend/girlfriend but indicates other friends who provide social support, then problems may be considered mild and scored 1. Occasional conflict with no stable or close friends yields a score of 2. If an adolescent reports problems with all peers and feels like he or she has no peer support system, then problems should be considered severe and scored 3.

Coding: 0 = No peer problems
1 = Mild problems with peers
2 = Moderate problems with peers
3 = Severe problems with peers

17. School/Legal Problems

Gould et al. (1996) report that "difficulties in school, neither working nor being in school, and not going to college, posed significant suicide risks" in the New York Psychological Autopsy Study (p. 1159). From that group of suicide completers, 17% were neither in school nor working at the time of death. The Pittsburgh Psychological Autopsy Study found conduct disorder to be a risk factor for suicide, particularly if an affective disorder was not present (Brent et al., 1993). Numerous studies have revealed that suicide risk is greater for incarcerated adolescents than for the general high school population (DiFilippo et al., 2003). Morris et al. (1995; cited in DiFilippo et al., 2003) examined suicidal behavior in 1,801 incarcerated adolescents who completed the Centers for Disease Control Youth Risk Behavior Surveillance System (YRBS). Compared to 7% of high school students who completed the YRBS, 15.5% of incarcerated adolescents had attempted suicide, with 8.2% resulting in serious injury. Only 2% of high school students who made an attempt suffered an injury.

Coding Guidelines / Suggested Questions

1. Do you attend school regularly?
2. Have you ever been expelled, suspended, or placed in in-school suspension?
3. Have you been in trouble with the police, such as an arrest, probation, or state custody?

If the adolescent is involved in substance abuse, the presence of any school or legal problems such as expulsion or incarceration indicates an increased risk and should be scored 3.

Coding: 0 = No school or legal problems
1 = Mild school or legal problems
2 = Moderate school or legal problems
3 = Severe school or legal problems

18. Contagion

When the mass media portrays suicide, a phenomenon known as contagion suicide can occur. Contagion is also referred to as imitation or cluster suicide. This phenomenon is very significant, as 1% to 13% of teenage suicides are estimated to occur in clusters within 2 weeks of the initial suicide (Gould & Kramer, 2001). Furthermore, when a celebrity commits suicide, this copycat effect is greatly increased due to massive, glamorized media coverage (American Foundation for Suicide Prevention and American Association of Suicidology Annenberg Public Policy Center, 2003). Imitation suicide also may result when a friend of the adolescent commits suicide (Rhode, Seeley, & Mace, 1997). Therefore, the contagion effect can be created by the media or peer groups.

Coding Guidelines / Suggested Questions

1. Has someone that you have known or admired committed suicide lately?
2. If yes to either 1 or 2: How does this make you feel?

Score 0 if there is no contagion present within the past 2 weeks. If contagion occurred within the past 2 weeks, score 3.

Coding: 0 = No contagion present
              (scores of 1 and 2 are not used)
            3 = Contagion present

Protective Factors

Protective factors are dynamic and significantly reduce the chance of an individual committing suicide. These factors lessen the risk of suicide by ameliorating existing risk factors. Because the absence of protective factors increases risk of suicide, reverse scoring is used for these items.

19. Reasons for Living

Adolescent suicide risk assessment cannot be complete without an evaluation of reasons for living (Overholser & Spirito, 2003). One assessment tool that is commonly used to evaluate if adolescents believe they have reasons to stay alive (protective factors) is the Brief Reasons for Living Inventory for Adolescents (BRFL-A; Osman et al., 1996). It contains four factors that are relevant to suicidal risk assessment. The first factor is Moral Objections, and a sample item is *"I believe only God has a right to end a life."* The second factor is Survival and Coping Beliefs; a sample item is *"I believe I can find other solutions for my problems."* Responsibility to Family is the third factor. Pertinent questions for this factor address adolescents' love for their family, and also their perception of their family's love for them. The fourth factor is Fear of Suicide: *"I am afraid of death."*

Coding Guidelines / Suggested Questions

1. How does your faith view suicide?
2. What are your expectations about your life problems improving?
3. Do you think things will get better for you?
4. How important is your family to you?
5. Are you afraid of dying?

A poor outlook on the future and no reasons for living is a severe indication of high risk. Score 0 if the individual provides one or more definite reasons for living. Score 1 if the individual provides one reason. If the individual has vague, unconvincing reasons for living score 2. No reasons for living indicate a score of 3.

Coding: 0 = Multiple clear reasons for living
1 = One clear reason for living
2 = Poorly defined reasons for living
3 = No reason for living

20. Current Treatment

Donaldson, Spirito, and Overholser (2003) state that therapy "can help to identify low levels of sadness or pessimism that can be confronted and managed before they reach unmanageable levels" (p. 318). In the Pittsburgh Psychological Autopsy Study, 85% of the suicide victims were not receiving psychiatric treatment within 1 month of death; more victims had been in treatment at some point than controls, but the vast majority were not currently in treatment (Brent et al., 1993). Current treatment provides opportunities for therapists to monitor current risk and to provide additional resources if needed (e.g., hospitalization, medication); therefore, current treatment is seen as a current protective factor.

Coding Guidelines / Suggested Questions

1. Are you currently seeing a therapist, counselor, or psychologist?
2. If yes, how long have you been in treatment?

If currently in treatment, a code of 0 should be given. If the adolescent is not in treatment, then a 3 should be coded.

Coding: 0 = In current treatment
(scores of 1 and 2 are not used)
3 = Not currently in treatment

Response Guidelines

After the evaluator scores the 20 separate items from 0 to 3, a total score (0-60) is obtained by adding the sum of the items. If the total score is from 0 to 15, the client falls in the *low-risk* range for suicidal behavior. A score from 16 to 19 places the individual in the *medium-risk* category, and a score of 20 and above places the individual in the *high-risk* category. The cutoffs are based on a pilot study of 60 adolescent outpatient evaluations by experienced clinicians, comparing their independent suicide risk ratings of low, medium, and high with total ASAP-20 scores. None of the low-risk group received an ASAP-20 score of greater than 15, while only 7% of the high-risk group scored below 15.

If the individual is in the low-risk category, then the original referral question should be pursued with less concern about suicidal risk at this time. The evaluator should continue to monitor for change in risk factors such as a recent loss, onset of depression or hopelessness, or contagion. However, the low-risk category overall suggests that suicidal behavior is not likely at this time.

If the adolescent is in the medium- or high-risk categories, then several additional actions should be taken. As outlined under Actions Taken, the evaluator should consider (a) referring for outpatient treatment, (b) referring for psychiatric consultation for possible medications, and (c) consulting with a colleague or supervisor regarding the risk assessment. At minimum these three steps are strongly encouraged for individuals in the medium-risk category. These steps would intensify treatment, provide additional resources such as medications, and ensure that the evaluator has consulted with another professional regarding this appraisal. Peer consultation demonstrates concern and sensitivity regarding the individual's risk and needs. Documenting the consultation is important to demonstrate appropriate professional action.

Additional actions that can be taken for clients at the medium- or high-risk levels are contracting for No Suicidal Behaviors. These No Suicide contracts are one of the many therapeutic strategies widely used; the contracts have strong clinical acceptance and demonstrate to the client the concern of the therapist for the client's welfare. However, the contract alone is not sufficient to ensure that the client may not impulsively harm himself or herself. Notifying the family and/or significant others of medium to high risk is strongly encouraged. However, if the danger is not imminent, it is desirable to ask the client's permission to notify family and significant others prior to breaching confidentiality. If the danger is clear and imminent, guidelines for confidentiality do not apply because the mental health professional must act to protect the life of the person at risk. The family/significant other could be informed of the risk and asked to help with social support, reduction of firearms, and assistance in obtaining treatment.

Reducing access to firearms is imperative for clients at medium to high risk. How this is accomplished would depend on where the firearms are stored. Involving family or significant others to reduce this access or remove these potential life-ending means would be the most conservative approach. Simply asking an adolescent to remove firearms would not be sufficient to confirm that this major step is taken. In short, reducing access to firearms requires the involvement of family or significant others.

Notifying legal authorities and/or Child Protective Services of risk to self or others should be considered if suicidal risk is arising from current maltreatment through neglect or abuse or if the client has angry/aggressive thoughts toward others in addition to himself or herself. Clinical guidelines require that mental health professionals carefully assess potential dangerousness to others and act with a "duty to protect" others who may be at risk. Notifying potential targets of risk and/or legal authorities are possible appropriate actions when danger extends to others (Fremouw et al., 1990). Finally, the mental health professional should consult with supervisors prior to notifying other agencies.

If an individual is considered high risk for suicidal behaviors, then increased therapeutic care is warranted. Referring the individual to day treatment or to voluntary or crisis hospitalization is strongly recommended. Individuals at high risk for suicidal behaviors are vulnerable to act on their suicidal ideation with little warning. Adolescents, in particular, are highly impulsive in terms of self-injurious behaviors. Any placement of an adolescent should involve the adolescent's family members. Placing adolescents in this more protected, intensive therapeutic environment would help monitor potential risk and provide treatment to lower that risk.

If the adolescent is unwilling to voluntarily commit to more intensive treatment and he or she is showing clear danger through ideation or behaviors toward self or others, then involuntary hospitalization should be considered. This decision to seek involuntary hospitalization would require consultation with a supervisor as well as family members and significant others for the adolescent. This action would be taken only if the adolescent was unwilling or unable to participate in voluntary intensive treatment. Involuntary hospitalization is always considered the last resort and the most restrictive alternative for treatment. Although in certain cases this placement is necessary, it is sometimes countertherapeutic as the individual does not want to be hospitalized.

The Actions Taken box on the ASAP-20 form lists 11 possible actions to be considered plus an "other" action. These actions are presented in hierarchical order for consideration but can be employed in any order provided that the professional has a rationale for the action taken. The major guideline is to *document* the actions taken and the rationale for each action. Furthermore, consultation with peers or supervisors is considered essential when dealing with high-risk individuals. The use of the ASAP-20, consultation, and documentation will demonstrate that the interviewer has exercised a high standard of professional judgment and has engaged in a "best practice" assessment and case management for adolescents.

Adolescent Suicide Assessment Protocol-20
(ASAP-20)

Client _____ Date _____

Agency _____ Age _____ Gender _____

HISTORICAL ITEMS:					Code (0-3)
Code: 0 = None 1 = Mild 2 = Moderate 3 = Severe					
1. History of suicide attempts			0 = None	3 = Definite	
2. History of physical/sexual abuse					
3. History of antisocial behaviors					
4. History of family suicide attempts/completions			0 = None	3 = Definite	

GENERAL CLINICAL ITEMS:					Code (0-3)
Code: 0 = None 1 = Mild 2 = Moderate 3 = Severe					
5. Depression					
6. Hopelessness					
7. Anger					
8. Impulsivity					
9. Substance Abuse					

SPECIFIC SUICIDAL ITEMS:	Code (0-3)
10. Currently, how often do you <u>think</u> about committing suicide? 0 = Almost never 1 = Occasional passing thoughts (monthly) 2 = Regularly (weekly) 3 = Almost daily	
11. Currently, do you have any <u>plans and methods</u> to commit suicide? 0 = None 1 = A general idea, but no specific plans 2 = A specific plan 3 = A specific plan with a method available and time schedule	
12. Do you <u>intend</u> to commit suicide? 0 = No intention 1 = Unlikely 2 = Likely, someday 3 = Likely, in the near future	

Subtotal Page 1 _____

CONTEXTUAL ITEMS:				Code (0-3)
Code: 0 = None 1 = Mild 2 = Moderate 3 = Severe				
13. Recent losses				
14. Firearm access				
15. Family dysfunction				
16. Peer problems				
17. School / Legal problems				
18. Contagion 0 = None 3 = Definite				

PROTECTIVE ITEMS:				Code (0-3)
19. Reasons for living 0 = Many 1 = One 2 = Vague 3 = None				
20. Current treatment 0 = Yes 3 = No				

Subtotal Page 2 _____

TOTAL 1-20 _____

OTHER CONSIDERATIONS:

RISK APPRAISAL	Low ☐ (0-15)	Medium ☐ (16-19)	High ☐ (20+)
TOTAL SCORE			

ACTIONS TAKEN (Check all that apply):
 1. Continue monitoring risk factors _____
 2. Notify family _____
 3. Notify/consult with supervisor _____
 4. Recommend/refer to outpatient treatment _____
 5. Recommend/refer to psychiatric consult/med evaluation _____
 6. Contract for NO SUICIDAL behaviors _____
 7. Recommend elimination of access to firearms _____
 8. Notify legal authorities of risk to self/or others _____
 9. Recommend/refer to day treatment _____
10. Recommend/refer to crisis unit/voluntary hospitalization _____
11. Initiate involuntary hospitalization _____
12. Other: _____ _____

Interviewer _____   Supervisor _____

CONTRIBUTORS

William Fremouw, PhD, received his doctorate from the University of Massachusetts in 1974. After an internship at the University of Rochester Medical School, he joined the West Virginia University faculty in 1975 where he has been the Director of Clinical Training and the Chairman of Psychology. Dr. Fremouw earned a Diplomate in Forensic Psychology from the American Board of Professional Psychology (ABPP) in 1989. His current research interests include stalking and malingering. Dr. Fremouw may be contacted at 1226 Life Sciences Building, 53 Campus Drive, Morgantown, WV 26506. E-mail: William.Fremouw@mail.wvu.edu

Julia M. Strunk, MS, is currently a doctoral student in clinical psychology at West Virginia University. She earned her bachelor's degree from Maryville College in Maryville, Tennessee, graduating Magna Cum Laude. Prior to graduate school, she taught English classes at Oak Ridge High School. Her special interest is forensic psychology, particularly in the areas of malingering, risk assessment, and juvenile offenders. Ms. Struck may be contacted at 1124 Life Sciences Building, 53 Campus Drive, Morgantown, WV 26505. E-mail: jstrunk@mix.wvu.edu

Elizabeth A. Tyner, MS, received her bachelor's degree from Western Michigan University and her master's degree at West Virginia University. She is currently a doctoral student in the clinical psychology program with a forensic emphasis at West Virginia University. Her research interests are in the areas of psychopathy, malingering, suicide risk assessment, forensic assessment, ethical/legal issues in clinical psychology, and criminal thinking styles. Ms. Tyner can be reached at 1124 Life Sciences Building, 53 Campus Drive, Morgantown, WV 26506. E-mail: etyner@mix.wvu.edu

Robert (Bob) Musick, MSW, is currently Director of Community Mental Health Services Development at Valley Health Care System in Morgantown, West Virginia. Mr. Musick also serves as the Executive Director of West Virginia's Counsel for the Prevention of Suicide. His background has been directing Crisis Service Programs, 24-hour crisis lines, walk-in crisis services, and the Crisis Residential Unit. Mr. Musick is an adjunct instructor at West Virginia University's Division of Social Work. Courses taught have been in Management/Supervision, mental health, and groups. In 2002 he was awarded NASW's Management Person of the Year in West Virginia. Mr. Musick can be reached at 301 Scott Avenue, Morgantown, WV 26508-8804. E-mail: bmusick@valleyhealthcare.org

RESOURCES

American Foundation for Suicide Prevention (AFSP) and American Association of Suicidology Annenberg Public Policy Center. (2003). *Reporting on Suicide: Recommendations for the Media*. Retrieved 11/16/03, from http://www.afsp.org/education/newrecommendations.html

Anderson, R. N., & Smith, B. L. (2003). Deaths: Leading causes for 2001. *National Vital Statistic Report, 52*, 1-86.

Bell, C., & Clark, P. (1998). Adolescent suicide. *Pediatric Clinics of North America, 34*, 365-380.

Brent, D. A. (2001). Assessment and treatment of the youthful suicide patient. In H. Hendin & J. Mann (Eds.), *The Clinical Science of Suicide Prevention* (pp. 106-131). New York: New York Academy of Sciences.

Brent, D. A., Perper, J. A., Kolko, D. J., & Zelenak, J. P. (1988). The psychological autopsy: Methodological considerations for the study of adolescent suicide. *Journal of the American Academy of Child and Adolescent Psychiatry, 27*, 362-366.

Brent, D. A., Perper, J. A., Moritz, G., Allman, C., Friend, A., Roth, C., Schweers, J., Balach, L., & Baugher, M. (1993). Psychiatric risk factors for adolescent suicide: A case-control study. *Journal of the American Academy of Child and Adolescent Psychiatry, 32*, 521-529.

Centers for Disease Control (CDC). (1995). Suicide among children, adolescents, and young adults—United States, 1980-1992. *Morbidity and Mortality Weekly Report, 44*, 239-291.

Centers for Disease Control (CDC). (1998). Youth-risk behavior surveillance—United States, 1997. *Morbidity and Mortality Weekly Report, 47*, 239-291.

DiFilippo, J. M., Esposito, C., Overholser, J., & Spirito, A. (2003). High-risk populations. In A. Spirito & J. C. Overholser (Eds.), *Evaluating and Treating Adolescent Suicide Attempters: From Research to Practice* (pp. 229-259). New York: Academic Press.

Donaldson, D., Spirito, A., & Overholser, J. (2003). Treatment of adolescent suicide attempters. In A. Spirito & J. C. Overholser (Eds.), *Evaluating and Treating Adolescent Suicide Attempters: From Research to Practice* (pp. 295-321). New York: Academic Press.

Douglas, K., Ogloff, J., Nicholls, T., & Grant, I. (1999). Assessing risk for violence among psychiatric patients: The HCR-20 violence risk assessment scheme and the Psychopathy Checklist: Screening Version. *Journal of Consulting and Clinical Psychology, 67*, 917-930.

Douglas, K., & Webster, C. (1999). The HCR-20 violence risk assessment scheme: Concurrent validity in a sample of incarcerated offenders. *Criminal Justice and Behavior, 26*, 3-19.

Eggert, L., Thompson, E., & Herting, J. (1994). A measure of adolescent potential for suicide (MAPS): Development and preliminary findings. *Suicide and Life-Threatening Behavior, 24*, 359-381.

Esposito, C., Johnson, B., Wolfsdorf, B. A., & Spirito, A. (2003). Cognitive factors: Hopelessness, coping, and problem solving. In A. Spirito & J. C. Overholser (Eds.), *Evaluating and Treating Adolescent Suicide Attempters: From Research to Practice* (pp. 89-112). New York: Academic Press.

Fremouw, W. J., dePerczel, M., & Ellis, T. (1990). *Suicide Risk Assessment and Response Guidelines*. Elmsford, NY: Pergamon Press.

Goldman, S., & Beardslee, W. R. (1999). Suicide in children and adolescents. In D. G. Jacobs (Ed.), *The Harvard Medical School Guide to Suicide Assessment And Intervention* (pp. 417-442). San Francisco: Jossey-Bass.

Goldston, D. B. (2003). *Measuring Suicidal Behavior and Risk in Children and Adolescents*. Washington, DC: American Psychological Association.

Gould, M. S., Fisher, P., Parides, M., Flory, M., & Shaffer, D. (1996). Psychosocial risk factors of child and adolescent completed suicide. *Archives of General Psychiatry, 53*, 1155-1162.

Gould, M. S., & Kramer, R. A. (2001). Youth suicide prevention. *Suicide and Life-Threatening Behavior, 31*, 6-31.

Gould, M. S., Shaffer, D., Fisher, P., Kleinman, M., & Morishima, A. (1992). The clinical prediction of adolescent suicide. In R. W. Maris, A. L. Berman, J. T. Maltsberger, & R. I. Yufit (Eds.), *Assessment and Prediction of Suicide* (pp. 130-143). New York: Guilford.

Horesh, N., Gotheif, D., Ofek, H., Weizman, T., & Apter, A. (1999). Impulsivity as a correlate of suicidal behavior in adolescent psychiatric inpatients. *Crisis, 20*, 8-14.

Kaplan, S. J. (1996). Physical abuse of children and adolescents. In S. J. Kaplan (Ed.), *Family Violence: A Clinical and Legal Guide* (pp. 1-35). Washington, DC: American Psychiatric Press.

Kashden, J., Fremouw, W. J., Callahan, T. S., & Franzen, M. D. (1993). Impulsivity in suicidal and nonsuicidal adolescents. *Journal of Abnormal Child Psychology, 21*, 339-353.

Litman, R. (1990). Suicides: What do they have in mind? In D. Jacobs & H. Brown (Eds.), *Suicide: Understanding and Responding* (pp. 143-156). Madison, CT: International Universities Press.

Marttunen, M. J., Henriksson, M. M., Isomesta, E. T., Heikkinen, M. E., Aro, H. M., & Lönnqvist, J. K. (1998). Completed suicide among adolescents with no diagnosable psychiatric disorder. *Adolescence, 33*(131), 669-681.

McKeown, R. E., Garrison, C. Z., Cuffe, S. P., Waller, J. L., Jackson, K. L., & Addy, C. L. (1998). Incidence and predictors of suicidal behaviors in a longitudinal sample of young adolescents. *Journal of the American Academy of Child and Adolescent Psychiatry, 37*, 612-619.

McNiel, D. E., Borum, R., Douglas, K. S., Hart, S. D., Lyon, D. R., Sullivan, L. E., & Hemphill, J. F. (2002). Risk Assessment. In J. R. Ogloff (Ed.), *Taking Psychology and Law into the Twenty-First Century* (pp. 147-170). New York: Kluwer Academic.

Miniño, A., Arias, E., Kochanek, K., Murphy, S., & Smith, B. (2002). Deaths: Final data for 2000. *National Vital Statistics Report, 50*(15), 1-120.

Myers, K., McCauley, E., Calderon, R., & Treder, R. (1991). The 3-year longitudinal course of suicidality and predictive factors for subsequent suicidality in youths with major depressive disorder. *Journal of the American Academy of Child and Adolescent Psychiatry, 30*, 804-810.

Negron, R., Piacentini, J., Graae, F., Davies, M., & Shaffer, D. (1997). Microanalysis of adolescent suicide attempters and ideators during the acute suicidal episode. *Journal of the American Academy of Child and Adolescent Psychiatry, 36*, 1512-1519.

O'Carroll, P. W., Berman, A. L., Maris, R. W., Moscicki, E. K., Tanney, B. L., & Silverman, M. M. (1996). Beyond the tower of Babel: A nomenclature for suicidology. *Suicide and Life-Threatening Behavior, 26*, 237-252.

Osman, A., Kopper, B. A., Barrios, F. X., Osman, J. R., Besett, T., & Linehan, M. M. (1996). The Brief Reasons for Living Inventory for Adolescents (BRFL-A). *Journal of Abnormal Child Psychology, 24*, 433-443.

Overholser, J., & Spirito, A. (2003). Precursors to adolescent suicide attempts. In A. Spirito & J. C. Overholser (Eds.), *Evaluating and Treating Adolescent Suicide Attempters: From Research to Practice* (pp. 19-40). New York: Academic Press.

Prinstein, M. J. (2003). Social factors: Peer relationships. In A. Spirito & J. C. Overholser (Eds.), *Evaluating and Treating Adolescent Suicide Attempters: From Research to Practice* (pp. 191-213). New York: Academic Press.

Rhode, P., Seeley, J. R., & Mace, D. E. (1997). Correlates of suicidal behavior in a juvenile detention population. *Suicide and Life-Threatening Behavior, 27*, 164-175.

Rudd, M. D., & Joiner, T. (1998). The assessment, management, and treatment of suicidality: Toward clinically informed and balanced standards of care. *Clinical Psychology: Science and Practice, 5*, 135-150.

Shaffer, D., Gould, M. S., Fisher, P., Trautman, P., Moreau, D., Kleinman, M., & Flory, M. (1996). Psychiatric diagnosis in child and adolescent suicide. *Archives of General Psychiatry, 53*, 339-348.

Spirito, A., & Overholser, J. C. (Eds.). (2003). *Evaluating and Treating Adolescent Suicide Attempters: From Research to Practice*. New York: Academic Press.

Substance Abuse and Mental Health Services Administration (SAMHSA). (2002). *SAMHSA Unveils Data on Youths Contemplating Suicide* [News release]. Retrieved 3/01/04, from http://www.samhsa.gov/news/news.html

Webster, C., Douglas, K., Eaves, D., & Hart, S. (1995). *HCR-20: Assessing Risk for Violence* (Version 2). Vancouver: Simon Fraser University.

Wolfsdorf, B. A., Freeman, J., D'Eramo, K., Overholser, J., & Spirito, A. (2003). Mood states: Depression, anger, and anxiety. In A. Spirito & J. C. Overholser (Eds.), *Evaluating and Treating Adolescent Suicide Attempters: From Research to Practice* (pp. 53-88). New York: Academic Press.

The Index of Race-Related Stress–Brief Version (IRRS-B)

Compiled by Tawanda M. Greer

SCALE DESCRIPTION

The Index of Race-Related Stress–Brief Version (IRRS-B; Utsey, 1999) is a 22-item measure designed to capture experiences of race-related stress among African American adults that are related to their encounters of racism. The IRRS-B represents a shortened version of the Index of Race-Related Stress (IRRS; Utsey & Ponterotto, 1996) which is comprised of 46 items. The IRRS was developed based upon the theoretical notions of daily hassles stress (Lazarus & Folkman, 1984), Jones' (1972) tripartite model of racism, as well as Essed's (1990) notion of persistent, everyday racism. Daily hassles stress can generally be defined as consistent pressures that are appraised by the individual to be taxing and/or exceeding their resources. When compared to infrequent life events, daily hassles stress has been found to be more detrimental to one's overall well-being (e.g., Kanner et al., 1981). Jones (1972) proposed that racism occurs on three levels: individual racism, institutional racism, and cultural racism. Individual racism refers to one's personal experiences of racism. Institutional racism refers to practices and policies that are embedded within institutions that serve to discriminate and marginalize those of a particular racial group. Institutional racism is intentionally or unintentionally designed to limit the rights of those belonging to a particular racial group. Cultural racism refers to the behaviors and communication within society that conveys the notion that one racial group is superior to another. Essed (1990) also coined the term *collective racism* to describe the collective, organized, or semi-organized efforts of Whites to deliberately seek to limit and/or destroy the rights of African Americans or other non-Whites. The IRRS measures these four domains of racism as experienced by African Americans, whereas the IRRS-B measures three domains (i.e., cultural racism, institutional racism, and individual racism).

SCALE DEVELOPMENT

The items for the original IRRS were derived from interviews of African American adults, personal experiences of one of the principal investigators (African American male), and reviewed literature. A pilot study was then conducted and consisted of 377 participants from various locations within the United States. The sample for the pilot study consisted of 203 women and 163 men (11 participants were not included due to missing data regarding gender). The mean age was 22.65. Utsey and Ponterotto (1996) conducted three additional studies to confirm the measure's structure, validity (discriminant and concurrent), and reliability. The final version of the IRRS yielded 46 items. In creating the shortened version of the IRRS, Utsey (1999) reported reanalyzing a data set consisting of 310 African American adult participants. This sample comprised 207 females and 92 males (11 participants were not included because of missing data). The participants were from various universities and colleges in an urban area of the northeastern United States. Participants ranged in age from 17 to 76 with a mean age of 23.38 years. Utsey (1999) reported that some items were eliminated based upon the results of an exploratory factor analysis and the finding that some items were relevant only by geographic location and that some items yielded extreme examples of racism. This process of item elimination generated a 22 item version of the IRRS. Utsey (1999) conducted a study to test the components of the shortened IRRS. The participants for this study were recruited from a Catholic university in the northeastern region of the United States, as well as from a substance abuse center and the general community. The sample consisted of 264 participants, 25 were European Americans and were included as a comparison sample to test the measure's validity. A total of 239 African American adults were included in this study (i.e., 138 females, 78 males, and 23 participants were not included due to missing data). The mean age for the total sample was 31.18 years, with an average of 13.78 years of education, and a mean annual income of \$23, 000. The shortened version of the IRRS was administered in conjunction with two subscales from another measure of racism-related stress, the Racism and Life Experiences Scales-Brief Version (RaLES-R; Harrell, 1997). Thus, the RaLES-R subscales of PER (i.e., the degree to which individuals feel that racism has impacted them personally) and GRP (i.e., the degree to which individuals feel that racism has impacted their racial group) were also administered to participants. Cronbach's alphas (Utsey, 1999) for each subscale of the IRRS-B were .78 for Cultural Racism, .69 for Institutional Racism, and .78 for Individual Racism. A confirmatory factor analysis showed adequate fit of the data for the shortened version of the IRRS. Convergent validity was demonstrated as the subscales of the shortened IRRS showed positive, significant correlations with subscales of the RaLES-R's PER and GRP subscales. The brief IRRS also showed adequate criterion-related validity as it effectively discriminated between African Americans and European Americans in the sample regarding experiences of racism.

SCALE ADMINISTRATION

The IRRS-B is appropriate for use with African American adults with similar ages of the validation sample (i.e., 16-91 years of age). The measure can be administered within 5 to 15 minutes and requires a 9th grade reading level. The items are endorsed using a Likert-type format with responses ranging from 0 to 4. Specifically, "0" indicates "This never happened to me," "1" indicates "This event happened, but did not bother me," "2" indicates "This event happened and I was slightly upset," "3" indicates "This event happened and I was upset," and "4" indicates "This event happened and I was extremely upset."

SCORING AND INTERPRETATION

The IRRS-B should be scored only if it is used as part of a research study. Its clinical utility is limited to acquiring a qualitative estimate of African American client experiences of persistent forms of racism. Therefore, the measure should not be scored after administration. Rather, the clinician should peruse the client's endorsements on the Likert scale and become keenly aware of responses that suggest that the client was impacted by his or her experiences of racism (i.e., response endorsements ranging from 2 to 4). Client endorsements can then be discussed with them and considered by the clinician in relation to their presenting physical and mental health concerns.

The Index of Race-Related Stress–Brief Version (IRRS-B)*

Shawn O. Utsey

INSTRUCTIONS

This survey questionnaire is intended to sample some of the experiences that Black people have in this country because of their "Blackness." There are many experiences that a Black person can have in this country because of his/her race. Some events happen Just Once, some more often, while others may happen frequently. Below you will find listed some of these experiences, for which you are to indicate those that have happened to you or someone very close to you (i.e., a family member or loved one). It is important to note that a person can be affected by those events that happen to people close to them; this is why you are asked to consider such events as applying to your experiences when you complete this questionnaire. Please circle [write] the number on the scale (0 to 4) that indicates the reaction you had to the event at the time it happened. Do not leave any items blank. If an event has happened more than once, refer to the first time it happened. If an event did not happen circle [write] 0 and go on to the next item.

0	=	This never happened to me.
1	=	This event happened, but did not bother me.
2	=	This event happened and I was slightly upset.
3	=	This event happened and I was upset.
4	=	This event happened and I was extremely upset.

1. You notice that crimes committed by White people tend to be romanticized, whereas the same crime committed by a Black person is portrayed as savagery, and the Black person who committed it, as an animal. _____

2. Sales people/clerks did not say thank you or show other forms of courtesy and respect (e.g., put your things in a bag) when you shopped at some White/non-Black owned businesses. _____

3. You notice that when Black people are killed by the police, the media informs the public of the victims criminal record or negative information in their background, suggesting they got what they deserve. _____

4. You have been threatened with physical violence by an individual or group of White/non-Blacks. _____

5. You have observed that White kids who commit violent crimes are portrayed as "boys being boys" while Black kids who commit similar crimes are wild animals. _____

6. You seldom hear or read anything positive about Black people on radio, TV, in newspapers, or history books. _____

7. While shopping at a store the sales clerk assumed you couldn't afford certain items (e.g., you were directed toward the items on sale). _____

8. You were the victim of a crime and the police treated you as if you should accept it as part of being Black. _____

9. You were treated with less respect and courtesy than Whites and other non-Blacks while in a store, restaurant, or other business establishment. _____

---

* Reprinted from *The Journal of Measurement and Evaluation in Counseling and Development*, Vol. 32, Issue 3, 1999, pages 149-167. Copyright © 1999 by the American Counseling Association. Reprinted with permission.

10. You were passed over for an important project although you were more qualified and competent than the White/non-Black person given the task. _____

11. Whites/non-Blacks have stared at you as if you didn't belong in the same place with them; whether it was a restaurant, theater, or other place of business. _____

12. You have observed the police treat White/non-Blacks with more respect and dignity than they do Blacks. _____

13. You have been subjected to racist jokes by Whites/non-Blacks in positions of authority and you did not protest for fear they might have held it against you. _____

14. While shopping at a store, or when attempting to make a purchase, you were ignored as if you were not a serious customer or didn't have any money. _____

15. You have observed situations where other Blacks were treated harshly or unfairly by Whites/non-Blacks due to their race. _____

16. You have heard reports of White people/non-Blacks who have committed crimes, and in an effort to cover up their deeds falsely reported that a Black man was responsible for the crime. _____

17. You notice that the media plays up those stories that cast Blacks in negative ways (child abusers, rapists, muggers, etc.), usually accompanied by a large picture of a Black person looking angry or disturbed. _____

18. You have heard racist remarks or comments about Black people spoken with impunity by White public officials or other influential White people. _____

19. You have been given more work, or the most undesirable jobs at your place of employment while the White/non-Black of equal or less seniority and credentials is given less work, and more desirable tasks. _____

20. You have heard or seen other Black people express a desire to be White or to have White physical characteristics because they disliked being Black or thought it was ugly. _____

21. White people or other non-Blacks have treated you as if you were unintelligent and needed things explained to you slowly or numerous times. _____

22. You were refused an apartment or other housing; you suspect it was because you're Black. _____

CONTRIBUTOR

Tawanda M. Greer, PhD, is an Assistant Professor in the Department of Psychology and Women's Studies at the University of South Carolina in Columbia, South Carolina. She received her doctorate degree in Counseling Psychology at Southern Illinois University at Carbondale in Carbondale, Illinois. Dr. Greer's areas of expertise include retention issues among African American college students, issues of race and racism, and multicultural counseling. Dr. Greer may be contacted at the Department of Psychology, Barnwell College, University of South Carolina, Columbia, SC 29208.

RESOURCES

Essed, P. (1990). *Everyday Racism: Reports From Women of Two Cultures.* Claremont, CA: Hunter House.

Harrell, S. P. (1997, May). *Development and Validation of Scales to Measure Racism-Related Stress.* Poster presented at the 6th biennial conference of the Society for Community Research and Action, Columbia, South Carolina.

Jones, J. M. (1972). *Prejudice and Racism.* Menlo Park, CA: Addison-Wesley.

Kanner, A. D., Coyne, J. C., Shaefer, C., & Lazarus, R. S. (1981). Comparison of two modes of stress measurement. Daily hassles and uplifts versus major life events. *Journal of Behavioral Medicine, 4,* 1-39.

Lazarus, R. S., & Folkman, S. (1984). *Stress, Appraisal, and Coping.* New York: Springer.

Utsey, S. O. (1999). Development and validation of a short form of the Index of Race-Related Stress (IRRS)-Brief Version. *The Journal of Measurement and Evaluation in Counseling and Development, 32*(3), 149-167.

Utsey, S. O., & Ponterotto, J. G. (1996). Development and validation of the Index of Race-Related Stress (IRRS). *Journal of Counseling Psychology, 43,* 490-502.

Eating Behaviors and Body Image Test for Preadolescent Girls*

Compiled by Eve M. Wolf

SCALE DESCRIPTION

The Eating Behaviors and Body Image Test for Preadolescent Girls (EBBIT; Candy & Fee, 1998a, 1998b) is a 42-item self-report questionnaire developed to measure body image satisfaction and eating behaviors and disturbances in preadolescent girls. Factor analysis of the EBBIT has yielded two factors. Factor one measures restrictive eating behaviors and body image dissatisfaction (Body Image Dissatisfaction/Restrictive Eating; BIDRE). Factor two is a measure of binge eating (Binge Eating Behaviors: BEB). Four items measuring compensatory behaviors were also included as an additional scale in order to enhance the EBBIT's clinical utility, though this scale has not been supported by factor analysis.

SCALE DEVELOPMENT

The scale was developed in an attempt to address a gap in the assessment of maladaptive eating behaviors in young girls. Research has also been conducted using the scale with preadolescent boys. Moreover, a Parent Eating Behaviors and Body Image Test for Preadolescent Girls is currently in the process of development. Psychometric properties of the EBBIT were investigated in research with 291 girls enrolled in the fourth, fifth, and sixth grades. This sample included 238 girls who identified as Caucasian, 48 African American, 2 Asian, 2 biracial, and 1 subject who did not report her race. Test items were generated based on content validity, and content domains were selected based on the primary symptom categories included in the *Diagnostic and Statistical Manual of Mental Disorders* (*DSM-IV*; American Psychiatric Association, 1994) diagnoses of anorexia nervosa and bulimia nervosa. In addition, open interviews were conducted with the mothers of two girls receiving eating disorder treatment, and experts in the field were asked to comment on the items. Finally, preliminary testing was conducted to assure that the scale could be read and understood by the target group, and comments were used to modify the instrument. In addition to administration of the EBBIT, Body Mass Index was estimated via assessment of height and weight, and body image was assessed by administering the Body Image Silhouettes (BIS) developed by Childress, Jarrell, and Brewerton (1993). Substantial internal consistency was evident for the EBBIT total score ($r = .89$) as well as the EBBIT factors: Factor One (BIDRE) had an internal consistency of .91; Factor Two (BEB) had an internal consistency of .75. Two-week test-retest reliability on the

---

* The Eating Behaviors and Body Image Test for Preadolescent Girls is reprinted with permission from Virginia E. Fee. For more information regarding the EBBIT, contact Dr. Fee at the Department of Psychology, P.O. Box 6161, Mississippi State University, Mississippi State, MS 39762. E-mail: vef2@ra.msstate.edu

total EBBIT score was .85: test-retest reliability for Factors One (BIDRE) and Two (BEB) were .90 and .79 respectively.

SCALE ADMINISTRATION

The EBBIT is appropriate for use with preadolescent girls between the ages of 9 and 12. After completing a brief cover page which includes the girl's name, age, grade, school, teacher, race, and any special diets or medical problems, subjects are asked to rate the degree to which they engage in a series of behaviors using a 4-point, Likert-type scale: 0 = never, 1 = rarely (once a month), 2 = often (once a week), and 3 = most of the time (everyday).

SCORING AND INTERPRETATION

Instructions for scoring the EBBIT can be found in the manual (Fee & Candy, 1998). A scoring form is provided on which the clinician is instructed to fill in item blanks with the number circled by the child. For each subscale, the ratings are summed to yield a total subscale score. There are 23 items on the BIDRE Subscale, 15 items on the BEB Subscale, and 4 items on the Compensatory Behaviors Subscale. The total score is a sum of the subject's totals on Subscale 1 (BIDRE) and Subscale 2 (BEB) and can be interpreted using the Mean and Standard Deviation by Age table which is attached (and can be found in the EBBIT manual). Note that the four items which comprise the Compensatory Behaviors subscale are not to be added into the total score, but rather are to be evaluated individually as critical compensatory behaviors indicated in the *DSM-IV*.

Eating Behaviors and Body Image Test
For Preadolescent Girls
(EBBIT)

Colette M. Candy and Virginia E. Fee

Name _____

Teacher _____   Age _____

School _____   Grade _____

Race: (Please circle)

African American/Black

Asian

Hispanic

White

Other

1. Do you have any medical problems that cause you to eat certain foods? (Please circle)

    No   Yes

    If yes, what is it?   _____

2. Does your family have a special diet (example, vegetarian, diabetic)? (Please circle)

    No   Yes

    If yes, what kind?   _____

Eating Behaviors and Body Image Test for Preadolescent Girls

3 Most of the Time (Everyday)	2 Often (Once a Week)	1 Rarely (Once a Month)	0 Never (Never)

Example

I eat a lot when I watch T.V.　　　　　　　3 .... ②......... 1 0

1. I diet (lose weight by eating less than normal) like my friends do.　3 ....2 ....1 0
2. My current weight bothers me.　3 ....2 ....1 0
3. I eat a lot of food all at once.　3 ....2 ....1 0
4. I try not to eat even when I am hungry.　3 ....2 ....1 0
5. I wish I was thinner.　3 ....2 ....1 0
6. I do not eat junk food or "fatty" food because I want to lose weight.　3 ....2 ....1 0
7. I try to lose weight by dieting.　3 ....2 ....1 0
8. I eat when I feel mad.　3 ....2 ....1 0
9. I collect food in my room and sometimes I eat it all at once.　3 ....2 ....1 0
10. I think I am fat.　3 ....2 ....1 0
11. I make myself throw up after eating.　3 ....2 ....1 0
12. I think I weigh more than most girls my age and height.　3 ....2 ....1 0
13. I eat what I want to eat, anytime I want to.　3 ....2 ....1 0
14. I eat until my stomach feels uncomfortable.　3 ....2 ....1 0
15. I worry about gaining weight.　3 ....2 ....1 0
16. I eat all of my Halloween candy at once.　3 ....2 ....1 0
17. I take diet pills to lose weight.　3 ....2 ....1 0
18. I feel really bad after I eat a lot of food.　3 ....2 ....1 0
19. I skip meals to lose weight.　3 ....2 ....1 0
20. I feel hungry when I am not eating.　3 ....2 ....1 0
21. I like my stomach to feel empty.　3 ....2 ....1 0

3 **Most of the Time** **(Everyday)**	2 **Often** **(Once a Week)**	1 **Rarely** **(Once a Month)**	0 **Never** **(Never)**

22. I eat junk food alone in my room, so no one sees what I am eating.   3 .... 2 .... 1 0

23. I take laxatives to lose weight.   3 .... 2 .... 1 0

24. I feel fat.   3 .... 2 .... 1 0

25. I really feel bad after I eat a lot of junk food, so I think about how
to get rid of what I just ate.   3 .... 2 .... 1 0

26. I eat a lot of food sometimes when I am not even hungry.   3 .... 2 .... 1 0

27. I worry that if I eat, I might gain weight.   3 .... 2 .... 1 0

28. I look at food labels to see the calorie and fat content.   3 .... 2 .... 1 0

29. After I eat a lot of food at one time, I try to skip the next meal or
the next two meals.   3 .... 2 .... 1 0

30. I would eat 10 candy bars at once if my parents would let me.   3 .... 2 .... 1 0

31. I sometimes sneak food.   3 .... 2 .... 1 0

32. I try not to eat foods with a lot of fat.   3 .... 2 .... 1 0

33. I look at the fat on my body and wish that it was not there.   3 .... 2 .... 1 0

34. I eat when I feel sad.   3 .... 2 .... 1 0

35. I eat when I feel bored.   3 .... 2 .... 1 0

36. I take diuretics to lose weight.   3 .... 2 .... 1 0

37. I exercise to burn off the food I eat.   3 .... 2 .... 1 0

38. I diet like my mother or sister does.   3 .... 2 .... 1 0

39. There are some foods I would eat way too much of if I had the chance.   3 .... 2 .... 1 0

40. I think about food a lot when I'm not eating.   3 .... 2 .... 1 0

41. I drink diet soda, instead of eating meals or snacks.   3 .... 2 .... 1 0

42. I do not eat dessert (cake, ice cream, cookies) because I want to lose weight.   3 .... 2 .... 1 0

I feel that I was able to answer these questions honestly?   Yes   or   No

EBBIT Scoring Form

Directions: For each item, fill in the blank with the number circled by the child. For each subscale, sum the ratings for a total subscale score. The three subscale scores can be added together to obtain the Total score. The scores can then be compared to the means and standard deviations attached.

BIDRE Subscale	**BEB** Subscale	**Compensatory** **Behaviors** Subscale
1. _____	3. _____	11. _____
2. _____	8. _____	17. _____
4. _____	9. _____	23. _____
5. _____	13. _____	36. _____
6. _____	14. _____	
7. _____	16. _____	
10. _____	20. _____	
12. _____	22. _____	
15. _____	26. _____	
18. _____	30. _____	
19. _____	31. _____	
21. _____	34. _____	
24. _____	35. _____	
25. _____	39. _____	
27. _____	40. _____	
28. _____		
29. _____		
32. _____		
33. _____		
37. _____		
38. _____		
41. _____		
42. _____		
Total _____	**Total** _____	**Total** _____

TOTAL SCORE (Subscale 1 + Subscale 2) _____

Note: The four items that make up the critical items should be evaluated individually. These items represent compensatory behaviors that are indicated in the *DSM-IV.*

EBBIT for Preadolescent Girls
Means and Standard Deviations by Age

		BIDRE Subscale		BEB Subscale		Total Score	
		Mean	*SD*	*Mean*	*SD*	*Mean*	*SD*
Age 9	63	24.19	16.71	8.43	6.98	32.93	20.39
Age 10	86	27.59	15.67	10.51	7.30	38.10	19.02
Age 11	88	26.81	17.23	11.22	8.51	38.11	20.47
Age 12	51	27.27	17.18	11.86	6.48	39.12	18.96
Total	288	26.40	16.65	10.49	7.58	36.92	19.91

CONTRIBUTOR

Eve M. Wolf, PhD, is an Associate Professor at the Wright State University School of Professional Psychology in Dayton, Ohio. For the past 20 years, she has been involved in clinical work and scholarship in the area of eating disorders. Currently, she supervises doctoral students in their clinical work at the University counseling center where eating problems and body image issues are common concerns. Dr. Wolf may be contacted at 220 Frederick A. White Health Center, 3640 Colonel Glenn Highway, Dayton, OH 45435. E-mail: eve.wolf@wright.edu

RESOURCES

Cited Resources

American Psychiatric Association. (1994). *Diagnostic and Statistical Manual of Mental Disorders (DSM-IV*; 4th ed.).Washington, DC: Author.

Candy, C. M., & Fee, V. E. (1998a). Reliability and concurrent validity of the Kids' Eating Disorders Survey (KEDS) Body Image Silhouettes with preadolescent girls. *Eating Disorders, 6*, 297-308.

Candy, C. M., & Fee, V. E. (1998b). Underlying dimensions and psychometric properties of the eating behaviors and body image test for preadolescent girls. *Journal of Clinical Child Psychology, 27*(1), 117-127.

Childress, A. C., Jarrell, M. P., & Brewerton, T. D. (1993). The Kid's Eating Disorders Survey (KEDS): Internal consistency, component analysis, and reliability. *Eating Disorders, 1*, 123-133.

Fee, V. E., & Candy, C. M. (1998). *Eating Behaviors and Body Image Test for Preadolescent Girls (EBBIT) Manual.* Unpublished manuscript.

Additional Resources

Childress, A. C., Brewerton, T. D., Hodges, E. L., & Jarrell, M. P. (1993). The Kids' Eating Disorders Survey (KEDS): A study of middle school students. *Journal of the American Academy of Child and Adolescent Psychiatry, 32*, 843-850.

Fee, V. E. (2004). *A Parent Report Measure of Problematic Eating Behaviors and Body Image in Preadolescent Girls: The Parent Eating Behaviors and Body Image Test (PEBBIT).* Unpublished manuscript.

Fee, V. E., & Meadows, T. J. (2004). *Psychometric Properties of the Eating Behaviors and Body Image Test (EBBIT) With Preadolescent Boys.* Unpublished manuscript.

Coping With Serious Illness*

Q. How important is it to treat the mind as well as the body during a serious illness?

A. When people are ill, it's important to deal with the illness on the physical, emotional, and spiritual levels. If you treat just the body, you short-change yourself.

We don't know exactly how the mind/body connection works, but we do have biochemical evidence that there's a connection.

Q. What are some areas where psychology can help those patients diagnosed with a serious illness?

A. There are six areas where psychology can help:

- finding the best fit in medical interventions
- forming a support group to help the patient
- dealing with the needs of family and friends
- reducing the side effects of medical treatments (like chemotherapy)
- managing pain
- helping patients cope with the "after-illness experience."

Q. How has psychology helped with specific illnesses?

A.

AIDS
Psychological interventions are helping gay, HIV-positive men better deal with their diagnosis, using stress management techniques, social support, and body relaxation training. The interventions are intended to counteract the fact that, for some people, finding out that they are HIV-positive may lead to social isolation and poor coping strategies that could suppress the immune system.

Heart Attacks
Psychological interventions can help before and after heart attacks. Brief psychological counseling before medical procedures produces shorter stays in the critical-care unit, less emotional distress, and shorter hospital stays. And after heart attacks, group therapy for recovering heart patients improves psychological well-being and cuts the death rate in the first three years of recovery. In addition, research has shown that two hours of psychological counseling per week for seven weeks reduces by 60 percent the rate of rehospitalization for heart patients.

Cancer
Cancer patients who have psychological interventions have shown an improved quality of life as well as improved their physical health. Targeted group therapy and relaxation training have been shown to improve patients' moods, lower their emotional distress, and improve their ability to cope with their illnesses.

Organ Recipients
Psychologists can also help medical teams identify the best transplant candidates. Psychologists are extensively involved in assessing who is most capable of dealing with the required medical regimen. Psycholo-

---

* With thanks to Sandra Haber, PhD, a psychologist in private practice in New York City, an associate clinical professor of psychology at the Derner Institute at Adelphi University and a fellow of the American Psychological Association; Michael Antoni, PhD, and Neil Schneiderman, PhD, of the University of Miami; and Mary Ellen Olbrisch, PhD, of Virginia Commonwealth University.

gists also intervene with those who are weak on such skills, but who can develop them through behavioral change strategies and support.

Q. Why is it so important for patients who are diagnosed with a serious illness to deal with their feelings at an early stage?

A. Being upset about having a serious illness is perfectly normal and reasonable.

Patients need to feel a sense of mourning, loss, and fear – all of that is reasonable. The goal is to let them experience it and move through it then they can emerge stronger and are more likely to manage their negative emotions. If they feel they have to cover up every negative emotion, they can't get beyond those feelings.

Q. What is the first reaction most patients have when they have been diagnosed with a serious illness such as cancer?

A. The first reaction with cancer is a fear for loss of life. "Cancer equals death" is the first thing people go through. Am I going to die? After that issues begin to differ for each person on what happens next. What treatment do I undertake? How do I make a choice? Will it be effective? What else can I do to conquer my illness?

Q. There are many options available as to what treatment patients should have. How can talking with a psychologist best prepare them for making that choice?

A. Overall, talking to a psychologist is an empowering process. Sometimes patients have to fight for what they want. Sometimes they need to push a bit. Most patients are uncomfortable pushing and asking questions because they're not the expert and it feels disrespectful.

Also, psychology is helpful for coping with the side effects of treatment. Some people give up chemotherapy, even though it may threaten their life, because they can't deal with the side effects.

Too often, a patient's psychological needs throughout the treatment regime are not taken into account. Making an educated choice with the patient means weighing both their psychological needs and their medical needs.

Q. How can psychology help people to manage their pain?

A. Psychologists can help people manage their pain by giving them language to describe the pain both to themselves and to physicians (is it shooting or numbing pain, for example) and can suggest helpful medications or use hypnosis as a pain management intervention.

Q. How are friends, family, and loved ones affected by a person's serious illness?

A. Serious illness can affect the whole family, not just the patient. Psychology deals not only with the patient, but also with his or her aging parents, children, spouse, or friends who are involved with that patient's treatments. The stress on a partner is enormous – they're taking over the other person's role, the financial burden, the burden of children, while simultaneously containing their own feelings. The stress on the caretaker cannot be understated. And children feel stress too. Parents mistakenly assume that they're hiding the illness from children in the family, but children often know when something is wrong.

The aging parents also are affected. Their child is dying. They may be in their 70s and their child may be 40, but it's still their child. There are many, many people affected when someone is seriously ill.

Q. Some believe that after that last physical therapy treatment, the illness is gone. Isn't it true that the battle is really just beginning?

A. The rest of the world may want the patient to go back to normal after the treatment is over, but the survivor of a serious illness will never return to who they were. They may still be upset, anxious, and worried. They've lost the protective umbrella of being under physician care. They're afraid they'll have a recurrence or they are left with bodily disfigurement. They're not back to themselves. They need to be reintegrated into the world. Psychology can help long after the physical therapy is over.

Q. Are there any positives that come out of dealing with a chronic illness?

A. One study shows that dealing with a serious illness such as cancer can make people reassess their life's priorities and get a better sense of who they are.

Ten Things Parents Can Do to Prevent Eating Disorders*

Examine closely your dreams and goals for your children and other loved ones. Are you overemphasizing beauty and body shape?

1. Consider your thoughts, attitudes, and behaviors toward your own body and the way that these beliefs have been shaped by the forces of weightism and sexism. Then educate your children about

   a. the genetic basis for the natural diversity of human body shapes and sizes, and
   b. the nature and ugliness of prejudice.

   Make an effort to maintain positive, healthy attitudes and behaviors. Children learn from the things you say and do!

2. Examine closely your dreams and goals for your children and other loved ones. Are you overemphasizing beauty and body shape?

   • Avoid conveying an attitude which says in effect, "I will like you more if you lose weight, don't eat so much, look more like the slender models in ads, fit into smaller clothes, etc."
   • Decide what you can do and what you can stop doing to reduce the teasing, criticism, blaming, staring, and so on that reinforce the idea that larger or fatter is "bad" and smaller or thinner is "good."

3. Learn about and discuss with your sons and daughters (a) the dangers of trying to alter one's body shape through dieting, (b) the value of moderate exercise for health, and (c) the importance of eating a variety of foods in well-balanced meals consumed at least three times a day.

   • Avoid categorizing foods into "good/safe/no-fat or low-fat" versus "bad/dangerous/fattening."
   • Be a good role model in regard to sensible eating, exercise, and self-acceptance.

4. Make a commitment not to avoid activities (such as swimming, sunbathing, dancing, etc.) simply because they call attention to your weight and shape. Refuse to wear clothes that are uncomfortable or that you don't like but wear simply because they divert attention from your weight or shape.
5. Make a commitment to exercise for the joy of feeling your body move and grow stronger, not to purge fat from your body or to compensate for calories eaten.
6. Practice taking people seriously for what they say, feel, and do, not for how slender or "well put together" they appear.
7. Help children appreciate and resist the ways in which television, magazines, and other media distort the true diversity of human body types and imply that a slender body means power, excitement, popularity, or perfection.
8. Educate boys and girls about various forms of prejudice, including weightism, and help them understand their responsibilities for preventing them.
9. Encourage your children to be active and to enjoy what their bodies can do and feel like. Do not limit their caloric intake unless a physician requests that you do this because of a medical problem.
10. Do whatever you can to promote the self-esteem and self-respect of all of your children in intellectual, athletic, and social endeavors. Give boys and girls the same opportunities and encouragement. Be careful not to suggest that females are less important than males, for example by exempting males from housework or childcare. A well-rounded sense of self and solid self-esteem are perhaps the best antidotes to dieting and disordered eating.

---

* This handout was written by Michael Levine, PhD, and Linda Smolak, PhD. Reproduced with permission from National Eating Disorders Association.

Tips for Kids on Eating Well and Feeling Good About Yourself*

It is no fun to worry all the time about how much you weigh, how much you eat, or whether you are thin. Here are some things you can do.

Be healthy and fit!
Have fun!
Feel good about how you look!

- Eat when you are hungry. Stop eating when you are full.
- All foods can be part of healthy eating. There are no "good" or "bad" foods, so try to eat lots of different foods, including fruits, vegetables, and even sweets sometimes.
- When having a snack try to eat different types. Sometimes raisins might be good, sometimes cheese, sometimes a cookie, sometimes carrot sticks or celery dipped in peanut butter.
- If you are sad or mad or have nothing to do – and you are not really hungry – find something to do other than eating. Often, talking with a friend, or parent, or teacher is helpful.
- Remember: Kids and adults who exercise and stay active are healthier and better able to do what they want to do, no matter what they weigh or how they look.
- Try to find a sport (like basketball or soccer) or an activity (like dancing or karate) that you like and do it! Join a team, join the YMCA, join in with a friend or practice by yourself – Just do it!
- Good health, feeling good about yourself, and having fun go hand in hand. Try out different hobbies, like drawing, reading, playing music, or making things. See what you're good at and enjoy these things.
- Remind yourself that healthy bodies and happy people come in all sizes, and that no one body shape or body size is a healthy one or the right one for everybody.
- Some people believe that fat people are bad, sick, and out of control, while thin people are good, healthy, and in control. This is not true and it is unfair and hurtful.
- Do not tease people about being too fat, too thin, too short, or too tall. And, don't laugh at other people's jokes about fat (or thin) people or short (or tall) people. Teasing is unfair and it hurts.
- If you hear someone (your mom or dad, a sister or a friend) say they are "too fat and need to go on a diet,"

TELL THEM – Please don't, because dieting to lose weight is not healthy – and no fun – for kids or adults.
TELL THEM – You think they look great just the way they are.
TELL THEM – Don't diet; eat a variety of foods and get some exercise.
TELL THEM – Remember, being "thinner" is not the same as being healthier and happier.

- Appreciate yourself for all you are – Everyone should respect and like themselves, enjoy playing and being active, and eat a variety of healthy foods.

---

* Reproduced with permission from National Eating Disorders Association.

Helping Yourself*

Be Your Own Best Resource

Are you concerned about the ways you deal with food? Or how you think about your body? If so, there are numerous ways you can help yourself and begin the practice of healthful living from the "inside out." Here are eight suggestions to get you started.

1. **Daily Check-In: Am I Eating to Feed Emotional Hungers?**

   Sometimes we resort to dieting, binging, excessive exercising, or other unhealthy "body" behaviors as an attempt to deal with psychological or emotional issues. It is all too common for us, especially for women living in a beauty-crazed culture, to transfer everyday life anxieties about jobs, relationships, and unexpected changes onto the shape and size of our bodies. We are under the mistaken impression that our bodies, unlike larger life and relational issues, are under control.

   Have you ever found yourself eating unconsciously or starting a new diet when you are feeling under pressure, upset, lonely, sad, mad, nervous, or bored? Everyone eats for emotional reasons now and then; this is normal. But when binge eating, dieting, or over exercising becomes your main coping strategy, this is a warning signal that you might be headed into unhealthy territory.

   If your stomach is not hungry but your mouth wants food, try to pause and figure out what is really "eating you." Are you angry with someone? An ice-cream cone might taste good and alter your mood in the short run, but it will not solve the real problem.

   Are you hungry for intellectual stimulation? A friend's company? Solitude? Emotional release? Creative expression? The challenge is to stay connected to all of our various appetites — emotional, spiritual, creative, relational, and physical — as we learn to nourish our whole selves.

2. **Practice Body Acceptance**

   This is a courageous and political act, especially in a culture that idealizes certain body sizes and types. Yet no matter how little you eat or how much you exercise, you will not be able to change your basic body type substantially because your optimal adult weight has been predetermined through genetics. Just as your height, hair type, and eye color are inherited, so is your physiologically healthiest adult weight.

   You can influence this to a small degree through healthy diet and exercise. But there is no avoiding the simple truth: Some people are genetically designed to be heavier than others, some to have broader shoulders and bigger bones, others to have a rounder middle. Because it wants to be strong and healthy, your body will work to maintain your "set point" weight.

   Your challenge is to maintain the healthiest body you can and to accept your body as it is meant to be, given your genetic predisposition. It also helps to learn about the ways bodies change throughout the life cycle. Did you know that it is normal and healthy for females to add an extra layer of body fat during puberty?

3. **Resist the Temptation to "Weigh" Your Self-Esteem**

   Sometimes people bond through "fat talk." For example, a fat talk conversation may sound something like this: "I hate my thighs!" "Yeah, I hate mine, too."

   Sometimes people bond by making food choice a moral issue and colluding in what might be called the "morality of orality." For example: "Let's be good and skip dessert" or "Let's be bad and order what we want."

---

* Reproduced with permission from Harvard Eating Disorders Center.

Your worth as a person is not determined by what you eat. Of course, it is important to learn how to eat healthfully, which means thoughtfully eating a variety of foods each day. Just as important, however, is learning how to take yourself seriously for who you are, what you care about, and the things you do to make the world a better place. When you wake up in the morning, affirm that your body is absolutely fine the way it is. What happens next? If "beauty" weren't such a cultural concern, what would you be doing with the energy you now put into changing your appearance?

4. Become Media Literate

This is a powerful means of keeping your body image in perspective. Fashion magazines, TV shows, movies, and ads plastered on billboards and buses all promote an unrealistic beauty standard for women. Realize that less than 5% of the female population is genetically predisposed to look like today's fashion model. This means that 95% of us are left out of the picture — and left feeling fat even if we are at a healthy weight.

Remember that models only look like cover girls after hours of make-up application, airbrushing, and often cosmetic surgery to remove any so-called imperfections (blemishes, skin discolorations, wrinkles, thin or uneven lips, and cellulite, for instance).

Don't let cultural images and messages devour you. If you feel worse about yourself after reading a fashion magazine, cancel your subscription. If you happen to glimpse [at] a magazine sporting a cover girl while standing in the supermarket check-out line, try talking back to the "perfect" image: "Get real! People come in all shapes and sizes."

5. Be Wary of "Magical Thinking"

It is tempting to. It is tempting to buy into the belief that problems will somehow become more manageable if we could only "manage" our bodies, as in the following: "If only I could lose/gain a few pounds, or trim my waist, or firm my thighs, or fit into a smaller size, I would feel/be better."

We get fed this message from a variety of sources, sometimes from friends and family members, often from fashion ads and the media which constantly beckon us to collude in a game called "Change Your Body: Change Your Life." But this game is a no-win endeavor. It is an example of disordered thinking that can set the stage for disordered eating (such as occasional dieting, binging, purging, over exercising, or laxative use) and full-blown eating disorders.

Think of a woman you know who is not buying into the pressure to "weigh" her self-esteem. What is it about her you admire most? Whatever your size, whatever your shape, your life is yours to live today. What are five things you're "weighting" to do until your body is somehow different? For example, are you waiting to wear shorts in the summertime, go swimming in public, fall in love, make a job change, dance, or begin a creative endeavor? The challenge is to stop waiting for our bodies to change to begin. Get rid of your scale and give yourself permission to begin today.

6. Combat "Weightism" in Yourself and in the World

Like racism, "weightism" is an unfair and cruel form of prejudice in which a person is judged or stereotyped not by body color, but by body shape or size. What are your attitudes toward people of differing body sizes and shapes? Do you ever feel better or less than someone because you think your body is superior or inferior to his or hers? How accepting or rejecting are you of your body? Have you or someone you know ever been discriminated against or hurt by comments made about body shape or size? How have you responded?

Think about how passionate you are about other social-justice issues; then bring the same amount of ardor to this one. Practice taking people in general, and women in particular, seriously for what they say and do, not for how slender or "well put together" they appear. Try not to greet friends with comments about how they look. Most importantly, do not tolerate anyone else putting you or another person down based on appearance. Remember, there is no such thing as a "joke" about someone's body.

7. Eat Healthfully. Do Not Diet — Unless You Want to Gain Weight

If you want to live healthfully in your body and stay in your body's healthy weight range, do not diet unless you have a health-related or medical reason to do so under a doctor's supervision. Non-medically supervised dieting leads to weight gain more often than not. If you do not eat enough, your body thinks it is starving and, to stay alive, adjusts its set-point higher and fights to defend its fat.

Many people become overweight due to yo-yo (repeated) dieting and irresponsible weight loss programs. The diet industry is unregulated; most promotions involve misleading advertising. The woman who claims to have lost "100 pounds in three months" likely does not maintain her lower weight over time. In fact, she typically gains back more weight than she initially lost and gains additional health risks from yo-yo dieting; however, she does lose money from the cost of the program and new clothes that will not fit in the long run.

Do not fall for fad diets. If you need to lose weight for health reasons, talk to your internist and ask for a referral to a nutritionist who can help you learn how to eat sensibly and create an all-around healthier lifestyle.

8. If You Think You Have a Problem . . .

Talk to someone you trust such as your doctor, a school counselor or nurse, clergy person, favorite aunt, parent, sibling, or friend. Do not stay in isolation when you are suffering. Instead, find out what kinds of help are available in your community. You deserve to get the help you need and the support of a professional who can "coach" you towards happiness and health.

Helping Your Child*

Please note: For ease in reading, we have used "she" and "her" in the description below even though eating disorders exist in men, women, girls, and boys. This advice is suitable for a child of either gender.

First, remain calm. Approaching a child with an eating disorder can be tricky. Naturally, it is very upsetting to discover that your child might have an eating disorder. If you are panicked, talk to your pediatrician, your partner, or a trustworthy family member or friend. Avoid letting your child overhear you or see you distraught.

Find resources. Before approaching your child, you need to find out what <u>resources</u> are available for your child and for your family, so you can offer her a helpful strategy. Talk with your pediatrician, internist, and school counselor or nurse for information and referrals. You might want to talk to another parent who has been in a similar situation for support and information about available resources. Learn as much about eating disorders as you need to feel like an informed parent and advocate.

Meet with a referred therapist initially – without your child, but with your partner – to learn how the therapist practices and to discuss the best strategy for approaching your child. If you are feeling strong emotions such as anger towards your child, you might want to work with a therapist on your own before approaching her.

Be prepared. Choose a cozy, safe, and private place to talk. Plan ahead for enough time so that you will not be interrupted.

Remember that her eating disorder is her desperate way of trying to cope with underlying problems. Even though you can see how unhealthy and unproductive her disordered eating is, your child may feel it is her only way of dealing with life. That is why it is common for children with eating disorders to be upset or mad if a parent tries to help them. They may fear that you are going to take away their only coping mechanism. A child may deny the problem, be furious that you discovered her secret, or perceive your caring to be a threat.

Raise your concerns, then give your child time and space to think about them. Begin by telling her how much you love her. Tell her that you are not angry; rather, that you are worried and concerned about her well-being. Gently offer some specific observations about her emotional well-being or lack thereof. For example: "You seem unhappy / preoccupied / anxious / fidgety / distant / jumpy / angry, and I'm worried about you."

Speak from your heart, using "I" statements. Avoid naming other people who are also worried about her, such as, "Your aunts, uncles, and grandparents are all worried too." That can feel like an overwhelming gang-up.

Make a few observations about your child's behavior to explain why you think she might have an eating disorder. For example: "I see you skip meals / I watch you run to the bathroom / I hear you talk all the time about being afraid of being fat, what you ate, how much you're going to exercise." Again, your child may feel threatened by your discovery or observations. Give her space to respond; listen to her and ask her to listen to you.

If your child gets upset, mad, or denies having a problem, stay calm. Do not panic or get angry. Do not get into a "Yes, you do / No, I don't" power struggle. Remind your child that parents tell children when they are worried about them.

---

* Reproduced with permission from Harvard Eating Disorders Center.

If she insists that she does not have a problem, that she will and can stop on her own, or that she stopped recently, you can say something like, "You know how it is with alcoholism and denial. The addiction makes it so hard to see you have a serious problem and that you need help. I'm worried that you're trapped in a similar kind of situation. Even though I hear what you're saying, I think you are really struggling, and you need help stopping. I believe in you, and I know you deserve to get help and get better."

Even if your child knows she has an eating disorder, she still may be afraid and resistant to getting help. The illness can lead sufferers to perceive help as very threatening. You may need to approach your child many times before she agrees to get help.

Let your child know that you are her parent, not an expert on eating disorders, and that you will stand by her and help her get the help she needs. It is important to realize that children generally feel safer with their parents in situations like this if they do not think that their parents are talking to everyone about their parenting crisis.

Try to avoid being the adult who tells your child news that she doesn't want to hear. Let the pediatrician be the bearer of hard news, so you can be the supportive parent, such as:

Doctor: "Yes, you have a serious eating disorder, and you might not be able to play sports."

Parent: "I see how upsetting it is for you to hear this. I'm so sorry you have to go through this. But we need to do what Dr. Smith says."

Sometimes it is better not to overwhelm your child with details about a treatment plan until she has had time to absorb the knowledge that you know about her eating disorder. On the other hand, some children feel relieved to learn that their parents have found a good person to help them. Trust your judgment about your child. If she refuses help, gently and firmly tell her that you see how upset or mad she is. Tell her that you see how she wishes that you'd leave her alone (or whatever matches her response to your initial approach), but that you are not going to stop being concerned. Do not get caught up in fighting about what she is or isn't eating.

Find a therapist, preferably one with experience treating eating disorders, and strategize how to get your child the help she needs. If your child is no longer living at home and you have less leverage and she refuses to get help, you might want to say something like, "Even if I can't convince you to get help now, I can't stop caring." That gives you a foot in the door without being too threatening and gives you time to strategize further.

Stay calm and avoid sounding as if your mission is to rescue or cure her. If your child is an adult, remember that she ultimately is the one responsible for getting help; you can't force her.

Eating disorders and disordered eating can be serious physical and psychological problems, but usually not emergencies. However, if your child is rapidly losing weight, not eating at all, fainting, depressed, suicidal, or otherwise in serious danger, get professional help immediately, and say something like, "I don't care if you're mad at me. Parents don't let their children suffer in danger and isolation."

Helping Your Friend*

Please note: For ease in reading, we have used "she" and "her" in the description below even though eating disorders exist in men, women, girls, and boys. This advice is suitable for a child of either gender.

If your friend doesn't admit to having a problem and/or doesn't want help, the best way to approach her is to help her see that she needs assistance. However, you'll need to prepare yourself well since approaching a friend with an eating disorder can be tricky.

Remember that her eating disorder is a desperate way of trying to cope with underlying problems. Even though you can see her disorder as unhealthy and unproductive, your friend may view her eating habits as a lifeline. That is why it is common for someone with an eating disorder to get upset or mad if you try to help her. She may fear that you are going to take away her only coping mechanism. She may deny the problem, be furious that you discovered her secret, or feel threatened by your caring. When you raise your concerns, give your friend time and space to think and respond.

Before approaching your friend, find out about resources for help in your community so that you can offer her a strategy to connect with that help.

You might first seek advice from someone else, like a counselor at school, or perhaps read more about eating disorders. Choose a cozy, safe, and private place to talk. Plan ahead for enough time to talk without being interrupted.

Begin by telling your friend how much you care about her. Next, gently offer some specific observations about her emotional well-being or lack thereof. For example: "You seem unhappy / preoccupied / anxious / fidgety / distant / jumpy / angry, and I'm worried about you." Speak from your heart, using "I" statements. Do not name other people who are also worried about her. That can feel like an overwhelming gang-up.

Then **give your friend a few observations about her behavior** to explain why you think she might have an eating disorder. For example: "I see you skip meals / I watch you run to the bathroom / I hear you talk all the time about being afraid of being fat, what you ate, how much you're going to exercise, etc."

If she gets upset or mad, stay calm. Do not get angry or panic. Do not get into a "Yes, you do / No, I don't" power struggle. Remind her that friends tell friends when they are worried about them.

If she insists that she doesn't have a problem, or that she can stop on her own, you can say something like, "You know how it is with alcoholism and denial. The addiction makes it so hard to see you have a serious problem and that you need help. I'm worried you're trapped in a similar kind of situation. Even though I hear what you're saying, I think you're really struggling and you need help stopping. I believe in you and I know you deserve to get help and get better."

Give your friend information about who can help her. Offer to go with her. It may take more than one approach before she will agree to get help. If she refuses to get help, tell her that you are not going to bug her, but that you are also not going to stop being concerned either. For example: "Even if I can't convince you [to] get help now, I can't stop caring." This gives you a foot in the door without being too threatening.

Stay calm and avoid sounding as if your mission is to rescue or cure her. Eating disorders are serious physical and psychological problems, but they are usually not emergencies. However, if your friend is fainting, suicidal, or otherwise in serious danger, get professional help immediately. These words may help: "I don't care if you're mad at me. Friends don't let friends suffer in danger and isolation."

---

* Reproduced with permission from Harvard Eating Disorders Center.

If your friend is getting help for her eating disorder, stay connected to her the same way you would with any friend. Call her, invite her to do things, hang out, and ask her for advice about your life.

When talking with her about herself, it is usually best to focus on daily life events, on her feelings about herself and her life, and on your concern about her. Do not focus on her eating disorder. Her eating disorder is a sign that other issues are troubling her and a way of trying to deal with those issues. Moreover, most people with eating disorders feel embarrassed about them and feel safer in friendships in which friends do not try to get involved in the details of the disorder.

Avoid all comments - even compliments - about looks, weight, food intake, or clothes. This includes hers, yours, and other people's. Avoid giving her advice on how she could change her behavior. Do not ask a lot of questions about her recovery. Remember that recovery takes time.

Introduction to Section IV: Selected Topics

This section includes contributions that do not fit neatly into any other sections of the volume.

The first contribution is written by Jeffrey Barnett, Lesley Johnston, and Deborah Hillard on the topic of psychotherapist wellness as an ethical imperative. Mental health professionals devote much of their professional lives to promoting their clients' mental health. But the years of training and efforts to provide quality care to clients may be insufficient if clinicians do not pay adequate attention to their own well-being and self-care. This contribution addresses the roles of distress, burnout, impairment, and self-care for mental health clinicians.

In the second contribution, Ron Bonner describes some of the professional and personal challenges that clinicians face who work in correctional centers. Clinician burnout is a high risk in correctional environments. This chapter describes some of the most frequent occupational hazards of working as a mental health provider in prison and provides suggestions for avoiding and treating burnout.

Psychotherapist Wellness As an Ethical Imperative

Jeffrey E. Barnett, Lesley C. Johnston, and Deborah Hillard

Mental health professionals devote much of their professional lives to promoting their clients' mental health. After years of arduous academic and clinical training, they typically dedicate themselves on an ongoing basis to keeping current with the relevant professional literature as well as participating in ongoing continuing education activities in an effort to provide the highest possible quality of care to their clients. But these years of training and ongoing efforts to provide quality care may all be insufficient if clinicians do not pay adequate attention to their own well-being and self-care.

This contribution addresses the roles of distress, burnout, impairment, and self-care for mental health clinicians. As will be illustrated, without adequate attention to these issues and an ongoing proactive program of self-care and wellness promotion, clinicians will find themselves at risk for the very difficulties they work to assist their clients with. This may likely lead to impaired competence, resulting in adverse consequences for clinician and client alike. But with adequate attention to their own wellness, clinicians will be better able to meet their goal of providing high-quality care to their clients. Helpful self-assessment questionnaires to assist you in meeting this goal may be found at the end of this contribution (see pp. 268-269).

DISTRESS AND IMPAIRMENT

The American Heritage Dictionary (1994) defines distress as "pain or suffering of the mind or body; severe psychological strain" (p. 248) and impairment as the noun form of the verb impair: "to diminish in strength, value, or quality" (p. 418). Distress and impairment are different but related concepts. For mental health professionals, the concept of distress focuses on the emotional reactions of the clinician in response to ongoing challenges, stressors, or demands in one's life. Impairment, however, refers to the impact or effect of the distress on the clinician's ability to function effectively. It is generally viewed as "the diminution or deterioration of therapeutic skill and ability due to factors which have sufficiently impacted the personality of the therapist to result in potential clinical incompetence" (Guy, 1987, p. 199).

Mental health professionals experiencing distress do not always become impaired. We each experience stress in our personal and professional lives and at times may manage these stressors quite well. But all mental health professionals are at risk of becoming distressed, and those who are distressed may at times become impaired if the stressors are too great and the clinician's coping resources are not sufficient. Distress and impairment are not dichotomous entities but should be viewed as falling on a continuum where there are progressive changes in symptomatology (Barnett, 1994). Therefore, as Hass and Hall (1991) advise, mental health professionals "should have the self awareness to know when they are functioning poorly and then pursue the options to resolve this problem" (p. 7).

UNDERSTANDING ETHICAL PRACTICE

The ethics codes of the mental health professions are all based upon a series of underlying virtues. These include *beneficence*, the duty to do good and help others; *nonmalfeasance*, the obligation to minimize harm in all actions we take as professionals; *fidelity*, the need to carry out and fulfill our professional obligations to those to whom we provide services; *autonomy*, the goal of promoting the independence of those we serve and not taking any actions that would increase their dependence on us; *justice*, the obligation to afford all individuals the opportunity for equal access to the same high-quality treatment; and *self-care*, the obligation to adequately attend to our own healthy functioning (Beauchamp & Childress, 2001; Thompson, 1990).

Although the first five virtues above are focused on actions by mental health professionals toward those we serve, the sixth virtue, *self-care*, is focused on the mental health professionals themselves. As will be seen, failure to take adequate care of oneself may very likely result in impairment in our ability to effectively implement the other virtues.

The mental health professions' ethics codes uniformly address the importance of actively addressing self-care as a means of fulfilling our professional obligations to help, but not harm, those we serve. The profession of psychology's ethics code, the Ethical Principles of Psychologists and Code of Conduct (American Psychological Association [APA], 2002), Principle A: Beneficence and Nonmaleficence, contains the statement, "Psychologists strive to be aware of the possible effect of their own physical and mental health on their ability to help those with whom they work" (p. 1062). Further, Standard 2.06, Personal Problems and Conflicts, states:

(a) Psychologists refrain from initiating an activity when they know or should know that there is a substantial likelihood that their personal problems will prevent them from performing their work-related activities in a competent manner.

(b) When psychologists become aware of personal problems that may interfere with their performing work-related duties adequately, they take appropriate measures, such as obtaining professional consultation or assistance, and determine whether they should limit, suspend, or terminate their work-related duties. (p. 1063)

Similar guidance is found in the American Counseling Association's Code of Ethics (ACA, 2005) in its standard on Professional Competence, which states in part, "Counselors are alert to the signs of impairment from their own physical, mental, or emotional problems and refrain from offering or providing professional services when such impairment is likely to harm a client or others. They seek assistance for problems that reach the level of professional impairment, and, if necessary, they limit, suspend, or terminate their professional responsibilities until such time it is determined that they may safely resume their work" (p. 9). In addition to addressing these issues similarly, the National Association of Social Workers' Code of Ethics (NASW, 1999) also addresses each social worker's responsibilities regarding impaired colleagues, stating:

(a) Social workers who have direct knowledge of a social work colleague's impairment that is due to personal problems, psychosocial distress, substance abuse, or mental health difficulties and that interferes with practice effectiveness should consult with that colleague when feasible and assist the colleague in taking remedial action.

(b) Social workers who believe that a social work colleague's impairment interferes with practice effectiveness and that the colleague has not taken adequate steps to address the impairment should take action through appropriate channels established by employers, agencies, NASW, licensing and regulatory bodies, and other professional organizations. (pp. 17-18)

THE MENTAL HEALTH PROFESSIONAL AND THE RISK OF IMPAIRMENT

One may wonder why the mental health professions place so much emphasis on addressing distress, impairment, and self-care. After all, mental health professionals are highly educated and well trained in the promotion of mental health. We are seen as experts in assisting others to more effectively cope with stressors and trauma in their lives. As a result, seeing ourselves as at risk for the same difficulties as those we regularly treat might seem inappropriate, and perhaps even insulting. Yet, mental health professionals are people too; susceptible to all the same life challenges and stressors and living with the same genetic predispositions to mental health conditions as nonmental health professionals. Additionally, there are some unique qualities of those who enter the mental health field as well as certain aspects of our professional work that make us especially vulnerable to the effects of distress and impairment. Viewing ourselves as caregivers may make it difficult for us to realize that we too need to take care of ourselves and that we are not immune from distress, mental illness, and stressful life situations. Further, we actually may be at a heightened risk for developing emotional disorders, substance abuse, and other forms of impairment due to the nature of our work (Orr, 1997).

Mental health clinicians regularly work with individuals who do not show signs of improvement, and depending on the work setting and population served, we may work with individuals who suffer from chronic conditions and who experience relapses despite our best efforts, at times including suicidal and homicidal behavior. Pope and Tabachnick's (1993) survey of mental health clinicians found that 97% of clinicians experienced a fear that clients would commit suicide, and over 50% acknowledged that their concerns about clients impacted their eating, sleeping, and concentration.

Psychotherapists also tend to work in relative isolation and may go through long periods of time without contact with colleagues. The very nature of our work requires us to focus on the needs of others, and we may fall into the trap of overlooking our own needs. We often work long hours without immediate feedback, are often "on call," and regularly may be contacted for emergencies and other crises. We also are under the pressure of being seen as experts and may feel the burden of responsibility for others' well-being and lives. We may feel at risk for ethics complaints and malpractice suits by dissatisfied clients and may feel unduly burdened by these pressures. Clinicians may also be affected by changes in their professional work due to managed care, including increased paperwork, reduced compensation, and working more hours. In fact, Sherman and Thelen (1998) found that malpractice claims, restrictions imposed by managed care, and changed work situations are among the work factors that lead to feelings of distress and resultant impairment.

Just who is attracted to a career as a mental health clinician may also be relevant to understanding our risk of distress and impairment. Many individuals are attracted to the mental health professions because of what Guy (1987) refers to as "dysfunctional motivators." These are inappropriate reasons for entering a helping profession, such as a desire to resolve one's own ongoing difficulties and unresolved emotional and interpersonal conflicts; a desire for power, control, and influence over others; and the belief that being a psychotherapist will somehow facilitate healthy living. Available data indicate that mental health clinicians have histories of physical and sexual abuse as children, parental alcoholism, psychiatric hospitalization of a parent, and family dysfunction in far greater numbers than those in other professions and in the general population, lending some credibility to the above-reported insights into many of those who are attracted to service as mental health clinicians (Elliott & Guy, 1993; Pope & Feldman-Summers, 1992).

Racusin, Abramowitz, and Winter (1981) found that alcoholism, child abuse, or both were reported in 50% of the families of psychologists they studied. These researchers also found that 50% of these psychologists reported performing a primary role in parenting in their family of origin, suggesting that these clinicians had taken on the role of caregiver due to absent or inadequate parental figures long before they became mental health professionals. These findings could suggest a possible link between a history of child abuse, alcoholism, or fulfilling parent-type roles in a family of origin and a desire to enter a helping profession (O'Connor, 2001). The mental health professions "allow a continuance of the care taking role as well as the potential for mastery of chaotic environments" (O'Connor, 2001, p. 346) that had also been experienced in childhood. Essentially, a significant portion of mental health clinicians may have been motivated to enter this field at least partially because they are well prepared for it. A traumatic childhood may allow greater identification with the client, and an opportunity to heal old wounds and work as a psychotherapist allows clinicians the opportunity to serve in the familiar caretaker role (O'Connor, 2001).

In addition to the above-mentioned factors that are specific to mental health professionals, clinicians also regularly experience personal life events that increase the level of distress in their lives and place them at further risk of impairment. Such life events include marital or relationship difficulties, death in the family, divorce, physical illness or legal problems for self or family members, and financial problems (DeAngelis, 2002; Freudenberger, 1990). The interaction of our personal histories and vulnerabilities, the very nature of the work we do as mental health professionals, and our ongoing life events and stressors all interact and create a significant vulnerability for clinicians and place us all at risk for distress and impairment.

For those clinicians who work with victims of trauma and abuse, an even greater risk of distress and impairment, in the form of vicarious traumatization, exists. It is not uncommon for clinicians working with trauma survivors to develop Secondary Traumatic Stress Disorder (Figley, 1995). This is a strong emotional reaction that results from the secondary exposure to the traumatic event and holds the great potential to impact the clinician as strongly as if it were lived through personally. The symptoms mirror those of Posttraumatic Stress Disorder and may include intrusive ideation related to the client's disclosures, avoidant responses, physiologic arousal, somatic complaints, distressing emotions, and addictive/compulsive-like behaviors, all of which may lead to impaired functioning by the clinician (Figley, 1995).

Additionally, the chronic nature of many of the stressors experienced by clinicians may lead to the experience of burnout, a general loss of concern, and loss of positive feelings for one's clients to the point where clients receive a substandard quality of care (Raquepaw & Miller, 1989). Freudenberger (1990) describes burnout as resulting in feelings of depersonalization and emotional exhaustion, along with feeling a lack of personal accomplishment and satisfaction. Chronic clients who do not improve, especially challenging clients such as those suffering from personality disorders and those who are suicidal, coupled with restrictive work requirements and demands such as when working within managed care and agencies, often are contributing factors to burnout.

Clinicians experiencing burnout may become less able to attend to the needs of their clients, to process new information, or to respond appropriately to the information. The clinician experiencing burnout may also demonstrate a decrease in problem-solving abilities, interest in their clients, empathy, and cognitive flexibility, all of which may have an impact on the clinician's ability to provide clients with effective treatment.

The modal clinician experiencing burnout is one who is young, is overcommitted, controls little of the treatment outcomes, and does little work in actual psychotherapy. They often work with sexual abuse and rape victims (or other victims of trauma), psychosis, and court-related cases, and they tend to have few growth-oriented clients. Additionally, clinicians who work for agencies, those who are generally inflexible, and those with poorer boundaries are also found to be more at risk for burnout (O'Connor, 2000).

Sanzone and Barnett (1996) reported several negative coping practices that clinicians may engage in that could lead to burnout. Working longer hours to compensate for lost wages due to managed care, cutting the therapy hour to less than 50 minutes, seeing multiple clients back-to-back with no breaks in between, and taking fewer vacations are such signs. Other factors that may contribute to the development of burnout include clinicians attending less to their own personal health needs by getting less sleep, getting less exercise, not maintaining a healthy dietary regimen, and spending less time engaging in pleasurable activities. See the self-assessment questionnaires on pages 268-269 to assess your own risk of burnout.

THE PREVALENCE OF DISTRESS AND IMPAIRMENT

One may wonder just how often clinicians demonstrate these difficulties and if there really is cause for concern. Thoreson, Miller, and Krauskopf (1989) found that of clinicians surveyed, 11% reported recurrent depression, 10% experienced recurrent physical illness, 9% experienced problems with alcohol, and 8% reported either marriage or relationship dissatisfaction, or loneliness in the past year. Further, the authors found that often, two or more of these aspects of distress co-occur, such as with relationship difficulties, loneliness, depression, and alcohol use, compounding the effects of each aspect of distress and greatly increasing the likelihood of professional impairment.

In a national study of psychologists, Guy, Poelstra, and Stark (1989) found nearly three-quarters of those surveyed to acknowledge experiencing distress in the preceding 3 years. More than one-third of this group further reported an awareness of a reduction in quality of client care as a result, and 5% reported that the treatment they provided was "inadequate" as a result of their distress. Further, in a study of psychologists who identify themselves as psychotherapists, Pope, Tabachnick, and Keith-Spiegel (1987) reported that 59.6% of those surveyed acknowledged working when too distressed to be effective.

Many female psychotherapists may be at greater risk for distress and impairment than their male counterparts. Sherman and Thelen (1998) reported that female psychotherapists reported greater amounts of distress and impairment surrounding their work situations than did male colleagues. Several possible explanations are suggested by these authors. First, women may actually experience greater distress and impairment surrounding their work situation, perhaps because of different attitudes toward, beliefs about, and experiences with work between men and women. Women may feel competing pressures to establish themselves professionally and to start a family. For those with families, many are often burdened with more domestic responsibilities than men, needing to expend more emotional and physical energy, and therefore being more vulnerable to emotional exhaustion and distress. Secondly, although men and women could actually experience the same level of distress, women may be more apt to report their experiences than men. Additionally, as increasing numbers of women enter the mental health professions, attention to the competing personal and professional roles of many women will be quite important in their efforts to better manage the distress in their lives and to minimize the risks of impairment.

In a study of psychotherapists' self-report of distress, Duetsch (1985) found that 57% reported problems with depression, 82% described recent relationship difficulties, and 11% reported alcohol abuse problems. In a more recent study of counseling psychologists, Good, Thoreson, and Shaughnessy (1995) found that 20% of the respondents reported daily or almost daily previous use of alcohol, while 16% indicated daily or almost daily use of alcohol at present.

Gilroy, Carroll, and Murra (2002) found that depression is one of the most prevalent symptoms of distress among psychotherapists and that most clinicians report the perception that their depressive symptoms negatively affect their work. Reported symptoms of depression include lack of enjoyment, sadness, memory problems, fatigue, poor concentration, and lack of energy and motivation to do therapeutic work. These symptoms, if left untreated, can easily lead to impairment of professional competence, resulting in harm to clients.

The results of distress left untreated may be devastating for clinicians as well. In one study of mental health clinicians, Pope and Tabachnick (1994) found that 29% of those surveyed acknowledged having felt suicidal, and almost 4% reported having attempted suicide in the past. Additionally, in Deutsch's (1985) study, 2% of those surveyed acknowledged having attempted suicide in the past. Ukens (1995) reports that the Occupational and Safety Hazard Administration (OSHA) lists male psychologists to have the highest suicide rate of any profession.

THE ROLE OF AWARENESS

Because all mental health professionals are at risk of experiencing distress and of developing burnout and impairment, awareness of risk factors and warning signs is greatly important for ensuring competent ethical practice. First, we must each be aware of our own unique signs of distress. Representative examples may include hoping that certain clients do not show up for their sessions, daydreaming or fantasizing about being elsewhere during treatment sessions, ending sessions early, missing or canceling treatment sessions, becoming bored or losing interest in clients' difficulties and what they have to say, becoming easily irritated by clients, feeling increasingly fatigued as the workday proceeds, and prematurely terminating clients' treatment. Such signs of distress may also show up in our personal lives such as in increased impatience and losing one's temper more easily, experiencing changes in mood, impaired sleep, and increased anxiety.

We must also be on guard against the use of negative coping practices such as the use of food, alcohol, and other substances to self-medicate for the distress we are experiencing. Additionally, the use of denial and minimization, avoidance, and isolation should also be avoided. Although they may seem to reduce distress initially, they only tend to compound our difficulties over time, in both our personal and professional lives.

Mental health clinicians should each take a personal inventory (such as those provided on pages 268-269) to become aware of our unique personal warning signs of distress and to ensure that we are not engaging in any negative coping behaviors. It is then important to become aware of the risk factors present in our personal and professional lives. Factors addressed earlier such as a history of trauma or abuse in our family of origin, ongoing relationship difficulties, work with chronic clients who are challenging and demanding, work within an agency or within managed care, and related factors all may place us at greater risk of impairment. It is also crucial to be on guard for signs and symptoms of burnout and vicarious traumatization and take preventive steps so they may be avoided.

Additional risk factors to be aware of and avoid include unrealistic expectations and feeling frequently disappointed in oneself and others, experiencing difficulties setting reasonable limits and ensuring that our boundaries are respected, minimizing or denying the presence of dissatisfaction or difficulties in our life, attending less to personal health needs, and an inability to enjoy previously enjoyable activities. Accepting our vulnerabilities and needs, being honest with ourselves about the stressors in our lives and their potential impact on us, and taking positive action to prevent and effectively respond to distress and impairment are all of vital importance for mental health practitioners.

Finally, Kramen-Kahn (2002) suggests the following 15 questions to determine ones current level of personal self-care. For those not able to respond affirmatively to each one, they provide helpful direction for corrective action in promoting self-care and minimizing the risks for distress, burnout, and impairment. Do you:

1) appear competent and professional?
2) appear warm, caring, and accepting?
3) regularly seek case consultation with another professional while protecting confidentiality.

4) at the end of a stressful day, frequently utilize self-talk to put aside thoughts of clients?

5) maintain a balance between work, family and play?

6) nurture a strong support network of family and friends?

7) use healthy leisure activities as a way of helping yourself relax from work? If work is your whole world, watch out! You do not have a balanced life.

8) often feel renewed and energized by working with clients?

9) develop new interests in your professional work?

10) perceive clients' problems as interesting and look forward to working with clients?

11) maintain objectivity regarding clients' problems?

12) maintain good boundaries with clients, allowing them to take full responsibility for their actions while providing support for change?

13) use personal psychotherapy as a means of maintaining and/or improving your functioning as a psychotherapist?

14) maintain a sense of humor? You can laugh <u>with</u> your clients.

15) act in accordance with legal and ethical standards? (p. 12)

THE ROLE OF SELF-CARE

Each mental health clinician must engage in an ongoing program of self-care. Self-care may include prevention activities, engaging in positive career-sustaining behaviors, and seeking professional assistance. A vital prevention activity for all clinicians is to learn to balance our professional and personal lives and achieve balance among the various activities in our lives. This may include taking regular breaks during the workday; taking time for lunch each day; getting out of the office for breaks periodically; scheduling a variety of clients in our case load and limiting the numbers of especially challenging or high-risk clients we treat at any one time; participating in peer consultation or support groups; taking time off and arranging for colleagues to provide coverage for us so we can forget about work temporarily and not have it interfere with our other activities; getting adequate exercise, diet, and rest; scheduling time for personal activities and time with family and friends; engaging in certain enjoyable activities "just for the fun of it"; practicing meditation and other relaxation types of activities; journaling; participating in hobbies; involvement in civic or professional organizations; travel; and attending to our religious or spiritual side (Barnett, Eiblum, & Blair, 2003).

Self-care is not an indulgence. It is an essential component of prevention of distress, burn-out, and impairment. It should not be considered as something "extra" or "nice to do if you have the time" but as an essential aspect of our professional identities. Without adequate attention to self-care, all clinicians and, eventually, their clients, will suffer. Coster and Schwebel (1997) speak of the goal of ongoing "well-functioning," which refers to a continuing excellence in one's functioning over time as a professional, including when faced with job-related and personal stress. Several themes are identified as important factors for maintaining well-functioning. These include engaging in relationships that provide ongoing peer support, having stable personal relationships in one's life, receiving supervision for challenging cases and when expanding practice into new areas, living a balanced life in which a wide range of personal and professional needs are attended to and hopefully met, obtaining personal psychotherapy at different points in our lives as needed to help us with the ongoing stressors and challenges we all face as well as to help us address the personal attributes that may place us at greater risk of impaired functioning, participating in ongoing continuing education activities to maintain competence as well as to interact with professional colleagues, being mindful of the ultimate costs of being impaired, and utilizing effective coping mechanisms and strategies on an ongoing basis. It has also been found that psychotherapists who engage in religious activities or who have a strong sense of spirituality may hold attitudes that allow distressful feelings and experiences to be viewed as chances for personal growth, lessening the feelings of distress and, ultimately, the chance of impairment. Positive patterns of religious coping appear to be related to benign outcomes from stress, fewer symptoms of psychological distress, and reports of personal psychological and spiritual growth of the clinician (Case, 2001).

Barnett and Sarnel (2003) suggest the following strategies to avoid distress, burnout, and impairment:

1. Make adequate time for yourself.
2. Do things you enjoy.
3. Take care of yourself physically and spiritually.
4. Say NO!
5. Don't isolate yourself.
6. Keep in mind that self-care is a good thing.
7. Watch out for warning signs, such as violating boundaries, self-medicating, wishing patients would not show up, finding it difficult to focus on the task at hand, boredom, fatigue, and missing appointments.
8. Watch out for distress, burnout, and impairment in your colleagues.
9. Conduct periodic distress and impairment self-assessments and seek help when it is needed.
10. Focus on prevention.
11. Make time for self-care!

Additionally, clinicians should seek out their own personal psychotherapy both as a preventive activity and in response to ongoing distress, and hopefully before becoming impaired. Unfortunately, available data suggest that mental health professionals may be more reluctant to seek out mental health services for themselves than members of the general public (Sherman, 1996), possibly due to a perceived stigma involved or a perception of it being incompatible with their role as caregiver and helper. Some clinicians may not seek out professional assistance for their distress and impairment due to a lack of awareness of the need for assistance due to denial or even resulting from the impairment itself. Yet, in one hopeful study, Pope and Tabachnick (1994) found that 84% of psychologists surveyed reported having recently been a client in psychotherapy.

Rather than wait until impairment impacts both themselves and their clients, it is recommended that clinicians seek out psychotherapy for assistance with distressing issues and life situations before they lead to impairment. Overall, psychotherapists report personal psychotherapy to be helpful to them. In Pope and Tabachnick's (1994) study, 85.7% of the psychologists who sought personal psychotherapy reported it to be very helpful or exceptionally helpful. Reported benefits include increased self-awareness or self-knowledge, improved self-esteem, and improved therapeutic skills.

Mental health clinicians must also be cautious about the attitudes and beliefs they hold about themselves and their work. For example, beliefs such as "I should be a model of mental health" and "When a client does not make progress it is my fault" can easily cause distress, especially in neophyte psychotherapists (Truell, 2001). Beliefs such as these create standards that can never be achieved and will tend to undermine the psychotherapist's self-esteem and professional capabilities. They may result in feelings of guilt, sadness, powerlessness, self-anger, and other emotional distress. Avoiding such tendencies is clearly of great importance.

It is also important for clinicians to reduce professional isolation, increase the use of peer support, and receive assistance with challenging clients. The use of peer consultation or support groups may be especially helpful in this regard. They may also be valuable for assisting clinicians to normalize signs of distress and use proactive coping strategies as well as to ensure realistic expectations of ourselves. Additionally, participation in peer consultation or support groups takes the clinician out of the office, provides a break from direct client care, and may serve as a very important source of emotional support when we are coping with both personal and professional challenges.

WHEN DISTRESS AND IMPAIRMENT ARE PRESENT

Those experiencing distress and impairment should consult with a trusted colleague to determine just what actions should be taken to promote self-care and to minimize the risk of harm to clients. Possible actions include personal psychotherapy, ongoing clinical supervision, restricting the scope of one's practice to include reducing the numbers of more challenging or stressful clients, and possibly suspending one's professional duties until impaired competence is remedied and well-functioning has returned. Many professional associations have colleague assistance committees and/or diversion programs to assist impaired practitioners. Such programs typically offer services such as assessment and case monitoring, referral and consultation, and educational workshops. Additionally, some also offer drug and alcohol screening, outreach to students and professionals, and treatment planning (Barnett & Hillard, 2001).

Clinicians also play an important role with distressed and impaired colleagues by seeking them out and discussing our concerns with them. Failure to do so may imply a tacit acceptance of any observed signs of distress and impairment and may further indicate to the colleague a lack of caring that can be interpreted to mean that they are not worth confronting or helping; something that can only lead to further distress and impairment and that will likely encourage continued impaired practice. Further, the ethics codes of each mental health profession highlight the need to confront unethical or potentially harmful behavior by colleagues and makes our colleagues' competence an ethical concern for us as well. Failure to actively address such concerns places their clients at further risk of harm and places the reputation of our professions in greater peril, possibly resulting in others not seeking out much-needed treatment services in the future due to a lack of confidence in mental health professionals.

O'Connor (2001) makes the following suggestions for improving clinicians' approach to impaired colleagues while, at the same time, hopefully protecting the public:

1. Reduce the stigma of distress and impairment. Provide collegial support and assistance and reduce these colleagues' sense of isolation.
2. Increase self-honesty. See that we are all vulnerable to distress and impairment. Be honest about the impact of distress on our competence and seek assistance before impairment results in harm.
3. Establish a professional environment of openness, sharing, peer support, and consultation. In this way we each may function as professional role models to colleagues and those in training.
4. Reduce professional isolation. Engage colleagues and get together outside the office. Participate in your community and nonprofessional relationships and roles.
5. Be a student and a teacher. Continue learning about distress and impairment and promote the training of colleagues and students in these important areas.
6. Reach out to colleagues in distress. Seek out colleagues showing signs of distress and impairment. Utilize our clinical skills to confront them in an effective manner.
7. Take responsibility for our actions and promote appropriate consequences for those who engage in unethical behavior and harm clients.
8. Educate oversight bodies. Be sure they understand the etiology of distress and impairment and the risk factors associated with work with certain client groups.

9. Attend to clients' issues. Remain alert to risk factors with clients and closely monitor our work with those likely to create riskier situations.
10. Work for prevention, diversion, and treatment programs for impaired colleagues. Ensure that oversight boards do not just respond punitively.

ONLINE RESOURCES*

Although it does not replace human contact and relationships, use of the Internet can help reduce isolation as well as provide easy access to a wide range of resources. The following are representative examples of online resources that may be of value to mental health clinicians seeking to prevent, respond to, and effectively manage distress, impairment, and burnout. Additional online resources may be easily found by using any of the many readily available search engines (e.g., Google, Dogpile, AltaVista, Lycos, MetaCrawler, and others) with search words such as burnout, burnout prevention, impairment, professional stress, self-care, stress, and stress management.

Inc.com. This is a website for entrepreneurs and small business owners. It can be accessed at www.inc.com. From there, click on Personal and Professional Growth, and then on Overcoming Burnout. There, readers will find a number of helpful resources. These include a series of personal accounts under the heading of "Been There, Burned Out: Personal Accounts of Entrepreneurial Exhaustion and How to Overcome It," a series of tips for avoiding burnout and achieving balance in one's life titled "Quick Tips: Professional and Personal Benefits of Taking Time to Rejuvenate," and a series of very practical brief articles entitled "Beating Burnout: Tried and True Strategies from Experts and Entrepreneurs."

For a humerous view of burnout prevention go to: http://web.mit.edu/afs/athena.mit.edu/user/w/c/wchuang/News/college/MIT-views.html. Here you will see a helpful list of steps for avoiding burnout along with the frowned on behavior to be avoided that goes along with each recommendation. So whether you want a recipe for preventing burnout or for achieving it, visit this site.

On the website of mentalhealth.about.com you will find a number of resources that address stress and stress management. For examples, there are brief articles such as "How Stressed-Out Are You?," "Women and Stress," "How to Meditate," and "Stress Management: A Review of Principles."

On the website mindtools.com at http://www.mindtools.com/pages/main/newMN_TCS.htm are a number of resources for stress management, burnout prevention, and increasing coping skills. Under the link for Stress Management Techniques are sections on stress management, the use of imagery and relaxation techniques, and a burnout self-test. An additional link on time management skills provides some useful resources as well.

iVillage.com. This is a general website providing a number of brief articles and checklists for personal and professional growth found in its Health and Wellbeing section. From there, click on Stress. There you'll find links to resources such as brief articles on stress and stress management, self-assessment quizzes on stress, and information on burnout. Additionally, in the Quizzes section of the site you can find additional self-assessments on your level of stress as well as on your use of effective stress management strategies.

At www.assessment.com you can find the brief article "13 Signs of Burnout and How to Help You Avoid It." Further, at http://homepage.mac.com/ktmanion/5minuteBurnoutAssessment.htm you will find the "5 Minute Burnout Self Asessment." This useful assessment addresses

---

* Although all websites cited in this contribution were correct at the time of publication, they are subject to change at any time.

issues such as cognitive factors, emotional overload, exhaustion, detachment, and reduced accomplishment.

FriedSocialWorker.com. This is a website that specifically focuses on the needs of mental health professionals and provides numerous helpful resources for the identification, prevention, and treatment of burnout, stress, distress, and impairment. It may be accessed at www.friedsocialworker.com. Available features include self-assessment quizzes for burnout, articles and tip sheets with helpful strategies for prevention and management of burnout, humorous resources for reducing stress and increasing coping, and an e-mail discussion list to provide support and discussion of relevant issues as well as to reduce professional isolation.

APA.org. This is the website of the American Psychological Association (APA) and can be accessed at www.apa.org. Here readers will find a number of relevant articles such as those in the section "Mentoring, Balance, and Self-Care – Especially for Women: A Collection of Articles and Resources." From the APA home page, click on Students, then on APAGS, then on Professional Development, and then on All About Mentoring and Self-Care (or just go to http://www.apa.org/apags/profdev/mentor.html). There readers will find brief articles on relevant topics such as mentoring, self-care, healthy habits, personal and professional identity, healthy relationships, and learning to find balance in one's life. Additionally from the APA, the article "Help for Coping With Stresses of Today's Practice" is found at http://www.apa.org/monitor/mar99/coping.html. It provides useful information about the stresses of being a practicing mental health professional and describes resources available to address them.

SUMMARY

Despite our best intentions, all mental health clinicians are at risk for distress, burnout, and impairment. In addition to risk factors associated with the nature of the work we do, we each bring with us our own personal vulnerabilities and professional blind spots that place us at greater risk for experiencing these difficulties. To be able to provide our clients with the high-quality services they deserve, to find our work gratifying, and to ensure that work-related stress does not adversely impact our personal lives and relationships, we must each engage in an ongoing program of self-care and wellness. This involves self-awareness and monitoring of our ongoing functioning (use the self-assessments provided on pages 268-269); knowledge of our professional and personal blind spots, vulnerabilities, and risk factors; maintaining a balance between work, personal relationships, and leisure time activities; regularly engaging in positive career-sustaining behaviors; minimizing the use of negative coping strategies; and utilizing colleagues and friends for professional and personal support. Such a program of ongoing self-care will help clinicians to prevent burnout and impairment of our competence. We must keep in mind that a focus on ongoing self-care is not an optional activity. It is an essential aspect of each clinician's professional competence and personal wellness.

Self-Assessment Questionnaires

These are not formal tests, and no specific cut-off scores are provided. They are to be used to highlight for you the presence of warning signs and risk factors for distress, burnout, and impairment; some positive coping behaviors to utilize; and some negative coping behaviors to avoid. They are intended to increase awareness and to promote positive action for prevention of, and response to, these potential difficulties that impact all mental health professionals.

Warning Signs Questionnaire for Distress, Burnout, and Impairment

Please check all that apply.

- ❐ I have disturbed sleep, eating, or concentration.
- ❐ I isolate myself from family, friends, and colleagues.
- ❐ I fail to take regularly scheduled breaks.
- ❐ I enjoy my work less than in the past.
- ❐ I find myself bored, disinterested, or easily irritated by clients.
- ❐ I have experienced recent life stresses such as illness, personal loss, relationship difficulties, financial problems, or legal trouble.
- ❐ I feel emotionally exhausted or drained after meeting with certain clients.
- ❐ I've become less empathic and caring toward my clients.
- ❐ I find myself thinking of being elsewhere when working with clients.
- ❐ I am self-medicating, overlooking personal needs, and overlooking my health.
- ❐ I find my work less rewarding and gratifying than in the past.
- ❐ I am feeling depressed, anxious, or agitated frequently.
- ❐ I am enjoying life less than in the past.
- ❐ I find myself experiencing repeated headaches and other physical complaints.

Checklist for Positive Coping Behaviors

Please check all that apply.

- ❐ I take regularly scheduled breaks.
- ❐ I take vacations periodically and *don't* bring work with me.
- ❐ I have friends, hobbies, and interests unrelated to work.
- ❐ I exercise regularly, have a healthy diet, and maintain an appropriate weight.
- ❐ I limit my work hours and caseload.
- ❐ I participate in peer support, clinical supervision, personal psychotherapy, and journaling as preventive strategies.
- ❐ I attend to my religious and spiritual side.
- ❐ I regularly participate in relaxing activities (e.g., meditation, yoga, reading, music).
- ❐ I regularly participate in activities that I enjoy and look forward to.

Checklist for Negative Coping Behaviors to Avoid

Please check all that apply.

- ❐ I self-medicate with alcohol, drugs (including over-the-counter and prescription), and food.
- ❐ I seek emotional support and nurturance from clients.
- ❐ I keep taking on more and try to just work my way through things.
- ❐ I try to squeeze more into the day, get more done, and measure success by how many tasks I complete and by how much I can accomplish in a day.
- ❐ I isolate, avoid colleagues, and minimize the significance of stresses in my life.
- ❐ I know that distress and impairment are for others and don't take seriously the warning signs I experience.
- ❐ I believe that everything will turn out fine just because I say so.

CONTRIBUTORS

Jeffrey E. Barnett, PsyD, is a licensed psychologist in practice in Arnold, Maryland, and is a Distinguished Practitioner in Psychology of the National Academies of Practice. He is also a Full Professor on the Core Faculty at Loyola College in Maryland's graduate programs in Psychology. Dr. Barnett is also a Past President and Past Ethics Chair of the Maryland Psychological Association and is active in the governance of the American Psychological Association. He regularly publishes and presents on ethics, legal, and professional practice issues in psychology. Dr. Barnett also enjoys running and cycling, coaching youth sports, mentoring graduate students and early career psychologists, and spending time with his family. Dr. Barnett may be contacted at 1511 Ritchie Highway, Suite 201, Arnold, MD 21012. E-mail: drjbarnett1@comcast.net

Lesley C. Johnston, MS, is currently a full-time doctoral student in Clinical Psychology at Loyola College in Maryland. Her interests mainly lie in assessing children and adolescents with learning disabilities and working with children with chronic illnesses and their families. She has previously published on ethical decision making in psychology. Ms. Johnston enjoys reading, cooking, and spending time with her husband and friends. She also sets aside specific time each day just for herself to reflect and contemplate about the day's events to keep her healthy and balanced. Ms. Johnston can be contacted at Department of Psychology, Loyola College, 4501 N. Charles Street, Baltimore, MD 21210. E-mail: lcjohnston@loyola.edu

Deborah Hillard, PsyD, is a licensed psychologist practicing in Baltimore, Maryland, at the Johns Hopkins University Faculty and Staff Assistance Program. She is also an Adjunct Instructor at Loyola College in Maryland's graduate program in Psychology and the Johns Hopkins School of Professional Studies in Business and Education. Areas of professional interest include professional ethics and diagnostic assessment. Dr. Hillard also enjoys tap dancing, spending time with her family, and playing with her favorite toy fox terrier, Ripken. Dr. Hillard may be contacted at 550 N. Broadway, Suite 507, Baltimore, MD 21117. E-mail: dhillard@jhu.edu

RESOURCES

American Counseling Association. (2005). *ACA Code of Ethics*. Alexandria, VA: Author.

American Heritage Dictionary (3rd ed.). (1994). New York: Laurel.

American Psychological Association. (2002). Ethical principles of psychologists and code of conduct. *American Psychologist, 57*, 1060-1073.

Barnett, J. E. (1994). Ethical principles and therapist judgment. *Psychotherapy Bulletin, 29*(3), 51-52.

Barnett, J. E., Eiblum, A., & Blair, A. (2003). Got self-care? *The Maryland Psychologist, 48*(4), 9, 11.

Barnett, J. E., & Hillard, D. (2001). Psychologist distress and impairment: The availability, nature, and use of colleague assistance programs for psychologists. *Professional Psychology: Research and Practice, 32*(2), 205-210.

Barnett, J. E., & Sarnel, D. (2003). No time for self-care? Retrieved May 30, 2004, from http://www.division42.org/StEC/articles/transition/no_time.html

Beauchamp, T. L., & Childress, J. F. (2001). *Principles of Biomedical Ethics* (5th ed.). New York: Oxford University Press.

Case, P. W. (2001). Spiritual coping and well-functioning among psychologists. *Journal of Psychology and Theology, 29*(1), 29-54.

Coster, J. S., & Schwebel, M. (1997). Well-functioning in professional psychologists. *Professional Psychology: Research and Practice, 28*(1), 5-13.

DeAngelis, T. (2002). *Normalizing Practitioners' Stress*. Retrieved May 30, 2004, from http://www.apa.org/monitor/julaug02/normalizing.html

Deutsch, C. J. (1985). A survey of therapists' personal problems and treatment. *Professional Psychology: Research and Practice, 16*(2), 305-315.

Elliott, D. M., & Guy, J. D. (1993). Mental health professionals versus non-mental health professionals: Childhood trauma and adult functioning. *Professional Psychology: Research and Practice, 24*(1), 83-90.

Figley, C. R. (1995). *Compassion Fatigue: Secondary Traumatic Stress From Treating the Traumatized*. New York: Bruner/Mazel.

Fruedenberger, H. J. (1990). Hazards of psychotherapeutic practice. *Psychotherapy in Private Practice, 8*(1), 31-34.

Gilroy, P. J., Carroll, L., & Murra, J. (2002). A preliminary survey of counseling psychologists' personal experiences with depression and treatment. *Professional Psychology: Research and Practice, 33*(4), 402-407.

Good, G. E., Thoreson, R. W., & Shaughnessy, P. (1995). Substance use, confrontation of impaired colleagues, and psychological functioning among counseling psychologists: A national survey. *The Counseling Psychologist, 23*(4), 703-721.

Guy, J. D. (1987). *The Personal Life of the Psychotherapist*. New York: Wiley.

Guy, J. D., Poelstra, P. L., & Stark, M. J. (1989). Personal distress and therapeutic effectiveness: National survey of psychologists practicing psychotherapy. *Professional Psychology: Research and Practice, 20*(1), 48-50.

Haas, L. J., & Hall, J. E. (1991). Impaired, unethical, or incompetent? Ethical issues for colleagues and ethics committees. *Register Report, 16*(4), 6-8.

Kramen-Kahn, B. (2002). Do you "walk your talk"? *The Maryland Psychologist, 44*(3), 12.

National Association of Social Workers. (1999). *Code of Ethics*. Washington, DC: Author.

O'Connor, M. E. (2000). Professional stress and burnout: Symptoms, sources, and solutions. *The Maryland Psychologist, 46*(1), 14.

O'Connor, M. E. (2001). On the etiology and effective management of professional distress and impairment among psychologists. *Professional Psychology: Research and Practice, 32*(4), 345-350.

Orr, P. (1997). Psychology impaired? *Professional Psychology: Research and Practice*, 28(3), 293-296.

Pope, K. S., & Feldman-Summers, S. (1992). National survey of psychologists' sexual and physical abuse history and their evaluation of training and competence in these areas. *Professional Psychology: Research and Practice, 23*(3), 353-361.

Pope, K. S., & Tabachnick, B. G. (1993). Therapists' anger, hate, fear, and sexual feelings: National survey of therapist responses, client characteristics, critical events, formal complaints, and training. *Professional Psychology: Research and Practice, 24*(1), 142-152.

Pope, K. S., & Tabachnick, B. G. (1994). Therapists as patients: A national survey of psychologists' experiences, problems, and beliefs. *Professional Psychology: Research and Practice, 25*(3), 247-258.

Pope, K. S., Tabachnick, B. G., & Keith-Spiegel, P. (1987). The beliefs and behaviors of psychologists as therapists. *American Psychologist, 42*, 993-1006.

Racusin, G., Abramowitz, S., & Winter, W. (1981). Becoming a therapist: Family dynamics and career choice. *Professional Psychology: Research and Practice, 12*(2), 271-279.

Raquepaw, J. M., & Miller, R. S. (1989). Psychotherapist burnout: A componential analysis. *Professional Psychology: Research and Practice, 20*(1), 32-36.

Sanzone, M. M., & Barnett, J. E. (1996). Market changes, burnout, and impairment: New challenges for psychologists. *The Maryland Psychologist, 41*(6), 11-12.

Sherman, M. D. (1996). Distress and professional impairment due to mental health problems among psychotherapists. *Clinical Psychology Review, 16*(4), 299-315.

Sherman, M. D., & Thelen, M. H. (1998). Distress and professional impairment among psychologists in clinical practice. *Professional Psychology: Research and Practice, 29*(1), 79-85.

Thompson, A. (1990). *Guide to Ethical Practice in Psychotherapy*. New York: Wiley.

Thoreson, R. W., Miller, M., & Krauskopf, C. J. (1989). The distressed psychologist: Prevalence and treatment considerations. *Professional Psychology: Research and Practice, 20*(3), 153-158.

Truell, R. (2001). The stresses of learning counseling: Six recent graduates comment on their personal experience of learning counseling and what can be done to reduce associated harm. *Counseling Psychology Quarterly, 14*(1), 67-89.

Ukens, C. (1995). The tragic truth. *Drug Topics, 139*, 66-74.

Ethical and Professional Issues for Mental Health Providers in Corrections*

Ron Bonner

Saakvitne (2002) outlined common pitfalls of being a psychotherapist and suggested methods either to prevent these occupational hazards from happening or to resolve them. As one examines various workplaces for mental health providers, it is apparent that unique occupational hazards may be found. Working in corrections is perhaps one of the most difficult workplaces for clinicians, presenting multiple tasks and challenges.

There are, no doubt, attractive benefits to joining a correctional environment (i.e., prison) as a clinician. The job provides opportunities for multiple tasks, from providing direct clinical services to inmates, to training, to providing Employee Assistance Program (EAP) services for staff members. In addition, mental health clinicians direct specialized programs, such as for suicide prevention, drug treatment, criminal lifestyle, hostage negotiation, and employee crisis management. Altruistic value is found in this work as the mental health provider is in the helping role to an underserved population with multiple life and mental health dilemmas. The opportunity to provide these services in a controlled and stable environment allows for service consistency, compliance, and continuity of care, as well as opportunities for behavioral management programs facilitated by the structure and controls of a correctional environment. For researchers, the correctional environment is uniquely suited for longitudinal investigations of large, stable populations over time. Finally, the benefit package for mental health providers in corrections often exceeds those found for work in community agencies and may include higher salaries, good health and life insurance, funding for continuing professional education, a greater number of days for personal and sick leave, and early retirement. These benefits vary, of course, across different systems (e.g., county, state, federal).

Mental health professionals who work in a correctional environment also face a number of professional and personal challenges, which, if left unaddressed, can hurt the clinician as well as his or her profession. The purpose of this contribution is to outline some of the most frequent occupational hazards of working as a mental health provider in prison and to provide suggestions for avoiding and treating burnout.

---

* The views expressed in this contribution are solely those of this author and do not necessarily reflect the past or current views or opinions of any of his institutional or organizational affiliations.

I want to thank Dr. Jim Davison, Pastor Doug Schader, Ms. Lisa Eddinger, Mr. Dennis Hammond, and Ms. Denielle Thomas who daily make this road easier and keep my soul from burning out. In addition, recognition and appreciation are expressed to Marc Lovecchio and Mike Zicolello who have been exceptionally strong advocates for staff by doing their very best to make the wrongs right or at least better. And to the many unnamed staff who have been seen as the "outsiders" or losers, you all have been a great inspiration to me, showing that in spite of the pain and alienation, you have come together in strength, perseverance, and solidarity. Finally, my deep respect and appreciation are expressed to Warden Mike Zenk and Associate Warden Tom Szulanczyk, true gentlemen who for me have risen to the very top of outstanding leadership, knowing how to run a good prison, working toward peace, and living the golden rule of treating others with respect and dignity.

It should be noted that the sources for this contribution come from consultations with colleagues, personal experiences, and a very limited research literature. As a result, such material may not always be generalizable to specific institutions or correctional systems. Wright (1994), for example, outlined a progressive prison leadership model, involving participatory management, emphasis on employee relationships, sensitivity to staff and inmates, and the supervisor serving as a good role model of a well-balanced, correctional worker. Although this ideal approach is practiced in some prisons, it is still unfortunately lacking for many settings. As one envisions the future direction of corrections, it is strongly hoped that such principles will become the norm and that much more research will be done to eliminate many of these hazards and greatly reduce the risk of burnout for mental health clinicians.

CHALLENGES OF THE CORRECTIONAL SYSTEM

Paramilitary Environment

In a correctional setting, authority is traditionally unilateral, with a clearly delineated chain of command (Van Voorhis, Braswell, & Lester, 1997). The warden is considered ruler and final decisionmaker. The nature of this environment is foreign to most mental health professionals, who prefer a democratic, participatory management style. Mental health clinicians can often be influenced or pressured by those higher up in the chain of command to make decisions that are system-friendly but not necessarily clinically sound. Efforts to operate under a collegial, team model may be met with resistance, if not punitive measures. The mental health provider will need to adjust to this environment in order to succeed, while still finding a way to assert clinical principles in a system-respectful manner, when possible, with minimal tension.

We Versus They

There is an overriding belief in many correctional facilities that inmates are the "bad guys" and staff are the "good guys" (Wright, 1994). This "we versus they" philosophy creates an unnecessary tension between inmates and staff which can break down communications, intelligence gathering, and overall inmate management. Respect begets respect in prison. Although boundaries are necessary, clinicians are more prone to see similarities and differences among and between inmates and staff and are more likely to view all persons with human compassion, while at the same time targeting problematic behaviors. The clinician's role is that of a helper, which many nonclinical staff members may not understand or may resent. The therapist must be able to operate in the prison as it is, while subscribing to humanistic and ethical principles in the treatment of both inmates and staff.

Treatment Model Versus Punishment Model

Van Voorhis et al. (1997) present an overview of the history and use of the treatment and punishment models in corrections. The punishment model of corrections views inmates as incorrigible and the purpose of the prison simply to secure and incapacitate inmates. It is best reflected in recent political messages of "getting tough" on crime. The treatment model, on the other hand, views inmates as a diverse population in which a number of inmates are capable of change and rehabilitation. Mental health treatment, counseling, and lifestyle programs are viewed as an integral part of inmate confinement and correcting criminal behavior.

Mental health providers have been trained in a wide array of interpersonal, dynamic, cognitive, pharmacological, and behavioral therapies as well as skill training to facilitate behavior change. Since the Crime Control Act of 1987, prisons have come to be warehouses for drug offenders, who are confined and incapacitated for many, many years. Although treatment programs do exist, the primary mission these days of many correctional facilities is to prevent escape and control inmates. The Rehabilitation Movement of the 1970s is gone. This paradigm shift can be very difficult for clinicians to accept because of their training, personal values, and professional ethics. It can be very difficult for a clinician to practice mental health care in an environment that is punitive and control driven. Inherent conflicts are present for clinicians who develop treatment plans that may be inconsistent or at odds with the overriding punishment model.

Treat All Inmates the Same

There is widespread belief in many correctional systems that inmates are all the same in terms of character, motives, and needs (e.g., all manipulators) (Allen & Bosta, 1981; American Correctional Association, 1992). Generally, the "treat all inmates the same" approach works to ensure consistency, firmness, and fairness for all inmates in the institution. The drawback to this approach is, however, the fact that all inmates are not the same, but vary in personality, lifestyle, strengths and weaknesses, and needs. Prisons have become the community mental health center for inmates with special needs, mental illnesses, and substance abuse (Harrington, 1999; Lunney, 2000). Ideally, different management approaches should be taken with different inmates. Many customary correctional procedures will be counterproductive—for example, with mentally ill inmates (e.g., placement in Segregation)—and for mental health purposes there must be flexibility to accommodate such needs. Mental health clinicians in prison spend a great deal of time assessing and identifying special needs inmates (Bonner, 2001b). There must be procedures to facilitate their adjustment; otherwise our work is futile. It can be extremely frustrating for the clinician to see correctional procedures actually lead to deterioration in special needs inmates.

Manipulation and Countertransference

Due to their character makeup, learning experiences, and the facility's reward system, many inmates manipulate the system to obtain secondary gains or special treatment (Allen & Bosta, 1981; American Correctional Association, 1992). Many clinicians operate from an honesty assumption about self-report. However, our training in objective personality scales that identify faking good or faking bad profiles teaches us that a person's response may be motivated by a number of different dynamics. Many mental health providers in prisons find themselves in situations in which an inmate is taking advantage of a situation and trying to obtain special treatment. This often comes in the form of exaggeration or production of mental health symptoms or self-destructive behaviors. When the provider realizes this has happened, it is not unusual for him or her to have a countertransference reaction with anger and ultimately rejection or avoidance of the behavior as well as the person. It goes without saying that this can be countertherapeutic and, in fact, may reinforce and increase the "manipulative" behavior (Bonner, 2001a). This is particularly a problem when an inmate's behavior is self-mutilation. Mental health clinicians and all correctional workers would improve inmate management by targeting behavior on some level as an effort to solve a problem in which an effective solution has yet to be found. A problem-solving approach avoids personalizing the behavior and leads to a study of the motives of the person's behavior and other possible solutions that might better solve the problem (Rich & Bonner, 2004). The wise words of an exceptional prison psychologist mentor, Dr. Al Smith (personal communication, U.S. Penitentiary, Lewisburg, PA, 1988), summarize the struggle: "The first biggest mistake you can make is to believe what an inmate tells you; and the second biggest mistake is to not believe what an inmate tells you."

Legal/Policy Directives and Staff Resources

Clinicians quickly learn that correctional mental health services are outlined in detail, usually based on legal precedence. The National Prisoner Rights Association, for example, has played a major role in advocating and litigating prison reform (Wright, 1994). Most positive change in corrections has come about because of inmate litigation. By policy, most correctional settings must conduct intakes on all inmates coming into the institution, complete 30-day mental status reviews for inmates held in Segregation, provide psychological and psychiatric treatment for mentally ill inmates, and provide drug treatment services for all inmates with substance abuse. However, with the increasing budget cuts and cost containment, mental health departments in prisons are often poorly staffed and cannot adequately complete the services required by policy and the law. This often leads to burnout for the clinician as well as the tendency to take shortcuts, and to the production of much paperwork with little clinical interaction. Unfortunately, no resource compass exists to identify which services can be reasonably expected for a given staffing level. This is probably intentional, as such a guideline would ultimately place the responsibility on the institution for not complying with legal directives and policy standards as the result of poor staffing.

Dual Roles and Definition of "Correctional Worker"

Some correctional systems view all employees, including professional staff, as "correctional workers" first. What this basically means is that security is everyone's responsibility, and all staff members are responsible to respond to security compromises or emergencies. Although, at first glance, this position may seem reasonable and promote a "team spirit," it is often taken out of context or to the extreme by using mental health clinicians to perform routine correctional officer responsibilities to save overtime and the hiring of more officers. So the mental health providers, for example, may find themselves working as a housing unit officer, with duties of supervising 150 inmates, conducting inmate counts, performing pat searches of inmates, and searching cells for contraband, to cover that vacated position. It goes without saying that this use of the "correctional worker"-first philosophy creates ethical dual role conflicts, not to mention a negative impact on mental health job duties, which are already minimized due to low staffing levels.

Type A Personality and the Mental Health Clinician

Corrections is a competitive business in which many levels of staff compete vigorously to move up the ladder. According to Wright (1994), "Where upward mobility dominates, approval replaces the group momentum and competition rather than cooperation becomes the norm (p. 63)." In this writer's experience, the business also seems to attract many nonclinical, highly driven, competitive, controlling individuals who can easily become angered when their control weakens. Under the punishment model, prison management is simply about the security and control of inmates. In working with employees in the employee assistance program, for example, it is apparent that many employees (primarily nonclinical) make corrections their first priority in life and expect to make multiple moves to be promoted. Anger, alcohol abuse, depression, and relationship problems are commonly seen in these employees. It is not uncommon for a warden, for example, to have worked at 15 or more different institutions across a state or the country. Such actions often take their toll on spouses, children, and family life. Mental health providers as a whole do not fit this model of a correctional worker because relationships are vitally important personally and professionally and self-balance is a primary goal. This difference between clinicians and other employees is sometimes mistakenly taken for lack of loyalty, motivation, or enthusiasm for the work. The provider must in time learn a very critical balancing act to maintain his or her wholeness and connectedness and serve as a role model for other staff to consider. On the positive side, the clinician's personality is often seen and appreciated as a source of calm and strength in the midst of emergencies and crises.

Ethical Compromises and the System

Weinberger and Screenivasan (1994) described the ethical and professional conflicts of a correctional psychologist. Some of the common ethical dilemmas include inmate (patient) confidentiality, clinical decision making, dual role duties, and informed consent. Perhaps the hardest struggle for the mental health clinician is to assert the ethical conflict to the administration, yet somehow try to avoid the perception of not being a "team player." It does not take much in the way of reporting a violation for one to be labeled "disloyal" to the warden and institution. Even providing direct mental health services to staff members with personal or disciplinary problems can be met with scorn, as one criticism illustrated: "He is defending and taking care of a bunch of losers . . . not loyal to this warden."

Weinberger and Screenivasan (1994) provided several case vignettes to illustrate specific ethical conflicts in prison for mental health workers. One of these will be discussed to demonstrate the ethical challenges: A clinician receives a call from the captain, directing him to fill a correctional officer post in a housing unit due to a shortage of correctional officers. In this role, the clinician will be responsible for supervising all inmates in the unit, "pat-search" inmates in the unit for contraband, and conduct regular scheduled counts. Policy at this institution, like many other facilities, states that clinicians are only to be used as officers in "emergency" situations.

The clinician now is in a bind. On the one hand, the therapist can bring these concerns to the attention of administrators. He can report that the situation is not a true emergency, presents dual role ethical conflicts, interferes with the professional role of being a mental health care provider, destroys his therapeutic image, and finally takes away one clinician, among few or none, to provide mental health service responsibilities. On the other hand, asserting these concerns to the captain or other administrators may be met with scorn, with their seeing the clinician as "not a team player" and "too good" for completing correctional responsibilities. The clinician then will likely suffer alienation, loss or respect, loss of credibility, and loss of cooperation in the provision of mental health services in the institution. This dilemma may be resolved if clinicians in general (but not one clinician alone) appeal to a higher authority regarding the implementation of policy regarding clinician responsibilities and if the organization leaders are encouraged to guide administrators in following policy directives and respecting the professional ethics of the mental health provider.

Employee Assistance Program, Dual Roles, and Confidentiality

Many prisons use institution mental health professionals to provide Employee Assistance Program (EAP) services to staff members (Cornelius, 1994). In addition to the previously noted staffing deficiencies and time constraints, this role is often experienced as "uncomfortable" for the clinician who works day to day beside the employee as a coworker or colleague. In addition, supervisors and administrators are often in a position where they desire personal information about employees that relate to job performance or conduct. This is a very delicate balance for the clinician, because obviously the employee's consent must be given for EAP services, and the possibility exists that such information may not be used in the best interest of the employee. For example, managers sometimes will ask an EAP counselor "How is the employee doing? What do we need to know?" With a signed release of information, the clinician may briefly describe the employee's struggles, any work-related issues, stress, or depression. Certain managers or administrators may then announce that the employee needs a "fitness for duty" evaluation, cannot work in a specific area of the institution, or require the employee to get a letter from his or her physician stating he or she is "stable" and "capable of work." Also, it is not uncommon for an administrator to pressure a clinician to give "off the record" insight and guidance on how to manage a troubled employee. In one instance, a colleague reported that an administrator requested that the clinician give the names of staff members receiving Employee Assistance Program services. Sometimes when staff members are discovered to be in treatment or on medication, they may inappropriately be removed from duty; as one administrator emphasized, "Not gonna have anyone on psycho drugs in my institution." Again, the ethical requirement of confidentiality must be asserted even with the possibility that administration will see this as a challenge to authority and the clinician will once again be labeled "disloyal." In addition, with some of these possible examples, the mental health provider may be bound by his or her professional and correctional code of ethics to report these violations. It is no wonder many staff members are paranoid and hesitant to seek EAP services. Fortunately, many systems now offer EAP services to staff by contract through outside agencies, taking institution staff out of the picture.

365 Days a Year, 24 Hours a Day

The prison never closes, and the clinician is expected to be on call for perceived mental health emergencies 365 days a year, 24 hours a day. If a department has only two mental health clinicians, then each one would take on-call duties 50% of the year. Although many times the cases can be easily handled on the phone, sometimes it is the expectation that the provider will come into the institution or be met with blame and shame should the problem appear to develop into a poor outcome. Pagers, cell phones, midnight calls, and the constant anticipation of getting a call all combine to create "noise" and pressure on the clinician's life. This stress not only impacts the clinician but also often negatively impacts his or her family. The prison mental health provider must be willing to accept this unpaid duty and find a way to still maintain balance and peace.

Who Is the Client?

Therapists will quickly learn in working in corrections that the client may be the administration, fellow employees, inmates, or a combination of them. Clinical decision making certainly does not occur in a vacuum and often is influenced by any of the above "clients." Mental health providers are sometimes pressured to find inmates "crazy" (particularly high-management, behavioral cases) so they can be moved to another institution. One extreme example comes to mind in which a clinician's evaluation report was changed significantly by a nonclinical, administrative staff member to make the inmate seem more psychotic and in need of involuntary hospitalization. Efforts to correct this staff member's action were met with avoidance and the response "just let it go," to threats of retaliation, all the way up the chain of command. The struggle in all of this for the clinician is to try to accommodate to the different clients' needs while maintaining integrity as a professional. The provider must have a clear picture of what requests or actions would be a direct violation of the code of ethics or licensure laws and be willing to stand up when a conflict arises, in spite of the direct and subtle consequences one may face in the system.

Environmental Conditions and Sensory Deprivation

Perhaps no greater risk factor has been associated with inmate mental breakdown and suicide than locked-down, sensory-deprived, isolated housing (Bonner, 2000; Toch, 1992). Terms to describe such housing vary in niceness and political correctness to include Special Housing Unit, Segregation, Protective Custody, Drunk Tank, Bullpen, Restricted Management Unit, and Special Management Unit. The bottom line for inmates is that such places simply refer to the "Hole." The "Hole" is devoid of social contact and stimulation, where inmates are locked down at least 23 hours a day in a small cell with heavy metal doors and a window to the outdoors which is often fogged or covered to prohibit sight to the outdoors and prohibit direct sunshine from coming in. The environment is sterile, often poorly lit, with sometimes a deadening silence or deafening noise of loud yells and door banging by an upset inmate.

For up to 5 days a week, due to legal dictates, inmates are provided "outdoor" recreation which amounts to an hour a day in a kennel-like structure with multiple recreation "pens." The rest of the time the inmate is trapped in a very small, sensory-deprived cell with little staff or inmate peer interaction. Although no doubt some inmates are so dangerous that some of such controls are necessary (i.e., SuperMax Control Units), the majority of inmates in the "Hole" are there for other reasons, such as minor infractions, being the victim of an assault, intoxication, classification (security and custody level scoring), captain's review (review of histories and previous institutional adjustment of incoming inmates), protective custody, fear of open population, or waiting for bed space in general population after arrival. Unfortunately, many mentally ill and special needs inmates end up in the "Hole" as the result of minor disciplinary infractions, which often come about because of an inability to regulate themselves for every rule or regulation, or problems with their psychotropic medication. This placement is a travesty, as these individuals are at high risk for breakdown already, and the "Hole" conditions have been shown to cause mental breakdown, depression, and, according to the courts, lead to a "morbid state of mind" which can be the cause of an inmate taking his or her life (Lee, 2002; O'Leary, 1989). The liberal use of the "Hole" runs counter to everything mental health clinicians have been taught, flies in the face of civil rights and humane treatment, and without a doubt is perhaps the most troubling part of working in mental health in the correctional system.

STRESS OF THE WORKPLACE, INSTITUTIONALIZATION, AND BURNOUT

Correctional work is highly stressful for many of the reasons discussed above (Cornelius, 1994). Inmates are often upset and angry over their confinement, particularly with the extreme sentences they have as a product of the "War on Drugs" and the Sentencing Reform Act. The Sentencing Reform Act at the federal level eliminated parole boards, reduced most "good time," and placed mandatory minimum sentences on various crimes (Alexander & Pratsinak, 2002). The drug war of recent years involves society's and law enforcement's view that drug use and trafficking are the major causes of most crimes and need to be dealt with in a harsh manner. As part of this war, federal antidrug laws were issued in 1988 which require minimum sentences for possession or distribution of specific street drugs.

There is an overall mood of negativity in prison. The fact that options for parole boards and "good time" have been eliminated or reduced for inmates causes many of them to have little hope for the future. These conditions make the work of a mental health provider extremely difficult, as they try to build prosocial skills and future orientation in the midst of negativity and despair. Staff members, too, sometimes can take on this negativity in dealing with inmates as well as with the work conditions of low number of staff, shift work, and authoritarian management. They frequently develop a "FI-WGAS" (F--- it, who gives a s---) attitude. Employees often become hardened and institutionalized, finding their only connection is to the job and other employees who are part of the system. Employees are at risk for abusing alcohol and losing their priorities, including their relationships with family members and friends outside the system. Divorce is quite common among correctional workers. Finally, these risks often add up for the employee, in which he or she feels alone with only the prison and its associates existing in the person's life.

The mental health clinician who works in a prison is especially prone to these struggles and eventual burnout (Grosch & Olsen, 1995). Freudenberger (1980) described burnout as charisma and commitment being replaced by exhaustion, fatigue, and psychosomatic ailments. Burnout was viewed as a risk experienced by the dedicated and highly committed clinicians who struggle with inner pressure to accomplish and succeed, while at the same time experiencing intense external pressure to serve the needs of people who suffer from overwhelming problems.

In terms of systemic burnout, Daniels and Rogers (1981) summarized a researcher's findings as follows:

I am forced by the weight of my research to conclude the problem is best understood in terms of social situational sources of job related stress. The prevalence of the phenomena and the range of seemingly desperate professionals who are affected by it suggest that the search for causes is better directed away from the unending cycle of identifying "bad people" and towards uncovering the operational and structural characteristics in the "bad situations" where many good people function. (p. 233)

To expand this analysis, the multimodal B.A.S.I.C. I.D. scheme of Arnold Lazarus (1995) illustrates that burnout is a transactional, multisystem process that is defined, determined, and maintained by some transaction of the following systems: **B**ehavior, **A**ffect, **S**ensations, **I**mages, **C**ognitions, **I**nterpersonal Systems, and **D**rugs (addiction, physiology, genetics). A BASIC ID analysis of prison burnout in mental health clinicians is presented on page 285. This analysis may be used by the mental health clinician to help determine if he or she or his or her colleague might be suffering burnout. Getting help then is simply applying relevant interventions for each modality of burnout.

Case Example

To illustrate the development and treatment of a burned-out correctional mental health clinician, the following hypothetical case vignette is provided:

A 48-year-old, male mental health clinician has worked in several correctional systems for many years under a number of administrations. Although he has periodically suffered the normal adjustment struggles of a mental health clinician in prison, he has managed to work exceptionally well with inmates and employees who have looked up to him as a strong resource for support and assistance. He has regularly been recognized as an excellent mental health clinician by outstanding performance evaluations and numerous performance awards. His family life has been very good with strong bonds between him and his wife and children. He is a proud husband, father, and clinician who has been able to share energy, compassion, wisdom, and humor with many others. He has felt good about who he was and what he did. Over the last 2 years, under a new administration, this clinician has experienced much stress, anxiety, and finally burnout alongside his fellow coworkers. Under this administration, employees have been constantly criticized and belittled and treated by the philosophy: "Either you are with me or against me, and if you are against me you can find a new zip code." During this time, employees who have spoken out or been perceived as "disloyal" have been met with retaliatory investigations and unfair discipline. Inmates have come to be seen as the "bad guys" in which "The more I have in Segregation the better. . . . I'll lock 'em all up."

The work environment is hostile and anxious with numerous employees coming to the mental health clinicians, including this clinician, through the Employee Assistance Program for guidance, support, and direction in coping with an unpredictable, paranoid atmosphere. This clinician also has experienced a number of professional attacks, including his decisions about starting or stopping suicide watches ("He wants something to happen, so it's on me!"), accusations about being disloyal and helping "losers," pressure to violate the confidentiality of the Employee Assistance Program by being asked for names of employees involved, threats that if staff are found to be on "psychodrugs" they will be out of the institution (ironically, an estimated 15% of the staff all the way up the chain of command were on antianxiety and antidepressant medication for severe symptoms of workplace stress), and actually changing a mental health report of the clinician on a highly political, difficult inmate management case so that the inmate appeared more psychotic and in need of involuntary hospitalization. The clinician believes one of the administrators is impaired mentally and tries to bring these concerns to the attention of other administrators in the system who respond with avoidance, statements such as "Just let it go," and actual indirect threats of retaliation if the issues are pushed.

The clinician in time becomes hypervigilant, anxious, paranoid, unsure whom to trust in the system, and preoccupied with the work conditions and suffering of numerous staff. He feels exhausted, emotionally drained, alienated from others, and shunned by various administrators. He has trouble sleeping and lies awake at night ruminating about the work conditions and his helplessness in the situation. He even questions his reality contact and if he has misperceived or imagined what is happening around him. The clinician experiences an overwhelming sense of despair, withdraws from his family, and is unable to concentrate or stop his mind from racing about these work conditions.

Due to physical and emotional discomfort and chest pains, the clinician seeks assistance from his family doctor, who finds his blood pressure very high and mood very tense, and to get his attention asks the clinician if he "wants to have a heart attack." He starts him on some medication and also makes a referral to a psychiatrist who diagnoses the clinician with Major Depression and Features of Posttraumatic Stress Disorder. He is started on a medication regimen which, after about 4 weeks, starts to reduce some of the symptoms. The clinician all along reaches out to a wonderfully supportive and inspiring colleague who is in the same situation, who reassures him he is grounded in reality, empathizes with his pain, and encourages the clinician to work together with him to try to remedy the situation. In time, the clinician's mood starts to improve, daily functioning improves, and he starts to repair the broken parts of his life, including normalizing his reaction to the hostile work environment, getting counsel on viable responses to try to improve the work environment, prioritizing family life, reaching out to God and the church, sharing more social events with friends and family, planning a number of wonderful vacations for his family and himself, and eventually accepting the injustice of the system, knowing all that could be done has been done. As this recovery unfolds, the clinician ultimately still does not discover justice or direct solutions to the problem, has to accept the reality that things are the way they are and that he has no control in the situation, and finally ironically learns that some of the problems will go away because the administrators are actually getting promotions to other settings!

The above case example demonstrates the multisystem nature of burnout, initiated by an accumulation of workplace stressors and aversive events. In time, the clinician loses his spirit and energy, becomes emotionally and physically exhausted, and becomes stuck in a self-defeating process of depression and agitation. In terms of system modalities, this case may be analyzed under the B.A.S.I.C. I.D. system as follows:

Behavior:	familial and social withdrawal, irritability and short temper, ineffective problem solving
Affect:	depression, anxiety, paranoia, fear, despair
Sensations:	chest pains, exhaustion, muscle tension, constant feeling of being "on edge"
Images:	the system does not work, I am a helpless victim, no one in authority cares or believes me, exposing the truth will result in retaliation, I am all alone and my supervisors and colleagues are shunning me, this is so wrong, and there is nothing I can do
Cognitions:	hypervigilance, obsessions and ruminations about the workplace situation and the injustice and unfairness of it all, belief I can't trust anyone in authority (as they are covering up), belief many staff are suffering and there is nothing I can do, belief there is so much wrong and out of sorts, I must be imagining it, belief certain people are out to get me
Interpersonal Systems:	withdrawal from others, professional and social alienation at work, just wanting to be alone, paranoia
Drugs:	muscle tension, chest pain, sleeplessness, sensation of nerves tingling/twitching, increased use of caffeine, increased use of over-the-counter medication for constant headaches

As the case description notes, treatment and recovery also involve a multimethod process whereby a variety of social, psychological, psychiatric, spiritual, family, and lifestyle interventions take place. These methods directly or indirectly target each system modality as it uniquely exists.

COPING WITH THE HAZARDS OF BEING A CORRECTIONAL MENTAL HEALTH PROVIDER

Recognition

Recognizing the many hazards and potential pitfalls in correctional mental health care is, of course, the first step in preparing for and learning to avoid or cope with these challenges. This requires an early self-inventory of professional values and ethics and a determination whether you want and can muster the fortitude to work as a career mental health provider in prison. Usually after the first 2 years of experience, the clinician will know whether the work is for him or her. If the answer is no, it is strongly advised that the provider "get out" and find another position, as the issues and struggles will only increase. You need to realize you have given a lot of your life to pursue the study, practice, and profession of mental health care. Your basic desire has been to help people with scientifically supported therapies. You should not waste your profession and this basic value to settle for other secondary benefits the system may provide. Numerous staff members have approached employee assistance services when they were miserable in their jobs and feeling "stuck" due to the time put in and remaining years until retirement. Many staff members simply live for retirement and miss all the wonderful family, spiritual, social, and recreational experiences along the way. Clinicians especially should be in tune with these issues and embellish a profession that contributes to the well-being of others and society, and one which gives back so much more. They need to be proud of their field and not compromise the basic tenets and ethical principles of their profession.

Outside Collegial Support

To maintain a healthy sense of balance and perspective, correctional mental health providers should actively seek support and dialogue with clinicians working in the outside community. In addition, if time is available, the clinician may want to get involved in a part-time clinical practice to keep his or her clinical skills sharp for mainstream clientele, or participate in teaching or research at a local university to keep knowledge and investigative skills current. Clinicians need to remember that prison work is not mainstream mental health care, and much of the work can be exhausting and alienating. Having support and connection to other professionals keeps the therapist balanced and may prevent burnout. Finally, when the clinician loses his or her sense of balance and perspective, getting involved in counseling or psychotherapy is highly recommended. Help for the helper is probably no more neglected than in the correctional environment.

Balance and Priorities

In spite of the multiple demands on prison clinicians, they must somehow establish a lifestyle of health, wellness, and balance. Prison work must simply be one part of their life and, in spite of the pressure, clinicians must find a way to make time and find energy for other parts of their life (e.g., wellness, family, recreation, spirituality, social relationships, etc.). As one teaches staff about self-care, the job is only one part of who you are so that you can take good care of those other parts that really matter. Family gatherings, marital dates, vacations, exercise, the arts, and community involvement all are critically important to the clinician's well-being and serve to refresh and renew the person of the correctional mental health professional.

Affect Expression and Connectedness

Authoritarian, paramilitary organizations are task and control oriented and by their nature do not support emotional expression and relationships with others. Obviously, this type of system is often foreign to clinicians whose values and profession are all about emotional expression and relationships with others. Restricted affect and disconnection are unhealthy ways to live; the provider must have outlets on the outside that support emotional catharsis and expression and develop and nurture relationships. This message is repeatedly emphasized in staff training and Employee Assistance Program services, yet clinicians do not always heed their own advice. Clinicians must surround themselves on the outside with good friends and loved ones who will ensure they experience the good feelings of love, joy, intimacy, excitement, and happiness, while at the same time having times to emote and eliminate the strains and tensions of mental health work in corrections.

Humor, Hope, Spirituality, and the Big Picture

Mental health clinicians working in prison would do well to often take several steps back from the chaos and craziness of the system to appreciate the absurdity and humor in it all. As the saying goes, "Life is too important to be taken seriously." Staff members need to hear this message as often as possible from the prison clinicians, who should emulate these sentiments. Therapists must live a well-balanced life with family and friends that provides hope in the midst of negativity, meanness, and despair. If you do not experience hope, your work in corrections with the hurting and hopeless people will be futile. Clinician burnout is a very high risk in prison. Providers need to quickly get professional treatment, and colleagues who work in prison need to have a strong understanding and support for burnout as being a major hazard. In spite of the strains, it is good for clinicians to practice and live spiritually and believe with all their being that their work and life fit into a much bigger picture, that of goodness, making the world a better place, and living a purpose-driven life of who and what matters. There are no words greater than those of the Great One who told his followers: "When I was in prison, you visited me . . . and what you do to the least of these you do unto me." In closing, in response to an earlier cited criticism of one mental health clinician, you should all feel happy and proud to take care of the "losers," as your work and reward will be great in the Big Picture.

Multimodal Signs of Burnout in Prison Clinicians

Use as a multimodal checklist of possible burnout symptoms for prison clinicians.

Behavior
Occupational, social, and familial withdrawal
Irritability and short temper with others (inmates, staff)
Poor task completion
Avoiding inmates and employees
Increased use of alcohol or sedatives
Engaging in self-destructive behavior
Blaming others

Affect
Anxiety
Fear
Depression
Anger

Sensations
Chest Pain
Sweating
Psychomotor agitation
Headaches
Fatigue
Tingling
Muscle tension
Exhaustion

Images
"Worn out."
"Others/System out to get me."
"People are trying to bother me."
"Just quit or run away from job."
"Losing it and telling others off."
"Retaliation for injustice."
"Helpless victim."

Cognitions
Poor concentration
Obsessions with work issues
Belief that nothing matters
Belief that nothing makes sense
Belief that you are ineffective
Cognitive overload (multiple burdens)

Interpersonal Systems
Avoidance and withdrawal from others
Alienating oneself
Rejecting others' help
Hostility and criticizing others
Cynicism toward clients
Wanting to be alone (people = burdens)

Drugs
Psychophysiological stress symptoms
Alcohol or drug abuse to sedate worries and anxieties
Increased reliance on over-the-counter medications for headache, backache, and stomach acid
Increased use of nicotine/caffeine to "keep going"

CONTRIBUTOR

Ron Bonner, PsyD, is a clinical psychologist who has worked for the last 18 years in jails or prisons. His research interests include depression, clinical suicidology, and correctional health care ethics. Dr. Bonner has presented his research to numerous professional meetings and has authored or coauthored about 50 publications. He has served as a consulting editor for *Suicide and Life-Threatening Behavior* for the last 15 years. Dr. Bonner may be contacted at 3 S. Market Street, Selinsgrove, PA 17870. E-mail: rbonner@bop.gov

RESOURCES

Alexander, R. B., & Pratsinak, G. J. (2002). *Arresting Addictions: Drug Education and Relapse Prevention in Corrections.* Lanham, MD: American Correctional Association.

Allen, B., & Bosta, D. (1981). *Games Criminals Play: How You Can Profit by Knowing Them.* Sacramento, CA: Roe John Publishers.

American Correctional Association. (1992). *Working With Manipulative Inmates.* Lanham, MD: Author.

Bonner, R. L. (2000). Correctional suicide prevention in the year 2000 and beyond. *Suicide and Life-Threatening Behavior, 30*(4), 370-376.

Bonner, R. L. (2001a). Rethinking suicide prevention and manipulative behavior in corrections. *Jail Suicide/Mental Health Update, 10*(4), 7-9.

Bonner, R. L. (2001b). Moving suicide risk assessment into the next millennium: Lessons from our past. In D. Lester (Ed.), *Suicide Resources for the New Millennium* (pp. 83-103). Philadelphia: Taylor & Francis.

Cornelius, G. F. (1994). *Stressed Out: Strategies for Living and Working With Stress in Corrections.* Lanham, MD: American Correctional Association.

Daniels, S., & Rogers, M. (1981, Fall). Burnout and the pastorate: A critical review with implications for pastors. *Journal of Psychology and Theology, 9,* 232-249.

Freudenberger, H. (1980). *Burnout: The High Cost of High Achievement.* New York: Doubleday.

Grosch, W. N., & Olsen, D. C. (1995). Therapist burnout: A self psychology and systems perspective. In L. VandeCreek, S. Knapp, & T. L. Jackson (Eds.), *Innovations in Clinical Practice: A Source Book* (Vol. 14, pp. 439-454). Sarasota, FL: Professional Resource Press.

Harrington, S. P. M. (1999). New bedlam: Jails, not psychiatric hospitals, now care for the indigent mentally ill. *Jail Suicide/Mental Health Update, 9*(1), 12-17.

Lazarus, A. A. (1995). Multimodal therapy. In R. J. Corsini & D. Wedding (Eds.), *Current Psychotherapies* (5th ed., pp. 322-355). Itasca, IL: Peacock.

Lee, D. W. (2002). Personal liability against correctional officials and employees for failure to protect an inmate. *Jail Suicide/Mental Health Update, 11*(1), 1-8.

Lunney, L. (2000). Nowhere else to go: Mentally ill and in jail. *Jail Suicide/Mental Health Update, 9*(3), 12-14.

O'Leary, W. D. (1989). Custodial suicide: Evolving liability in corrections. *Psychiatric Quarterly, 60,* 31-71.

Rich, A. R., & Bonner, R. L. (2004). Moderators, mediators, and social problem solving. In E. C. Chang, T. J. D'Zurilla, & L. J. Sanna (Eds.), *Social Problem Solving: Theory, Research, and Training* (pp. 29-45). Washington, DC: American Psychological Association.

Saakvitne, K. W. (2002). How to avoid the occupational hazards of being a psychotherapist. In L. VandeCreek & T. L. Jackson (Eds.), *Innovations in Clinical Practice: A Source Book* (Vol. 20, pp. 325-341). Sarasota, FL: Professional Resource Press.

Toch, H. (1992). *Mosaic of Despair: Human Breakdowns in Prison.* Washington, DC: American Psychological Association.

Van Voorhis, P., Braswell, M., & Lester, D. (1997). *Correctional Counseling and Rehabilitation.* Cincinnati, OH: Anderson Publishing Company.

Weinberger, L. E., & Screenivasan, S. (1994). Ethical and professional conflicts in correctional psychology. *Professional Psychology: Research and Practice, 25*(2), 161-167.

Wright, K. N. (1994). *Effective Prison Leadership.* Binghamton, NY: William Neil Publishing.

Subject Index

A

Abortion and selective reduction, 67
Abuse,
    sexual, of children with disabilities, 131-142
    suicide assessment and, 210
Adolescence, eating disorders of, 107-109, 121 (*also see* specific disorders)
Adolescent Suicide Assessment Protocol-20 (ASAP-20), 207-224
Anger,
    cardiac patients and, 93
    suicide assessment and, 212-213
Anonymity of online clients, 189-190
Anorexia nervosa, 107, 116 (*also see* Eating disorders in children and adolescents)
Antisocial behavior, suicide assessment and, 210
Anxiety disorders,
    breast cancer and, 44-45
Assessment,
    of breast cancer patients, 43
    of cardiac patients, 90-93
    of child and adolescent eating disorders, 111-118
    of chronic medically ill patients, 25-26
    of eating disordered patients, 111-118
    of quality of life, 11-15
Autonomy, 258

B

Beneficence, 258
Binge eating disorder, 107, 108, 110-112, 114 (*also see* Eating disorders in children and adolescents)
Biological therapy, breast cancer and, 39
Breast cancer, 33-55
Breathing, diaphragmatic, for cardiac patients, 97
Bulimia nervosa, 107-108, 111, 117, 121-122 (*also see* Eating disorders in children and adolescents)
Burnout, 257-271, 279-280, 285

C

Cancer,
    breast, 33-55
    quality of life and, 6-7
Cardiac patients, 23-24, 85-104
    psychosocial issues with, 85-104
    quality of life and, 9-10
    statistics of, 85
Caregivers, breast cancer and, 50-51
Chemotherapy, breast cancer and, 37-38
Child/Adolescent Food Diary (form), 127
Childhood, feeding and eating disorders of, 105-107
Children with disabilities, sexual abuse of, 131-142
Children's Body Image Scale (CBIS), 113, 114, 125-126
Chronic medical illness (*also see* specific illnesses),
    assessing cognitive and psychological deficits of, 21-32
    quality of life and, 5-20
Chronic obstructive pulmonary disease, 24-25
Client, identifying, in correctional system, 278
Cognitive assessment of cardiac patients, 90
Cognitive-behavioral therapy for,
    breast cancer, 47
    eating disorders, 121-122
Cognitive deficits, chronic medical disease and, 21-32
Cognitive/Neuropsychological History (form), 27-28
Cognitive processing theory, 41-42
Cognitive restructuring interventions for cardiac patients, 98-100
Confidentiality,
    in correctional system, 277-278
    online therapy and, 178-179, 192-193

Contagion, suicide assessment and, 217-218
Coping,
  assessment of, in cardiac patients, 91-92
  with breast cancer, 40-41
  strategies for, in correctional system, 282-284
Coping With Serious Illness (handout), 239-241
Correctional system, issues for mental health providers in, 273-286
Countertransference,
  breast cancer and, 52
  in correctional system, 275
Couples issues, breast cancer and, 48-49
Crisis situations, online therapy and, 193
Cultural factors,
  in eating disorders, 109-111
  in mental health interventions, 145-158

D

Depression,
  breast cancer and, 44
  heart disease and, 88-89
  suicide assessment and, 211-212
Developmental issues, eating disorders and, 110-111
Diabetes, quality of life and, 8-9
Disabled children, sexual abuse of, 131-142
Distress, therapist, 257-271
Dual roles in correctional system, 276-278
Duty to protect, online therapy and, 180-181

E

Eating Behaviors and Body Image Test for Preadolescent Girls (EBBIT), 231-238
Eating disorders in children and adolescents, 105-130
  anorexia nervosa, 107, 116
  binge eating disorder, 107, 108, 110-112, 114
  bulimia nervosa, 107-108, 112, 116
  feeding disorder of infancy or early childhood, 105-107, 120-121
  pica, 105-106, 118-119
  rumination disorder, 106, 119-120
Employee assistance programs in correctional system, 277-278
Endocrine disorders, psychological and neuro-psychological manifestations of, 22-23

Environmental conditions in correctional system, 278-279
Ethics,
  for mental health providers in corrections, 273-286
  online therapy and, 180-181
  therapist wellness and, 257-271
Ethnic identity, eating disorders and, 110 (*also see* Cultural factors)

F

Family dysfunction, suicide assessment and, 216
Family response, breast cancer and, 49-50
Family therapy for eating disorders, 122-123
Fee collection, online therapy and, 179, 191
Feeding disorder of infancy or early childhood, 105-107, 120-121
Fidelity, 258
Firearm access, suicide assessment and, 215
Forms and Instruments
  Adolescent Suicide Assessment Protocol-20 (ASAP-20), 221-222
  Child/Adolescent Food Diary, 127
  Children's Body Image Scale (CBIS), 125-126
  Cognitive/Neuropsychological History, 27-28
  Eating Behaviors and Body Image Test for Preadolescent Girls (EBBIT), 233-237
  Index of Race-Related Stress–Brief Version (IRRS-B), 227-228
  Multimodal Signs of Burnout in Prison Clinicians (Checklist), 285
  Neuropsychological Referral Worksheet, 29-30
  Planning a Website: Worksheet, 183-184
  Quality of Life Rating (QOLR) Instrument, 203-205
  Quality of Life (QOL)-Specific Clinical Interview, Additional Domains for (form), 18
  Race and Cultural Issues With Racial and Ethnic Minorities, Key Questions in Addressing, 157
  Self-Assessment Questionnaires (for therapist distress and coping behaviors), 268-269
  Self-Rating of Life Quality (form), 204

G

Genetics, breast cancer and, 34
Group therapy, breast cancer and, 47
Guided imagery for cardiac patients, 96

H

Handouts
    Coping With Serious Illness, 239-241
    Helping Your Child, 251-252
    Helping Your Friend, 253-254
    Helping Yourself, 247-249
    Ten Things Parents Can Do to Prevent Eating
        Disorders, 243
    Tips for Kids on Eating Well and Feeling Good
        About Yourself, 245
Health disparities between racial and ethnic
        minorities and whites, 145-158 (*also see*
        Cultural factors)
Heart disease (*also see* Cardiac conditions),
        psychosocial aspects of, 74-75
        quality of life and, 9-10
Helping Your Child (handout), 251-252
Helping Your Friend (handout), 253-254
Helping Yourself (handout), 247-249
HIV/AIDS, quality of life and, 7-8
Hopelessness, suicide assessment and, 212
Hormonal therapy, breast cancer and, 38-39

I

Impairment, therapist, 257-271
Impulsivity, suicide assessment and, 213
Index of Race-Related Stress–Brief Version
        (IRRS-B), 225-229
Individuals with Disabilities Education Act (IDEA),
        137
Infancy, feeding and eating disorders of, 105-107
Infertility, psychosocial aspects of, 64-67
Interpersonal therapy for eating disorders, 123

K

Key Questions in Addressing Race and Cultural
        Issues With Racial and Ethnic Minorities
        (form), 157

L

Legal issues of online therapy, 193-194
Legal/policy directives in correctional system, 276
Liver failure, 75
Losses, recent, suicide assessment and, 214-215

M

Manipulation in correctional system, 275
Meditation, mindfulness, 97-98
Menopause, 59-60
Mental status assessments, online therapy and, 191
Metabolic conditions, 22-23
Mindfulness meditation for cardiac patients, 97-98
Minorities (*also see* Cultural factors),
        eating disorders and, 110
        health disparities of, 145-158
Miscarriage and stillbirth, 67-68
Multimodal Signs of Burnout in Prison Clinicians
        (Checklist), 285
Multiple sclerosis, 22

N

Neuropsychological Referral Worksheet (form), 29-
        30
Neuropsychological status,
        heart disease and, 89
        in patients with chronic medical illness, 25-30
Nonmalfeasance, 258
Nonverbal communication, online therapy and, 190

O

Obstetrics, gynecology, and fertility, 57-71
Online therapy,
        practical and ethical issues of, 177-181
        problems and solutions of, 187-197
Organ failure and transplantation, 73-84

P

Paramilitary environment in correctional system,
        274
Peer problems, suicide assessment and, 216-217

Perimenopause, 59-60

Pica, 105-106, 118-119 (*also see* Eating disorders in children and adolescents)

Planning a Website: Worksheet (form), 183-184

Postpartum psychiatric illnesses, 61-64

Pregnancy, 60-61

Premenstrual disorders, 57-59

Progressive muscle relaxation, 94-96

Protective factors, suicide assessment and, 218-219

Psychoeducation, breast cancer and, 46

Psychopharmacological treatment for eating disorders, 123-124

Q

Quality of life, chronic medical illness and, 5-20

Quality of Life Rating (QOLR) Instrument, 201-206

Quality of Life (QOL)-Specific Clinical Interview, Additional Domains for (form), 18

R

Race and Cultural Issues With Racial and Ethnic Minorities, Key Questions in Addressing (form), 157

Race, issues of (*see* Cultural factors)

Race-Related Stress–Brief Version (IRRS-B), Index of (form), 227-228

Radiation, breast cancer and, 38

Renal failure, 74

Risk factors,
    for breast cancer, 33-34
    for heart disease, 86-89

Rumination disorder, 106, 119-120 (*also see* Eating disorders in children and adolescents)

S

School/legal problems, suicide assessment and, 217

Self-Assessment Questionnaires (for therapist distress and coping behaviors) (form), 268-269

Self-care, therapist, 263-265

Self-monitoring, eating disorders and, 117

Sex therapy, 159-168

Sexual abuse of children with disabilities, 131-142

Sexual difficulties, breast cancer and, 48-49

Social support,
    breast cancer and, 42
    heart disease and, 88, 92

Stress,
    in correctional system, 279-280
    heart disease and, 87, 91
    Index of Race-Related, 225-229
    in transplant teams, 81

Substance abuse, suicide assessment and, 213-214

Suicide,
    Adolescent, Assessment Protocol-20, 207-224

Supportive psychotherapy, breast cancer and, 46

Surgery, breast cancer and, 36-37

T

Ten Things Parents Can Do to Prevent Eating Disorders (handout), 243

Tips for Kids on Eating Well and Feeling Good About Yourself (handout), 245

Transplants (*see* Organ failure and transplantation)

Treatment versus punishment model in correctional system, 274-275

Type A personality,
    in correctional system, 276-277
    and hostility, heart disease and, 87-88, 93

W

Website (*also see* Online therapy)
    design of, for mental health professionals, 169-185
    Planning a (Worksheet), 183-184

Wellness,
    approach to sexual abuse, 139-140
    as an ethical imperative in therapists, 257-271

Continuing Education
Available for Home Study

The most recent volumes of *Innovations in Clinical Practice* are available as formal home-study continuing education programs. This best-selling, comprehensive source of practical clinical information is complemented by examination modules which may be used to earn continuing education credits.

Credits may be obtained by successfully completing examinations based on those contributions in each volume which have been selected by the editorial advisory board. Each of these contributions explores a timely topic designed to enhance your clinical skills and provides the knowledge necessary for effective practice. After studying these selections, a multiple-choice examination is completed and returned to the Professional Resource Exchange for scoring. Upon passing the examination (80% of test items answered correctly), your credits will be recorded and you will receive a copy of your official transcript.

At the time of publication of this volume, continuing education modules are available for Volumes 17 through 20 of *Innovations in Clinical Practice: A Source Book*. Each module contains examination materials for 20 credits (equivalent to 20 hours of continuing education activity). Twelve-credit programs are available for *Innovations in Clinical Practice: Focus on Children and Adolescents* and *Innovations in Clinical Practice: Focus on Violence Treatment and Prevention*. Fourteen-credit programs are available for *Innovations in Clinical Practice: Focus on Adults* and *Innovations in Clinical Practice: Focus on Health and Wellness*.

The *Innovations in Clinical Practice* Continuing Education (CE) Programs are one of the most efficient ways to stay current on new clinical techniques and obtain formal credit for your study. If your professional associations and state boards do not currently require formal CE activities, you may still wish to consider these programs as an excellent means of receiving feedback on your professional development. These self-study programs are . . .

- *Relevant* - selections are packed with information pertinent to your practice.
- *Inexpensive* - typically less than half the cost of obtaining credits through workshops and these expenses may still be tax deductible as a professional expense.
- *Convenient* - study at your own pace in the comfort of your home or office.
- *Useful* - the volumes will always be available as a practical reference and resource for day-to-day use in your professional practice.
- *Effective* - as a means of staying up to date and obtaining feedback on your knowledge acquisition and professional development. In most states with continuing education requirements, credits earned from American Psychological Association (APA) approved sponsors are automatically approved for licensure renewal. Consult your profession's state board for their policies regarding the status of programs offered by APA approved sponsors.

Specific learning objectives are available upon request.

To receive additional information on these CE programs, please see next page. ⟶

Do You Want More Information?

Yes! Please Send Me . . .

❐   Information on the other volumes in the *Innovations in Clinical Practice* series (Tables of Contents for all volumes and ordering information).

❐   Information on your Home-Study Continuing Education Programs.

❐   Your latest catalog.

Name: _____
(Please Print)

Address: _____

Address: _____

City/State/Zip: _____

Telephone: (_____) _____

E-Mail: _____

My Primary Profession Is: _____

For Fastest Response . . .

Fax to Our 24 Hour FAX Line at **1-941-343-9201**

OR

E-mail to **orders@prpress.com**

OR

Visit Our Website at **http://www.prpress.com**

Or Mail This Form To . . .

Professional Resource Press
PO Box 15560 • Sarasota FL 34277-1560